IMAGING IN MEDICAL SCIENCES

Farid Ezat

ALLIED
HEALTH
PRESS

Imaging in Medical Sciences

Author: **Farid Ezat**

Allied Health Press
4164 Lakeshore Road
Burlington ON L7L 1A4
Canada
www.alliedhealthpress.com
Email: orders@arclereducation.com

ISBN: 978-1-77956-271-5

ABOUT THE AUTHOR

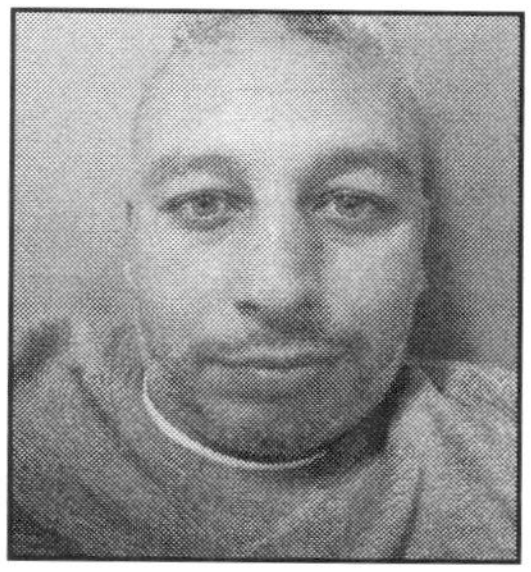

Farid Ezat is a dedicated medical doctor with a diverse background in radiology, general practice, and research. Currently serving as a consultant teleradiologist for teleradiology solution , Bangaluru , India , He meticulously analyzes radiological images and engages in research. Previously, Farid honed his clinical skills as a General Practitioner in Alexandria main university hospitals. Farid's academic journey includes earning his Master degree from the Alexandria university ", Faculty of Medicine in Egypt. Committed to continuous learning, Farud actively participates in extracurricular activities and preparing for final FRCR exam.

Word Roots, Prefixes, and Suffixes by Chapter

Chapter 1 Advances in Imaging from the First X-ray Images

a-, an-: negative, without

ab-: away from

ad-: towards

anti-: against

ante-: before

bi-: two, both

brachy-: short

brady-: slow

dors-: back

Chapter 2 Computed Tomography

neo-: new

para-: beside or below

peri-: around

poly-: many

post-: after

sub-: below

super-: above

tachy-: fast

-pathy: disease

Chapter 3 Magnetic Resonance Imaging

-itis: inflammation

-osis: abnormal condition

micr: small

-scopy: to look, observe

-graphy: recording an image

-gram: the image (X-ray)

-ology: study, specialize in

Chapter 4 Positron Emission Tomography

-ad: toward dorsad

-al: pertaining to lateral

-algia: pain myalgia

-amnios: amnion, amniotic fluid oligohydramnios

-centesis: surgical puncture to aspirate fluid amniocentesis

-crine: to secrete exocrine

Chapter 5 X-ray Detectors

CXR: chest x-ray

radi/o: (x-ray) radiation

rheumat/o: discharge, flow, joint

gram: the image (X-ray)

graphy/ graph: recording an image (X-ray, CT or MRI scan or a written recording)

gastr/o: stomach

osis: abnormal condition

Chapter 6 Dental Radiography

-algia: ain odontALGIA = tooth pain

a-: without Acellular = having no cells

arth-: joint ARTHOscope=an instrument to see inside a joint

dent-, odont-: tooth or teeth ODONToma = tumor composed of tooth structures

-ectomy: excision append ECTOMY = excision of the appendix

-emia: blood hyperEMIA = above normal amount of blood in tissue

Chapter 7 Ultrasound Imaging

Carcin/o-: Cancer

Cardi/o-, Coron-: Heart

hem/o -: Blood

Hist/o-, Histio-: Tissue

Chapter 8 Digital Radiography

-ia: condition

pulmon: lung

path: disease

nephr: kidney

Chapter 9 Raman Spectroscopy in Medicine

- gastr-: tomach
- chrom- or chromato-: color
- cry/o-: cold
- homo-: same
- -osis: condition; usually abnormal
- -stasis: level; unchanging

Chapter 10 Angiography

- abdom-: the abdomen
- angi-: blood vessels
- arteri-: arteries
- axill-: armpit region
- brachi-: the arm
- cardi-, coron-: the heart
- cerebr-: the brain
- clav-, cleid-: collar bone
- cran-: the skull
- cut-, derm-: the skin
- cyt-: cell

Table of Contents

LIST OF FIGURES

LIST OF TABLES

PREFACE

Medical imaging has become indispensable in numerous areas of biomedical research and clinical practice. Biologists use it to study cells and generate 3D confocal microscopy datasets, while virologists create 3D reconstructions of viruses from micrographs. Radiologists rely on medical imaging to identify and quantify tumors from MRI and CT scans, and neuroscientists utilize it to detect regional metabolic brain activity from PET and functional MRI scans.

Image processing plays a crucial role in the analysis, enhancement, and display of images captured through various medical imaging technologies. Techniques like image reconstruction and modeling enable the instant processing of 2D signals to produce 3D images. Moreover, image processing and analysis can determine the diameter, volume, and vasculature of a tumor or organ, flow parameters of blood or other fluids, and microscopic changes that may not be otherwise apparent.

Several medical imaging techniques have been developed, including X-rays, computed tomography (CT) scans, magnetic resonance imaging (MRI), ultrasound, and nuclear medicine imaging. These advanced techniques have numerous applications in diagnosing myocardial diseases, cancers of various tissues, neurological disorders, congenital heart disease, abdominal illnesses, complex bone fractures, and other serious medical conditions.

While these imaging techniques offer significant benefits, they also carry some risks. Steps can be taken to minimize the risks of radiation exposure associated with certain imaging techniques. Advanced medical imaging modalities, such as PET/CT hybrid, three-dimensional ultrasound computed tomography (3D USCT), and simultaneous PET/MRI, provide high resolution, improved reliability, and safety in diagnosing, treating, and managing complex patient abnormalities.

Continued innovation and technological advancements in medical imaging systems are expected to lead to the development of more accurate imaging tools with improved resolution, sensitivity, and specificity. In the future, the field of medical diagnostics is likely to see regular measurements of various complex diseases, offering improved healthcare solutions.

The book "Imaging in Medical Sciences" is intended to provide a comprehensive overview of the various imaging modalities used in the field of medicine. The book covers a wide range of imaging techniques, including radiography, CT, MRI, ultrasonography, nuclear medicine imaging, and molecular imaging. Each modality is discussed in detail, highlighting its principles, indications, contraindications, advantages, and limitations. Advanced imaging techniques, such as functional MRI, diffusion tensor imaging, and positron emission tomography (PET), are also explored, providing readers with a comprehensive understanding of the latest developments in the field.

Additionally, the book addresses the role of imaging in various medical specialties, including cardiology, oncology, neurology, orthopedics, and pediatrics. It discusses how imaging techniques are used to diagnose, stage, and monitor disease progression, as well as to guide treatment planning and interventions. Special emphasis is placed on the importance of multidisciplinary collaboration in interpreting imaging findings and providing optimal patient care.

By providing a thorough overview of imaging in medical sciences, this book aims to enhance the knowledge and skills of healthcare professionals involved in the use and interpretation of medical imaging. It serves as a valuable resource for both beginners and experienced practitioners, helping them stay abreast of the latest advances and best practices in the field.

Chapter 1

ADVANCES IN IMAGING FROM THE FIRST X-RAY IMAGES

Contents

Introduction

X-rays and other forms of radiation continue to be essential in both medical and experimental science. With the advancements in computer technology, it is now possible to create detailed 3D images by combining multiple 2D X-ray slices. This has greatly improved the accuracy in detecting tumors, fractures, and other internal issues within the human body. X-rays are not only used in the medical field but also in a variety of other applications. Due to their wavelength being similar to the size of atoms, X-rays are ideal for examining the structural arrangement of atoms and molecules in different materials. This chapter is organized in a logical order, starting with the discovery of X-rays, detailing experimental processes, and concluding with the physics of diagnostic radiology and other non-medical uses. While Roentgen's contributions are well-known, many other individuals who laid the groundwork for radiology remain relatively unknown, especially to younger physicists and physicians.

Orientation and Directional Terms

Term	Definition	Illustration
Diagnostic radiology	Diagnostic Radiology is a group of various modalities of medical imaging by using X-rays.	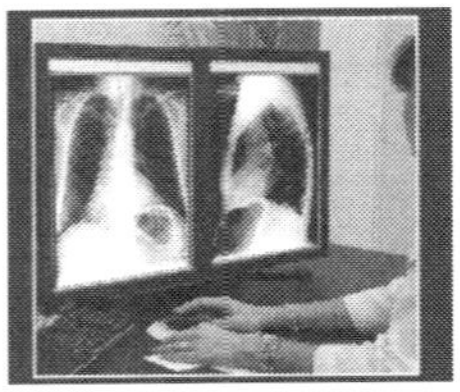
Medical imaging	Medical imaging is the technique and process of imaging the interior of a body for clinical analysis and medical intervention, as well as visual representation of the function of some organs or tissues.	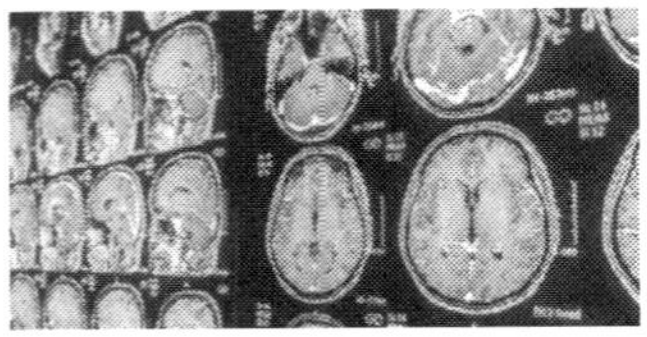
Radiant energy	Radiant energy is energy that is transferred by electromagnetic radiation, such as light, X-rays, gamma rays, and thermal radiation.	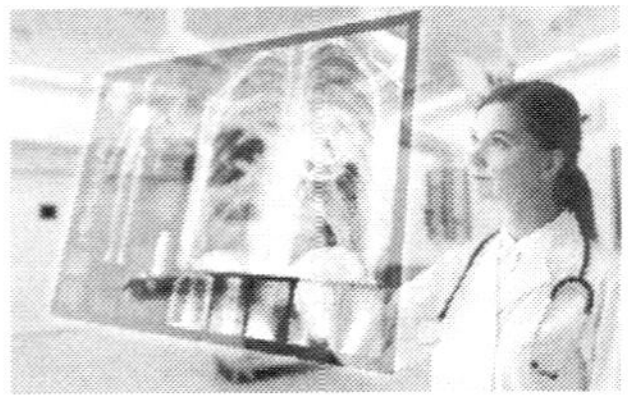
X-rays	X-rays are a form of electromagnetic radiation, similar to visible light.	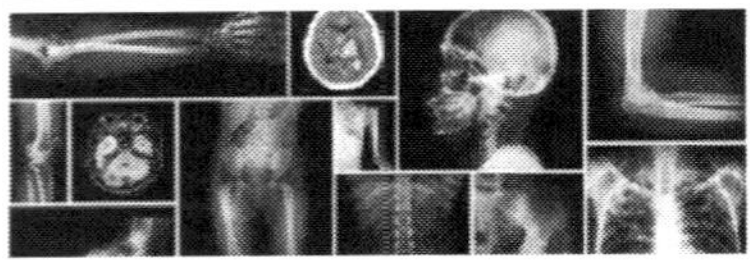
2D X-ray	A 2D x-ray is an x-ray examination that captures images of the mouth. This includes the teeth, upper and lower jaws, and surrounding structures and tissues. These types of X-rays can range from simple intraoral to extraoral full mouth X-rays.	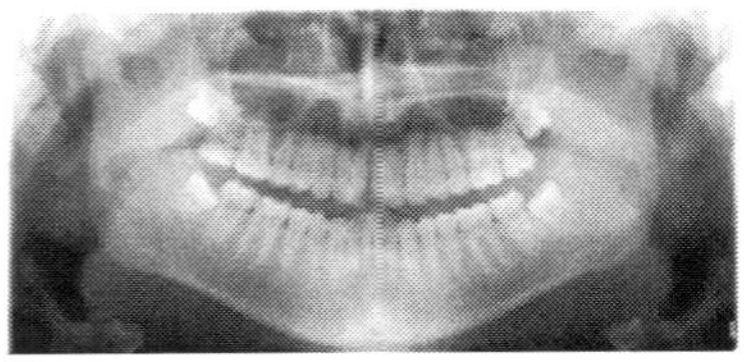
3D image	A 3D X-ray image is a comprehensive representation of an object in three dimensions, including length, width, and height. It's created by post-processing medical scan data using a collection of techniques and tools.	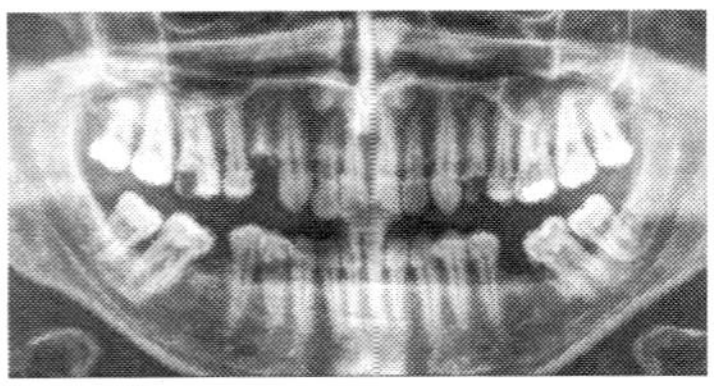

1.1. Definition of X-rays

X-rays are a type of electromagnetic radiation, meaning they adhere to the same principles as other forms of electromagnetic waves. This type of radiation, also known as radiant energy, carries energy through space in the form of waves or photons, similar to radio waves, visible light, and microwaves. It can be described using either a photon or wave model.

The wavelength can also be represented by frequency f_p and the waves propagation speed, i.e., the speed of light c_0

$$\lambda_p = \frac{c_0}{f_p} \tag{1.1}$$

In Eq. (1.2), where h denotes Planck's constant (≈6.626 069 × 10^{-34} J s) and c_0 is the speed of light (≈2.997 92 × 10^5 m s^{-1}). The energy is directly related to the photon's wavelength λ_p or its frequency f_p and is given by the unit electron volt [eV]

$$E_p = \frac{h\,c_0}{\lambda_p} = f_p\,h \tag{1.2}$$

Additionally, electromagnetic radiation is classified into various groups using this energy, i.e., radio waves, microwaves, visible light, ultraviolet (UV) light, infrared (IR), X-rays, and γ-rays. Figure 1.1 displays these groups in relation to their distinctive wavelength and frequency ranges. It should be noted that most X-rays have wavelengths between 0.01 and 10 nm. This means that the energy range is from 100 keV to 100 eV.

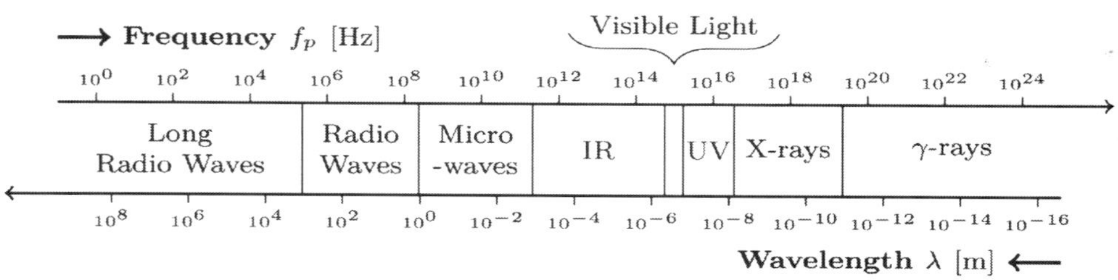

Figure 1.1. *Wavelengths and frequencies in electromagnetic radiation.*

Source: Berger, M., Yang, Q., & Maier, A. X-ray Imaging. 2018 Aug 3. In: Maier, A., Steidl, S., Christlein, V., et al., editors. Medical Imaging Systems: An Introductory Guide [Internet]. Cham (CH): Springer; 2018. Chapter 7. Available from: https://www.ncbi.nlm.nih.gov/books/NBK546155/ doi: 10.1007/978-3-319-96520-8_7 /.

Similar to visible light, X-rays lose energy as they travel through various materials. The material's absorption behavior determines the amount of energy lost. For instance, X-rays lose less energy passing through 10 cm of water than they do passing through 10 cm of bone. The fundamental idea of conventional X-ray imaging is absorption, which results in the reduction of energy. X-ray radiography, in general, measures the quantity of energy lost. We can see a certain contrast in the image because this energy loss varies depending on the material. An X-ray image, for instance, reveals lower intensities where the radiation entered bones and higher intensities for soft tissue. Keep in mind that the dose given to the patient during an acquisition has a direct impact on the amount of energy absorbed (Buzug, 2008).

1.2. X-rays—Early History

The discovery of the X-ray by Roentgen on November 8, 1895, in his Wurzburg laboratory, marked the beginning of imaging as we know it today. Imaging techniques based on Wilhelm Conrad Roentgen's discovery of the X-ray were put into practice worldwide almost immediately after the discovery was announced.

For instance, chest radiography emerged as one of those pioneering uses, even though the apparatus appears antiquated in light of modern technology and there was undoubtedly no awareness of the possible harmful consequences of X-ray ionizing radiation. Roentgen's creation signaled the beginning of the contemporary medical imaging era (Figure 1.2).

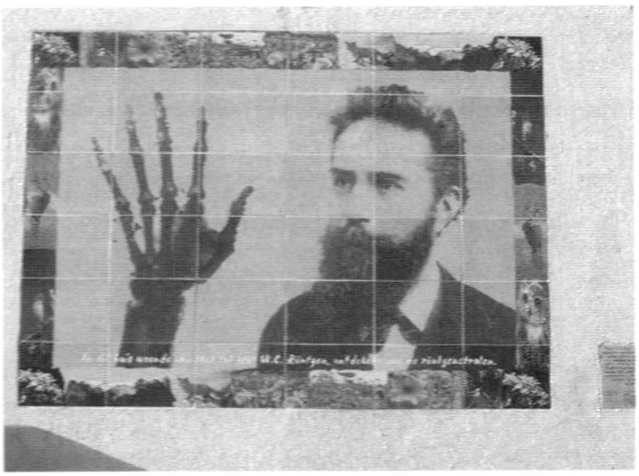

Figure 1.2. *Wilhelm Conrad Roentgen and the famous x-ray image of his wife's hand.*

Source: By Brbbl – Own work, CC BY-SA 3.0, https://commons.wikimedia.org/w/index.php?curid=22577806.

In 1895, German physicist Wilhelm Conrad Roentgen discovered X-rays while conducting electricity experiments. Initially unsure of what these rays were, he gave them the name X-rays. By 1900, doctors were utilizing X-rays to capture radiographs of bones, aiding in the more efficient treatment of injuries.

Roentgen's discovery of this short-wave ray won him the first-ever Nobel Prize in physics in 1901. He gave his university the entire prize money. The recently found rays were given the name "X-rays" against his will (the letter "x" is typically used to indicate the unknown entity). He wanted everyone to be able to benefit from X-rays, so he declined to file a patent for this discovery. He even prohibited these rays from being named after him. The reader can find excellent articles by Linton, Assmus, and Mould, to name a few, that provide historical details about events that occurred around the time of Roentgen's discovery. Before drafting a paper that was submitted for publication to a local scientific publication on December 28, 1895, Roentgen conducted tests on his new rays to determine their properties and made a number of observations. Because of Roentgens' high standing in the community, his paper was accepted without a review and released right away.

In a new section of Scientific American, a bulletin titled "Professor Roentgen's Wonderful Discovery" was published, discussing the X-ray. The first mention of the X-ray in Science magazine came in a letter from Harvard University physics professor Hugo Munsterberg on January 31, 1896. Nature later published a full translation of Roentgen's paper. Despite his shyness, Roentgen's discovery quickly progressed from a physics experiment to a common medical practice.

It is possible to observe what physics was capable of before the advent of the technological revolution, which involved not only computer applications but also the demise of independent small X-ray companies and their replacement by multinational corporations. These days, research and development are simply too costly for many independent, financially supported high-tech contributions.

1.3. X-ray Generation

A classical X-ray tube is shown in Figure 1.3. In essence, an X-ray tube is a glass evacuated tube that contains a solid metal anode and a cathode. The heated filament at the cathode is the source of thermonuclear emission. Because the thermal energy applied to the filament material is greater than its binding energy, heat-induced electrons (e^-) are produced. The acceleration voltage of the tube between the positive anode and the negative cathode then accelerates the electrons. The anode's atoms' electric field causes the fast electrons to slow down and deflect when they come into contact with it. Electromagnetic waves are produced whenever particles that are loaded accelerate. The slowing down also occurs, i.e., the electrons' negative acceleration in the metal anode. It produces radiography.

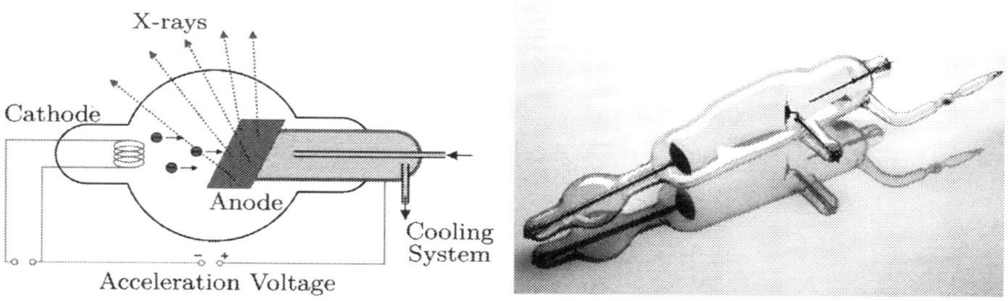

Figure 1.3. *Vacuum X-ray tube: The image on the left shows a schematic how electrons are accelerated from the cathode to the anode to generate x-ray photons. The image on the right shows a historic vacuum x-ray tube.*

Source: Berger, M., Yang, Q., & Maier, A. X-ray Imaging. 2018 Aug 3. In: Maier, A., Steidl, S., Christlein, V., et al., editors. Medical Imaging Systems: An Introductory Guide [Internet]. Cham (CH): Springer; 2018. Chapter 7. Available from: https://www.ncbi.nlm.nih.gov/books/NBK546155/ doi: 10.1007/978-3-319-96520-8_7.

To aim the X-rays that emerge in the proper direction, the anode is inclined at a specific angle. Every electron is usually accelerated or deflected multiple times, resulting in the production of multiple photons. Nevertheless, an electron may also lose all of its energy and velocity in a single step. Here, the electron's whole energy is contained in a single photon that is produced.

As seen in Figure 1.4, two distinct processes lead to the production of X-rays. First, characteristic X-radiation may be generated if the electron interacts with an inner-shell electron of the target. This type of X-ray is produced when an interaction is strong enough to completely remove the inner-shell electron, ionizing the target atom. An electron from the outer shell fills the resulting "hole" in the inner shell. An X-ray photon with an energy equal to the difference in the binding energies of the involved orbital electrons is emitted when an orbital electron moves from an outer to an inner shell. Consequently, a line spectrum, also known as a discrete spectrum, is produced by the distinctive radiation. This type of radiation is obviously material dependent. The accelerated electrons interact with the electrons of the target material to produce both thermal energy and characteristic X-rays.

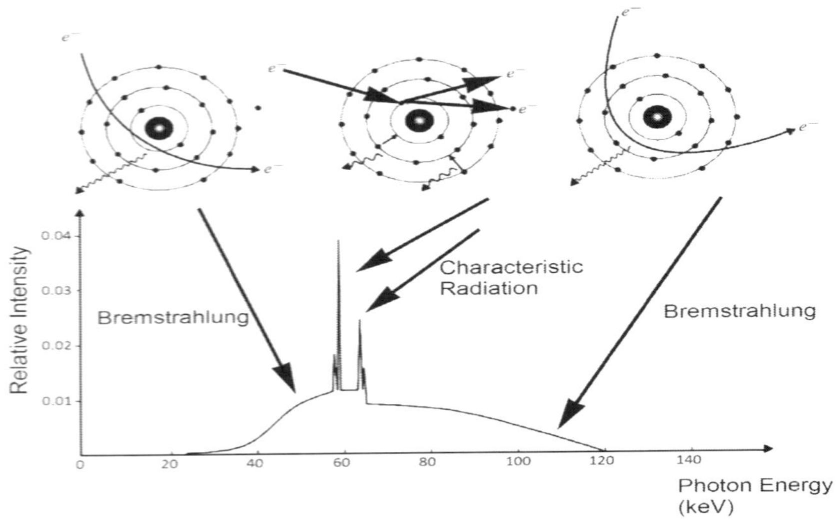

Figure 1.4. *X-ray spectrum of a tungsten tube. The peaks correspond to the characteristic radiation; the continuous part of the spectrum represents the Bremsstrahlung.*

Source: Berger, M., Yang, Q., & Maier, A. X-ray Imaging. 2018 Aug 3. In: Maier, A., Steidl, S., Christlein, V., et al., editors. Medical Imaging Systems: An Introductory Guide [Internet]. Cham (CH): Springer; 2018. Chapter 7. Available from: https://www.ncbi.nlm.nih.gov/books.

The second process of X-ray production is brought about by an electron interacting with a target atom's nucleus, which is another kind of interaction in which the electron may lose its kinetic energy. The colliding electron is deflected and slowed down as it passes by the anode atom's nucleus, exiting with less kinetic energy in a different direction. The kinetic energy is lost and reappear as an X-ray photon. The term "bremsstrahlung" refers to this kind of X-ray, where "Bremsen" is the German verb for "to slow down." This can result in kinetic energy losses ranging from zero to the total incident energy. The Bremsstrahlung produces a continuous spectrum, but the characteristic radiation produces a discrete X-ray spectrum with characteristic peaks. Even at very low photon energies, the quantity of X-rays released rapidly decreases. Figure1.4 illustrates the spectrum of a tungsten source. Before interacting with a patient in medical imaging, very low energies of the X-ray spectrum are usually eliminated by placing a thin metal plate between the patient and the X-ray source. This is because the patient would absorb nearly all of the low-energy photons, increasing the patient dose without significantly improving the quality of the image. The mathematical filters used for image processing are not to be confused with the metallic plate, which is also known as an X-ray filter.

1.4. X-ray Matter Interaction

X-rays can pass through materials, but the quantity of X-ray photons that do so depends on the material. Actually, their capacity to pierce human tissue is what makes them useful for obtaining details about internal organs. Higher or lower energy X-ray spectra are produced by varying the tube voltage between the cathode and the anode. X-rays passing through matter can result in three different types of relevant interactions in the energy range used for medical imaging:

- interaction with atomic electrons,
- interaction with nucleons,
- interaction with electric fields associated with atomic electrons and atomic nuclei.

As a result, the X-ray photons undergo inelastic scattering, elastic scattering, or complete absorption.

The method used in medical imaging involves reducing the intensity of radiation, meaning fewer photons reach the detector. This process, known as attenuation, is influenced by various physical effects such as changes in photon count, direction, or energy. These effects result from interactions between individual photons and the material they pass through, with attenuation varying based on the energy involved. It is important to note that pair production does not apply to typical diagnostic X-ray energies, as it requires a minimum photon energy of 2 × 511 keV to produce a positron and an electron.

1.4.1. Absorption

When a monochromatic X-ray beam traverses a homogeneous object with absorption coefficient μ, according to Lambert-Beer's law, the observed intensity I is related to the intersection length of the object x and the ray (Figure 1.5):

$$I = I_0 \cdot e^{-\mu x}. \quad (1.3)$$

Here, I_0 is the X-ray intensity at the x-ray source.

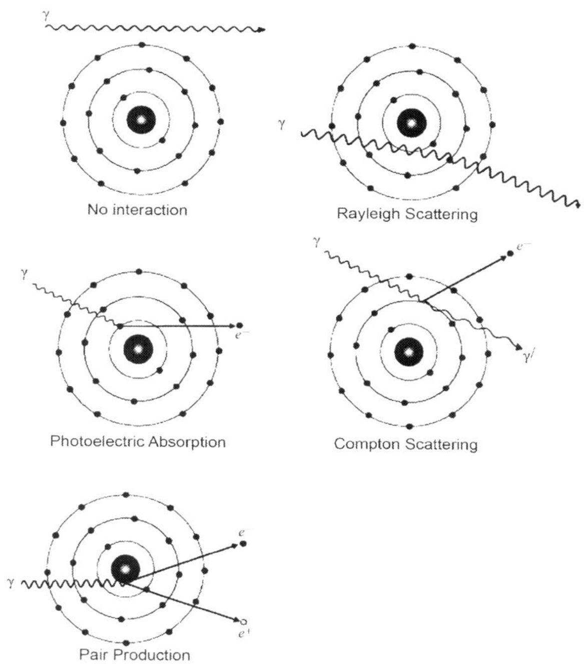

Figure 1.5. *Principles of photon-matter interactions.*

Source: Berger, M., Yang, Q., & Maier, A. X-ray Imaging. 2018 Aug 3. In: Maier, A., Steidl, S., Christlein, V., et al., editors. Medical Imaging Systems: An Introductory Guide [Internet]. Cham (CH): Springer; 2018. Chapter 7. Available from: https://www.ncbi.nlm.nih.gov/books.

In X-ray CT, the fractional transmitted intensity I/I_0 is used to measure a large number of ray paths through the object. The logarithm of this ratio is used to obtain a set of line integrals as an input to reconstruction algorithms.

When the ray passes through inhomogeneous objects, factor $\mu(x)$ is the linear attenuation coefficient at each point on the ray path

$$-\ln \frac{I}{I_0} = \int \mu(x) \mathrm{d}x \ . \quad (1.4)$$

However, in practical setups, the emitted X-ray photons have various energies, resulting in polyenergetic energy spectra as shown in Figure 1.4. The measured intensity of a polychromatic beam I on the detector can be written as the sum of monochromatic contributions for each energy E in the X-ray spectrum ($E \in [0, E_{max}]$). The attenuation coefficient μ is also energy dependent. When polychromatic X-rays are taken into account, we get;

$$I = \int_0^{E_{max}} I_0(E) \exp\left(-\int \mu(x, E) \mathrm{d}x\right) \mathrm{d}E \qquad (1.5)$$

where $I_0(E)$ is the normalized energy spectrum, i.e., $I_0(E)\mathrm{d}E=1$.

1.4.2. Photoelectric Effect

When Einstein first established the quantized nature of light, he also described the photoelectric effect. It characterizes an instance where the energy of the incident X-ray photon surpasses the binding energy of an electron within the atom of the target material. The incident X-ray photon releases an electron from an inner-shell by using up all of its energy. We refer to the released electron as a photoelectron. At that point, the incident photon vanishes. Where the ejected electron was previously located, the inner shell of the atom is frequently left vacant by the photo-electric effect. An electron from the outer shell fills the "hole" that is consequently made in the inner shell. A characteristic radiation is produced because the electron in the outer shell is in a higher energy state. As a result, a positive ion, a photoelectron, and a photon of distinctive radiation are produced by the photoelectric effect. The K-shell electrons' binding energy is extremely low for materials that resemble tissues. As a result, the photoelectron gains practically all of the X-ray photon's energy.

1.4.3. Compton Scattering

The Compton scattering, named for Arthur Holly Compton, who was awarded the Nobel Prize in 1927 for his discovery, is the second kind of matter interaction. Compton scattering is the predominant interaction mechanism in tissue-like materials at high X-ray energies. The incident X-ray photon's energy is significantly greater than the electron's binding energy. Consequently, an electron is struck by the incident X-ray photon and is ejected from the atom. When a photon enters Compton scattering, it is partially loss of its initial energy and is deflected or scattered through an angle θ. The electron, also known as the Compton electron or "recoil electron," receives some of the energy from the incident photon. As a result, a positive ion, a "recoil electron," and a scattered photon are produced by the interaction. There are 0 to 180-degree angles at which the scattered photon can be deflected. The scattered photon retains the majority of its energy after Compton interaction, which corresponds to a small deflection angle.

1.4.4. Rayleigh Scattering

Rayleigh scattering is the main type of scattering that occurs at low X-ray energies and involves the interaction of the incident wave with outer shell electrons. When a low-energy photon interacts with the atom's electrons, there is no ejection of electrons, but instead the atom vibrates in response to the photon's wavelength. The excess energy from this vibration is transferred to another photon with the same wavelength, potentially in a different direction. This process does not result in the ejection of electrons or the conversion of energy into kinetic energy, preventing ionization from occurring. Rayleigh scattered photons are mostly emitted forward in the same direction as the incident photon. In X-ray imaging, Rayleigh scattering typically makes a small contribution to total attenuation compared to other factors (Buzug, 2008).

1.5. X-ray Imaging

Electromagnetic waves are used in X-ray imaging to produce images of the interior of the body. Different body parts absorb X-rays in different ways as they pass through the body. For instance, bones appear white in the pictures because they absorb X-rays the most. The body parts are depicted in the pictures in various tones of black and white.

We will now concentrate on various detection techniques in this section to turn the X-rays that have already passed the patient into an actual image. Modern detection systems convert X-rays to light and then to electrons, as opposed to the old X-ray films that used X-rays directly to alter the chemical properties of the X-ray film material.

1.5.1. Image Intensifiers

The vacuum tubes used in X-ray image intensifiers transform X-rays into visible light, i.e., an image. Figure 1.6 illustrates the process's schematic principle. First, a substance known as the input phosphor is used to change the incoming X-ray photons into light photons. Using a photocathode's internal photoelectric effect, the light is further converted to electrons. An electron optic system is then used to accelerate and concentrate these electrons toward the output phosphor. The electrons are transformed back into visible light in the output phosphor, which is subsequently captured by film or television camera tubes.

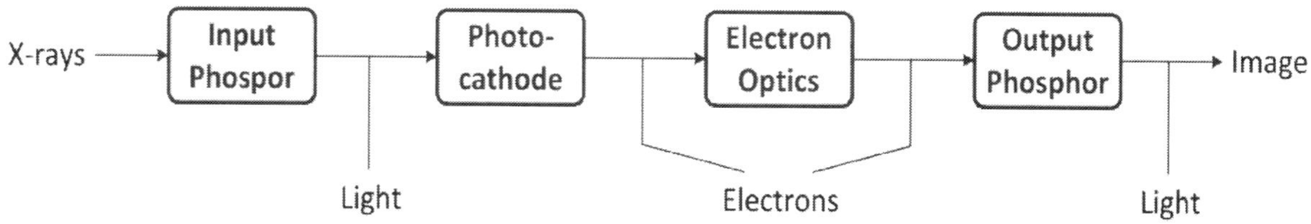

Figure 1.6. *Schematic principle of an image intensifier detector. The X-rays are first converted to light, which is converted to electrons. An optic accelerates the electrons towards a fluorescent screen which converts the electrons to light, which eventually results in an image.*

Source: Berger, M., Yang, Q., & Maier, A. X-ray Imaging. 2018 Aug 3. In: Maier, A., Steidl, S., Christlein, V., et al., editors. Medical Imaging Systems: An Introductory Guide [Internet]. Cham (CH): Springer; 2018. Chapter 7. Available from: https://www.ncbi.nlm.nih.gov/books.

Fluoroscopic detection systems used a single phosphorus material that directly converted X-rays into light before image intensifiers were invented in the late 1940s. However, very dark images and high radiation exposure resulted from the mismatch between the high amount of needed X-ray quanta and the low amount of emerging visible light quanta. Consequently, the radiologists had to view the images in dimly lit environments and after their eyes had had time to adjust to the darkness. The ability to adjust the brightness of the output image by varying the amount of acceleration provided by the electron optics is the primary benefit of image intensifier systems. The input field diameter of contemporary X-ray image intensifiers ranges from 15 to 57 cm. Conversion factors, which show how effectively X-rays are converted to visible light, are what define them.

1.5.1.1. Function

Figure 1.7 provides a more thorough breakdown of each component that makes up an image intensifier. The incoming X-rays first pass through the input window, which is usually made of an aluminum plate with a convex shape and a thickness of about 1 mm. In addition to improving mechanical stability, the convex shape is used to close the distance to the patient, thereby expanding the useful entrance field size.

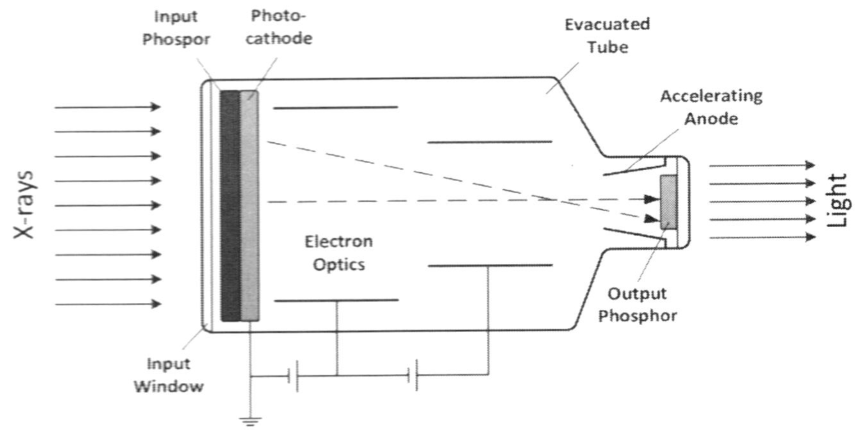

Figure 1.7. *Detailed principle of an image intensifier detector. The X-rays are first converted to light, which is converted to electrons. An optic focuses the electron beam to a fluorescent screen or film material, which converts the electrons to light, i.e., the image.*

Source: Berger, M., Yang, Q., & Maier, A. X-ray Imaging. 2018 Aug 3. In: Maier, A., Steidl, S., Christlein, V., et al., editors. Medical Imaging Systems: An Introductory Guide [Internet]. Cham (CH): Springer; 2018. Chapter 7. Available from: https://www.ncbi.nlm.nih.gov/books.

The X-rays strike the input phosphor, which transforms X-ray photons into light photons after they have passed through the input window. The light photons that are produced cause the photocathode to undergo a photoelectric effect, which releases (photo-)electrons. Usually, the photocathode and input phosphor are layered into one unit. The intermediate layer and the photocathode layer come after the input phosphor, which is made up of a second aluminum plate coated with the phosphor layer.

Let's take a closer look at the input phosphor layer. The thickness of the input phosphor layer is a crucial factor that affects its effectiveness. Greater phosphor layer thickness results in increased absorption of X-ray photons, which in turn produces more light. As a result, fewer X-ray photons are needed, lowering the patient's radiation exposure. But as the layer gets thicker, more light photons scatter inside the phosphor layer, which essentially lowers the spatial resolution.

The mass attenuation coefficient that results from the chemical composition of the input phosphor material is another property that is used to raise conversion factors. It is ideal to modify the attenuation coefficient of the input phosphor in accordance with the remaining incoming X-ray spectrum. Cesium iodide (CsI) has taken the place of zinc-cadmium sulfide (ZnCdS), which was once employed as phosphor material in detector systems. CsI is superior to ZnCdS in two ways.

In Figure 1.8, we display the mass attenuation coefficients for ZnCdS (dotted, light blue line) and CsI (dashed, dark blue line) with respect to the photon energy. A solid, orange line represents the estimated spectral distribution of a typical X-ray spectrum after it has passed through the patient. The better the conversion efficiency, the larger the overlap area between the attenuation characteristics and residual X-ray spectrum. It is obvious that the mass attenuation coefficient of CsI is advantageous because it more closely matches the predicted residual X-ray spectrum.

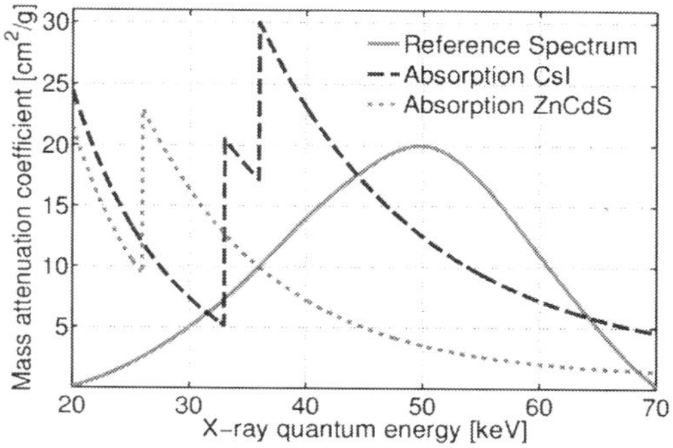

Figure 1.8. *Mass attenuation coefficient of CsI and ZnCdS and the estimated X-ray spectrum after transmission through the patient.*

Source: Berger, M., Yang, Q., & Maier, A. X-ray Imaging. 2018 Aug 3. In: Maier, A., Steidl, S., Christlein, V., et al., editors. Medical Imaging Systems: An Introductory Guide [Internet]. Cham (CH): Springer; 2018. Chapter 7. Available from: https://www.ncbi.nlm.nih.gov/books.

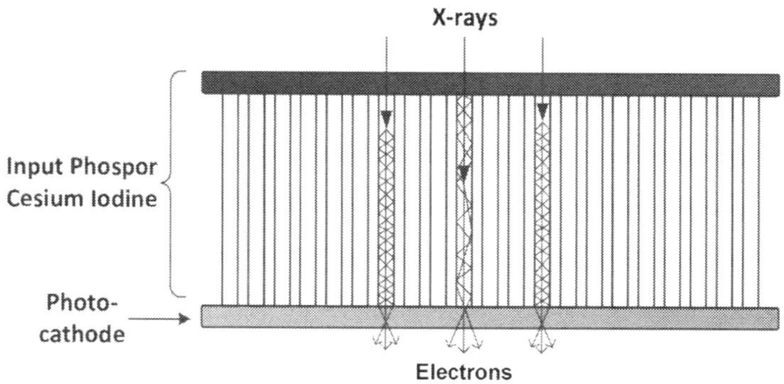

Figure 1.9. *Cesium-iodine layer has a cylindrical structure and acts as optical fibers. Thus, the scattering of the light photons is reduced significantly.*

Source: Berger, M., Yang, Q., & Maier, A. X-ray Imaging. 2018 Aug 3. In: Maier, A., Steidl, S., Christlein, V., et al., editors. Medical Imaging Systems: An Introductory Guide [Internet]. Cham (CH): Springer; 2018. Chapter 7. Available from: https://www.ncbi.nlm.nih.gov/books.

Furthermore, the CsI manufacturing process enables the phosphor layer to be constructed as a group of localized, tiny cylindrical structures, as seen in Fig.1.9. The cylinder wires function as optical fibers that have a high degree of spatial accuracy in guiding the light that is released toward the photocathode. Consequently, there can be a significant reduction in the light photons' scattering within the phosphor material. Approximately 300 μm to 500 μm thick, the input phosphor in modern detectors can absorb up to 70% of the incoming X-ray photons. A solitary 60 keV X-ray photon can generate up to 2600 light photons, of which about 62% arrive at the photocathode (Figure 1.9).

Usually, antimony-cesium ($SbCs_3$) makes up the photocathode layer. As with the input photon layer, the incoming light must match the photocathode's sensitivity spectrum. The sensitivity spectrum of an $SbCs_3$ photocathode is displayed in Figure 1.10, along with the distinctive light spectra from a ZnCdS phospor layer and a CsI. Here, too, as we can see, CsI appears to produce a light spectrum that is more compatible with the photocathode, which results in a higher efficiency of light photon conversion to electrons.

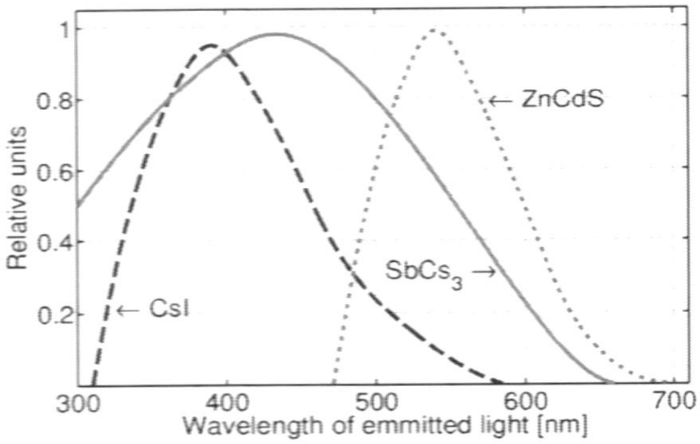

Figure 1.10. *Sensitivity of a $SbCs_3$ photocathode and characteristic light spectra emitted from a CsI as well as a ZnCdS phosporlayer.*

Source: Berger, M., Yang, Q., & Maier, A. X-ray Imaging. 2018 Aug 3. In: Maier, A., Steidl, S., Christlein, V., et al., editors. Medical Imaging Systems: An Introductory Guide [Internet]. Cham (CH): Springer; 2018. Chapter 7. Available from: https://www.ncbi.nlm.nih.gov/books.

The anode accelerates the electrons as they exit the photocathode. Additionally, the electron optic's electrostatic fields are used to focus the accelerated electrons onto the output phosphor. This process only accelerates and deflects the already present electrons in the system; no new electrons are introduced. When the electrons strike the output phosphor, they release more light photons due to the increased kinetic energy that results from the acceleration process. Thus, adjusting the acceleration voltage can change the output phosphor's brightness or intensity. Silver-activated zinc-cadmium sulfide (ZnCdS: Ag) is the usual component of the output phosphor, which is extremely thin (4 μm to 8 μm). For every 25 keV electron, approximately 2000 light photons are produced. This also indicates a brightness increase of a factor of 2000 because in the photocathode, one light photon emits one electron.

1.5.1.2. Known Problems

In addition to universal restrictions that all imaging systems have, e.g., image intensifier systems are most renowned for their vignetting and distortion artifacts, despite their superior spatial resolution and contrast ratio. Vignetting, as shown in Figure 1.11, is the term used to describe a decrease in brightness that happens at the screen's edges. It results from light scattering, which moves light photons in the output phosphor from its exterior to its interior. But there isn't any scattering from the outside of the material to the phosphor's outer regions, which results in brighter central areas. Image distortion, a common artifact, is seen in Figure 1.12. It is understood that external magnetic or electric fields can affect the electron optics of image intensifiers. Even the earth's magnetic field can create significant distortions in the resulting image. To fix these artifacts, frequent calibration is necessary, where the distortion field is determined by measuring specific calibration objects. The distortion can be fixed by adjusting the electron optics or through image processing if the images have been digitized.

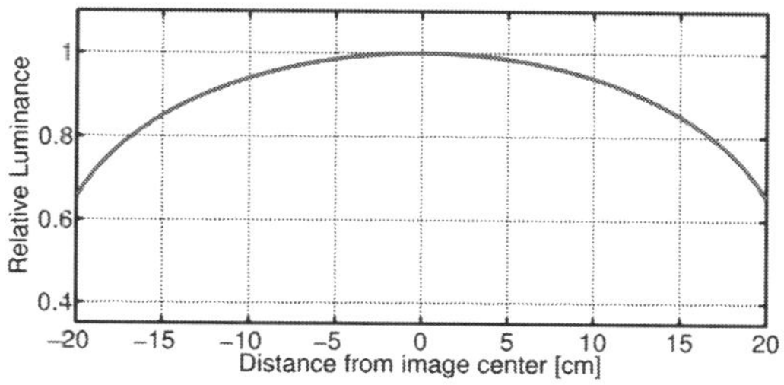

Figure 1.11. *Vignetting artifact, i.e., luminescence drops at the image periphery.*

Source: Berger, M., Yang, Q., & Maier, A. X-ray Imaging. 2018 Aug 3. In: Maier, A., Steidl, S., Christlein, V., et al., editors. Medical Imaging Systems: An Introductory Guide [Internet]. Cham (CH): Springer; 2018. Chapter 7. Available from: https://www.ncbi.nlm.nih.gov/books.

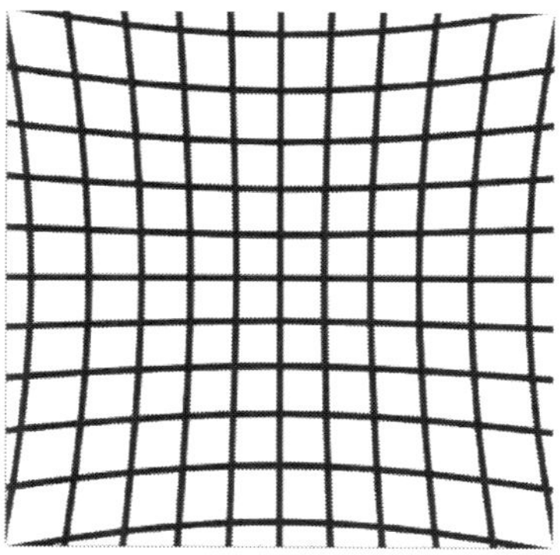

Figure 1.12. *Distortion artifacts due to an external electric or magnetic field.*

Source: Berger, M., Yang, Q., & Maier, A. X-ray Imaging. 2018 Aug 3. In: Maier, A., Steidl, S., Christlein, V., et al., editors. Medical Imaging Systems: An Introductory Guide [Internet]. Cham (CH): Springer; 2018. Chapter 7. Available from: https://www.ncbi.nlm.nih.gov/books.

1.5.2. Flat Panel Detectors

In recent years, flat panel detectors (FPDs) have emerged as the cutting-edge technology in X-ray detector technology for various medical applications such as radiography, angiography, and C-arm CT. Introduced in the mid-1990s, FPDs offer the benefits of direct digital readout of X-ray images and improved spatial resolution. These detectors are typically classified as either direct or indirect conversion FPDs.

- **Indirect Conversion FPDs:** Like the image intensifier system described previously, the FPD also utilizes a layer of cesium iodide (CsI) to convert X-rays to light photons. The tubular structure of the CsI in the FPD is the same as the input layer in an image intensifier system. However, the FPD differs in its detection process. Image intensifiers convert light photons to electrons which are then accelerated for increased and controlled illumination. This extra conversion step is not needed for flat panel detectors. Instead, a matrix of photodiodes is directly connected to the CsI layer, converting light photons to electric charges stored in capacitors for each pixel. Each pixel also includes a thin-film transistor (TFT) that functions as a switch for reading out the stored charges.
- **Direct Conversion FPDs:** A homogeneous layer of X-ray sensitive photoconductors is present on the TFT matrix in direct conversion FPDs in place of an explicit conversion to light photons. An electric field is created across the photoconductor by the high-voltage bias electrode in the top layer. If the photoconductor absorbs X-rays, so-called charge-carriers— i.e., pairs of electrons. Following their separation into positive and negative charges,

these pairs are then carried to the electrodes of the pixel by the global electric field. Positive charges are kept in capacitors at the bottom of each individual pixel electrode after traveling there.

- **Data Readout and Properties:** Pixels are read out row-wise using a specific readout frequency for both the indirect and direct conversion FPDs. Selecting a row involves "turning on" the TFTs of its pixels, i.e., through the application of a voltage to the gate of the TFT. Each pixel's stored charges are fed into a charge integrating amplifier, which transforms them into a digital representation. The digital pixel values are serialized and sent to the imaging computer via a bus system. Typical FPDs used in medical imaging can have a pixel size of between 100 and 150 μm and a side length of up to 40 cm. They come in wide and quadratic format options. Twelve-to-sixteen-bit quantization is used in the analog to digital conversion. During the readout process, multiple pixels are frequently combined to create a larger pixel, a technique known as binning, to increase the signal-to-noise ratio. 2x2 or 4x4 binning are common binning modes that reduce the image size by a factor of 2 or 4, respectively. The binning factor causes the frame rate to increase because binning doesn't need any extra time. The frame rate can range from 7.5 seconds to 30 frames per second, contingent on the specific medical application, dosage specifications, and binning factors.

One of the main benefits of flat panel detectors is that they require a lot less weight and space for the detection unit. While this may seem insignificant, the advantages become evident when we take into account that space is usually at a premium, particularly in interventional settings, and that the rotation speeds of CT or C-arm CT devices are directly correlated with increased weight. An additional benefit is its resilience to mild to moderate electrical and magnetic fields, which presented a significant challenge for image intensifiers. Additionally, the images are immediately available in digital format, improving the efficiency of patient care and data storage.

1.5.3. Sources of Noise

Probabilistic noise and artifacts are the two types of undesired effects in medical imaging systems. Like noise, artifacts are degradations in images that originate from physical effects that occur during the scanning process. But noise differs from artifacts in that noise effects vary according to a probabilistic scheme, whereas artifacts are precisely reproduced when a scan is repeated with the same object and scan parameters. We concentrate on the causes and spread of noise in X-ray imaging in the sections that follow.

As demonstrated in Figure 1.13, an X-ray photon can exist in multiple states. This chain has steps that either follow a binomial distribution or a Poisson distribution. We compare the two distributions in In Figure 1.14. There is a Poisson distribution in the process of producing X-ray photons. A binomial distribution governs both the matter interaction and the detection phase. Along the X-ray's path, both processes interact to produce a different Poisson distribution. Because of this, Lambert-Beer's law can also be interpreted in terms of probability, and in the case of monochromatic data, each detector observation is Poisson distributed.

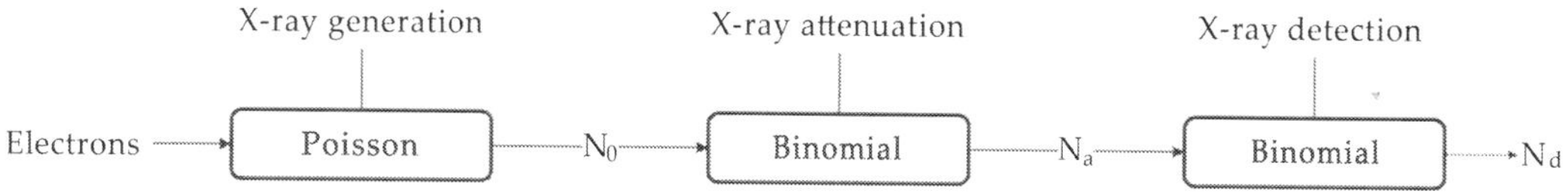

Figure 1.13. *Noise-related processes in X-ray imaging.*

Source: Berger, M., Yang, Q., & Maier, A. X-ray Imaging. 2018 Aug 3. In: Maier, A., Steidl, S., Christlein, V., et al., editors. Medical Imaging Systems: An Introductory Guide [Internet]. Cham (CH): Springer; 2018. Chapter 7. Available from: https://www.ncbi.nlm.nih.gov/books.

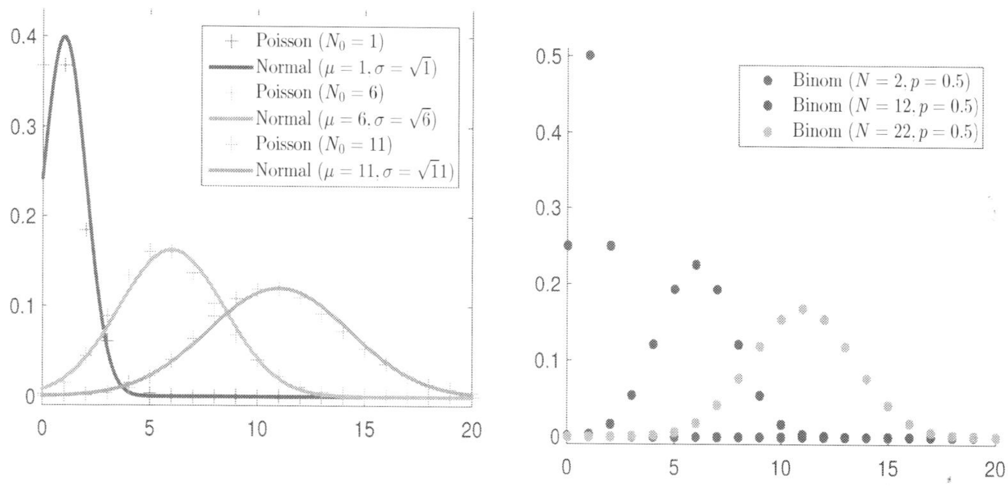

Figure 1.14. *Mass distribution functions of Poisson and binomial distributions.*

Source: Berger, M., Yang, Q., & Maier, A. X-ray Imaging. 2018 Aug 3. In: Maier, A., Steidl, S., Christlein, V., et al., editors. Medical Imaging Systems: An Introductory Guide [Internet]. Cham (CH): Springer; 2018. Chapter 7. Available from: https://www.ncbi.nlm.nih.gov/books.

The signal-to-noise ratio is a frequently used quality metric in imaging (SNR). It is not specifically defined across all application domains.

$$SNR(\mathcal{N}) = \frac{\bar{n}}{\sigma} = \frac{E(\mathcal{N})}{\sqrt{E((\mathcal{N} - \bar{n})^2)}} . \tag{1.6}$$

For random variables N that follow a normal distribution, $\bar{n}$ is the mean value and σ represents the standard deviation. More generally speaking, the two variables define the first moment ($\bar{n}$) and the second central moment (σ) of the underlying distribution. The first moment of the Poisson distribution is given by its expectation value $\bar{n} = E(\mathcal{N})$, whereas the second central moment is the square root of the expectation value of the squared difference between the random variable and its expectation value $\sigma = \sqrt{E((\mathcal{N} - \bar{n})^2)}$. Hence, no matter distribution, σ provides a measure of variation, i.e., a measure of noise. As a result, the SNR gives a measure for the signal quality by dividing the expectation value with the second central moment. If the measured data would not contain any noise, σ would be zero and the SNR would approach infinity. If the noise level increases, also σ increases, thus the SNR decreases. The expectation value $\bar{n}$ in the numerator makes the SNR stable to scaling that means if we measure very high values at the detector a small amount of noise is less critical as if we measure small values that contain the same amount of noise. For X-rays, we can demonstrate that the $SNR(\mathcal{N}) \propto \sqrt{N_0}$. As a consequence, SNR only doubles if we use four times as many photons for N_0. Note this estimation is simplified and neglects some effects such as detector read-out noise (Buzug, 2008).

1.6. The Use of X-rays for Analysis

X-rays are electromagnetic radiations with wavelengths that fall approximately between 0.05 and 100 Angstroms. Because of their similarity to light, the established wave optics tests of polarization, diffraction, reflection, and refraction were conducted. Roentgen could find no evidence of these, despite the limited facilities for experiments. Perhaps there was another reason he referred to them as "x" rays.

Only short wavelength X-rays (hard X-rays) between a few Angstroms and 0.1 Angstrom (1 keV - 120 keV) are used for diffraction applications. X-rays are perfect for examining the structural configuration of atoms and molecules in a variety of materials since their wavelength is similar to that of an atom. Deep penetration of the materials by the intense X-rays allows them to reveal details about the bulk structure.

This year marks the 100th anniversary of the discovery of X-ray diffraction and its use as a probe of the structure of matter. Sixteen years after Wilhelm Conrad Rontgen announced in 1895 his discovery of "X" rays that can penetrate the body and photograph its bones, Max von Laue, a professor of physics at the University of Munich in Germany, worked on a theory of the interference of light in plane parallel plates. Laue was Plank's favorite disciple. His interest covers the whole of physics. If, as some argued, X-rays were not made up of particles but were a form of electromagnetic radiation similar to ordinary (visible) light, and then it should be possible to repeat well-known optical experiments using X-rays instead of beams of ordinary light.

In 1911, von Laue proposed that Walter Friedrich, one of his research assistants, and Paul Knipping, a doctoral student, experiment with X-rays on crystals. He reasoned that since X-rays and crystals have wavelengths that are comparable, the crystal ought to function as a diffraction grating. Von Laue was always the theorist and never carried out the necessary experiments. Friedrich and Knipping conducted a single sophisticated experiment in which von Laue simultaneously demonstrated the space-lattice structure of crystals and the wave-like nature of X-rays (Figure 1.15). When he received the Nobel Prize for what the Committee said was his "epoch-making discovery," Max von Laue gratefully acknowledged Friedrich and Knipping for their roles in the discovery; and for him it went without saying that he shared his prize money with them. Einstein hailed von Laue's discovery as one of the most beautiful in the history of physics.

After X-rays were used to image the internal anatomy of the human body, the Laue experiment made the internal structure of crystals accessible on a nanoscale. Before the Laue experiment, did anyone dream of tools allowing one to explore the structure of matter on the molecular scale and use this information for deriving structure–property relationships of materials – or for understanding the molecular basis of life?

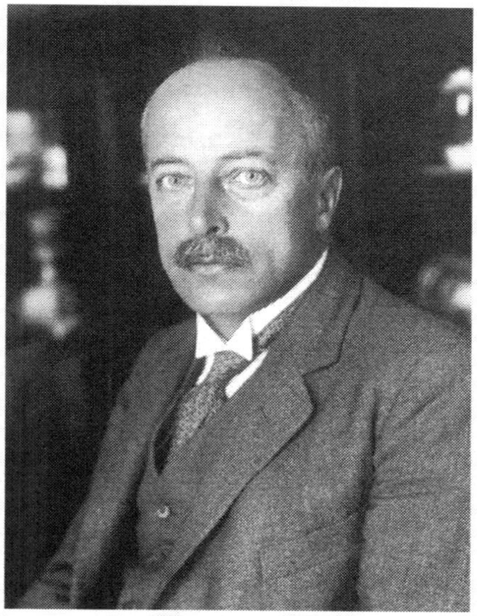

Figure 1.15. *Maxvon Laue*

Source: By Bundesarchiv, Bild 183-U0205–502/ CC-BY-SA 3.0, CC BY-SA 3.0 de, https://commons.wikimedia.org/w/index.php?curid=5437448.

Due to Laue's groundbreaking work in X-ray crystallography, two very significant advances in physics were made possible. Firstly, it established the electro-magnetic nature of X-ray radiation and allowed for highly accurate X-ray wavelength determination. Secondly, it provided chemists and physicists with a new instrument to study the atomic structure of matter. The structure of nucleic acids, or DNA and RNA, was discovered in the 1950s thanks to X-ray diffraction studies, which also helped to find the new field of molecular biology.

The English physicists Sir William Henry Bragg and Sir William Lawrence Bragg (Figure 1.16) contended that if the difference in the wavelengths of X-rays reflected off two successive planes of atoms in the crystal, the interference would be constructive. The Bragg condition is:

$$n\lambda = 2d \sin\theta.$$

They have developed the above relationship to explain why the cleavage faces of crystals appear to reflect X-ray beams at certain angles of incidence (θ). The variable d is the distance between atomic layers in a crystal, and the variable λ is the wavelength of the incident X-ray beam; n is an integer. This observation is an example of X-ray wave interference, commonly known as X-ray diffraction (XRD), and was direct evidence for the periodic atomic structure of crystals. A year after they had invented the technique, in 1913, X-ray crystallography was a common procedure. The findings provided information about crystal structure. The Braggs' work in determining crystal structures, starting with NaCl, ZnS, and diamond, earned them the Nobel Prize in physics in 1915 (Buzug, 2008).

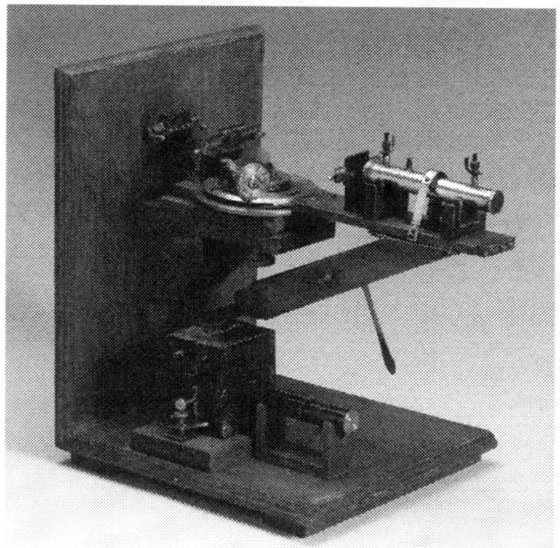

Figure 1.16. *This X-ray spectrometer was used by Sir William Henry Bragg and his son William Lawrence Bragg (1890–1971) to investigate the structure of crystals.*

Source: V By Science Museum London/Science and Society Picture Library – X-ray spectrometer, 1912. Uploaded by Mrjohncummings, CC BY-SA 2.0, https://commons.wikimedia.org/w/index.php?curid=28024339.

Bragg's law, which explains the process of X-ray diffraction, was a crucial discovery that served as the foundation for the field of crystallography as it exists today (Figure 1.17).

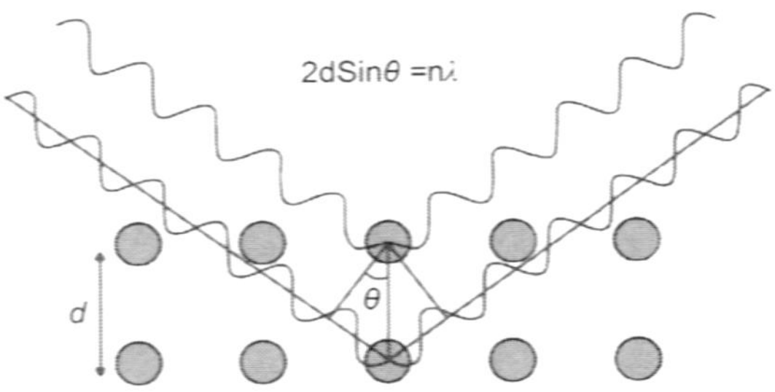

Figure 1.17. *Bragg's law: a representation*

Source: Mikla, V. I., Rusin, V. I., & Boldizhar, P. A. Advances in imaging from the first X-ray images. Journal of Optoelectronics and Advanced Materials. Vol. 14, No. 7–8, July–August 2012, pp. 559–570.

In atoms, X-rays mostly interact with electrons. Certain photons from the incident beam will be deflected away from their original direction of travel when X-ray photons collide with electrons. The process is referred to as elastic scattering because only momentum has been transferred during the scattering process if the wavelength of these scattered X-rays remained constant, indicating that X-ray photons did not lose any energy. Since the scattered X-rays reveal details about the electron distribution in materials, these are the X-rays that are measured in diffraction experiments. However, in the process of inelastic scattering, X-rays impart part of their energy to electrons, resulting in scattered X-rays that differ in wavelength from the incident X-rays.

Different atoms can interfere with one another through diffractive waves, and this interaction strongly modulates the resulting intensity distribution. Sharp interference peaks with the same symmetry as the atom distribution will make up the diffracted waves if the atoms are arranged in a periodic pattern, as in crystals. Thus, we can infer the atom distribution in a material by measuring the diffraction pattern. The atomic distances are directly correlated with the peaks in an X-ray diffraction pattern.

In the same year, Moseley demonstrated that the wavelengths matched the atomic numbers in sequence in addition to being characteristic of the element the target was composed of. This made it possible to definitively determine atomic numbers for the first time.

X-ray crystallography has been a fundamental technique in solving crystal structures for over a century since the discovery of X-rays. Advancements in data collection, instrumentation, and data reduction methods have been continuously evolving. The recent introduction of synchrotron radiation sources, area detector-based data collection instruments, and high-speed computers have greatly improved the efficiency of crystallographic structural determination. Synchrotron radiation, emitted by electrons or positrons traveling at near-light speed in a circular storage ring, is significantly more intense than traditional X-ray tubes. These powerful sources have become essential tools for a variety of structural investigations, leading to advancements in numerous fields of science and technology.

X-ray crystallography is now commonly employed in both materials science and biological studies.

X-ray crystallography utilizes the integrated intensities of diffraction peaks to create an electron density map within the crystal's unit cell. Fourier transforming the diffraction intensities with the correct phase assignment is essential for accurate reconstruction. To achieve this high level of accuracy, it is necessary to have a high degree of data completeness and redundancy, meaning that all reflections must be measured multiple times to minimize errors. One effective method for accomplishing this is by using an area detector, which can collect diffraction data over a large solid angle.

The primary application of powder diffraction is in chemical analysis. It is used for tasks such as identifying phases, studying high or low temperature phases, examining solid solutions, and determining the unit cell parameters of new materials. Inorganic and organic polymers with crystalline inclusions display sharp, narrow diffraction peaks, while the amorphous component produces a broad peak. By analyzing the ratio between these intensities, one can determine the proportion of crystalline phase present in the material.

These days, X-ray diffraction (XRD) can be used to determine a variety of things, such as glass content, quality control techniques, phase quantification, and crystalline material phase identification, to name a few.

Not too long after, it was also determined that any material exposed to primary X-ray beams could produce secondary fluorescent X-rays. This sparked research into the potential applications of fluorescence X-ray spectroscopy in elemental analysis, both qualitative and quantitative.

1.7. Industrial Radiology

In the industrial setting, X-rays are also widely used as a nondestructive testing technique to measure a specimen's volume. A specimen's radiographs revealed any thickness variations, internal and external flaws, and assembly details that are hidden from view.

Ionizing radiation is becoming more widely used worldwide, especially in industry and medicine, and this trend is expected to continue as new technological advancements from research lead to greater applications. Industrial radiography, which employs gamma and X radiation to examine the structural integrity of machinery and buildings, is one of the oldest known uses of ionizing radiation. Almost all developed nations use industrial radiography extensively. It is essential to the quality control needed in contemporary engineering practice and is used by both small and large corporations.

Samples are collected for analysis or a non-destructive test (NDT) is performed to confirm a product's quality. Nondestructive testing must be done, especially with fabricated (welded) assemblies, where a high level of constructional skill is required.

The majority of NDT systems are intended to identify flaws, following which a determination is made regarding the defect's significance in terms of operational safety and/or reliability. Standards have established acceptance criteria for weld defects in newly constructed buildings. Nevertheless, NDT is also employed in research, maintenance inspections of process installations, the development of manufacturing processes, the verification of assembled parts, and the detection of corrosion or other types of deterioration.

Industrial radiography has a wide range of applications. The necessary equipment is easy to use and reasonably priced. It might be incredibly portable and able to be used by one person in a variety of settings, including complicated fabrication facilities, remote construction sites, offshore locations, and cross-country pipelines. Safe working practices must be established to reduce the potential risks to radiographers and anyone else who might be nearby the work due to the associated hazards. The amount of radiation exposure from work is greatly decreased by using shielded enclosures, or fixed facilities, equipped with reliable safety devices.

Several factors have been identified as contributing to the likelihood of accidents in industrial radiography. These include the demands and rewards of the field, the accessibility of necessary equipment, the variety of working conditions, and the fact that the techniques used typically involve the routine manipulation and exposure of powerful gamma-emitting sources and X-ray machines. Individual industrial radiographers are the most likely group of workers to receive doses approaching relevant dose limits. On average, industrial radiographers receive radiation doses that surpass those of other occupationally exposed workers, even in the highly developed regulatory infrastructures of the United States of America and EU-Member States. Thus, industrial radiography safety and radiation protection are crucial in both developed and developing nations.

There are many different types of industrial radiography equipment, image formation methods, and examination techniques available today. The best technique must be chosen with skill and experience for a given application.

The final decision will depend on many variables, including the object's location for examination, the size of the NDT equipment, the required image quality, the inspection time allotted, and, last but not least, financial considerations.

1.8. Airport Security

To find bombs in luggage, airports started using metal detectors in the 1960s and added X-ray screening equipment. They have since become a common sight in many government buildings as well as airports.

Because security scanners can identify both metallic and non-metallic objects carried on a person, they provide a useful substitute for current screening techniques and a practical way to screen passengers. The need for manual searches of passengers, crews, and airport workers may be greatly reduced by the quickly advancing scanner technology.

Only security scanners without X-ray technology have been added recently to the list of approved techniques for passenger screening in airports across the European Union to reduce the risk to the health and safety of traveling citizens (Buzug, 2008).

1.9. The Use of X-rays for Medical Purposes

1.9.1. Retrospective Glance

The remarkable potential of X-rays for diagnostic purposes was recognized by the medical community right away and was further developed over time. When doctors read about X-rays showing bones, they immediately saw the potential for medical use. The patient, who had a fractured ulna and had the first medical X-ray ever recorded in the United States, was brought to Edwin Frost by his brother, a physician. Several applications in the decades that followed showed, for the first time, that it was possible to look inside the body without dissecting it in order to study internal anatomy. The greater sensitivity and fidelity of the recording films have led to considerable advancements in the X-ray technique over time, albeit not always in the fundamental methodology.

This section aims to provide a concise overview of the development of internal body visualization for medical purposes, concentrating primarily on current developments. We'll extrapolate from current developments to potential future advancements to make a few predictions. Many citations will not be used because the majority of this treatise is based on the author's forty years of personal experience and opinion, as well as the past, present, and future topics covered in this perspective. Medical imaging began with direct visualization through dissection in anatomy theaters in the early 12th and 13th centuries, if we limit our attention to the historical development of the field and ignore the notable parallel advancements in biological imaging made possible by the invention of the microscope. For nearly 600 years, this was the main method of imaging, which involves direct visualization through dissection. However, toward the end of the 19th century, a new method of imaging known as X-ray imaging was developed to help visualize the body without dissection. Over the following few decades, this technique's sensitivity and recording quality increased.

X-ray fluoroscopic examinations were conducted in a dark room using images on a fluorescent screen that glowed in response to X-rays that had passed through the patient's body for many years following the discovery of X-rays.

The fields of diagnostic and therapeutic medical physics were founded on Roentgen's groundbreaking discovery. Since then, scientists have been working tirelessly to make new discoveries in physics that will advance radiation therapy and medical imaging technology. Higher speed imaging systems, electronic amplification devices, scintillation cameras, ultrasonographic (US) devices, sophisticated high-capacity X-ray tubes, and rapid film processors were developed in the first 70 years following Roentgen's discovery. But as computers have advanced even further, new technologies have been made possible, including sophisticated interventional fluoroscopy, magnetic resonance imaging (MRI), and computed tomography (CT).

Early radiology equipment was very basic, with exposed metal high-voltage cables hanging across the ceiling and little to no shielding surrounding the X-ray tube (Figure 1.18). Often the physician responsible for the "X-ray laboratory "served as the technologist, service engineer, and medical physicist to ensure that the equipment was functional.

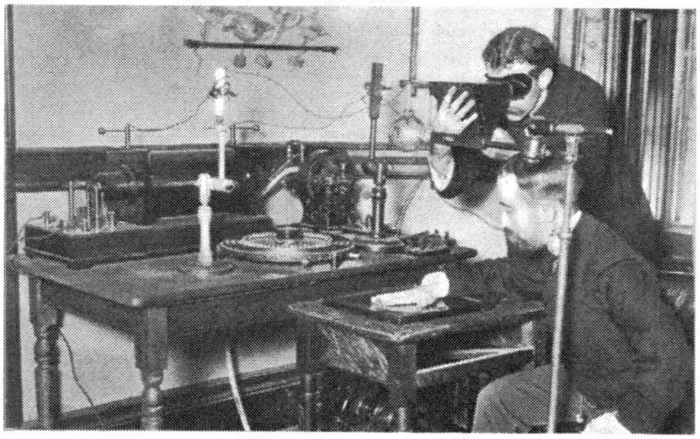

Figure 1.18. *An X-ray examination room with bare high-voltage cables.*

Source: By William J. Morton – Downloaded 2007–12–23 from William J. Morton and Edwin W. Hammer (1896) The X-ray, or Photography of the Invisible and its value in Surgery, American Technical Book Co., New York, fig. 54 on Google Books, Public Domain, https://commons.wikimedia.org/w/index.php?curid=3272036.

Chronologically speaking, a significant advancement in fluoroscopy was achieved in the 1950s when an electronic device based on television technology took the place of the fluorescent screen. The brightness of the image is significantly increased as a result.

With the advent of the CT scanner in the early 1970s, significant modifications to medical physics practice began. Gray remembers being in the equipment exhibit hall at the 1972 Radiological Society of North America (RSNA) meeting held at the Palmer House Hotel in Chicago, just after the exhibits opened. When the author saw the original EMI CT scanner on display, she immediately concluded that the radiology community would not accept it because it produced images with pixels the size of checkerboards (Figure 1.19). Why a radiologist would be interested in anything that produced images with such low spatial resolution baffled the author. Since then, medical physicists have discovered that diagnostic imaging requires consideration of other image quality factors in addition to spatial resolution.

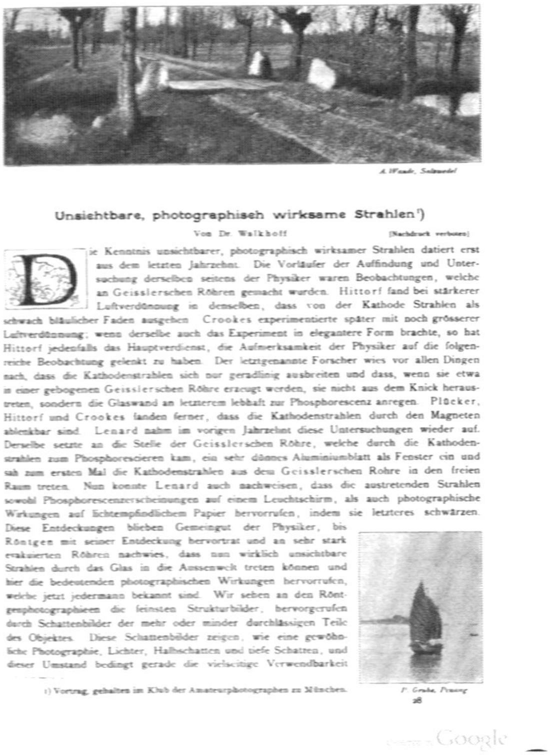

Unsiehtbare, photographiseh wirksame Strahlen[1])

Von Dr. Walkhoff [Nachdruck verboten]

Die Kenntnis unsichtbarer, photographisch wirksamer Strahlen datiert erst aus dem letzten Jahrzehnt. Die Vorläufer der Auffindung und Untersuchung derselben seitens der Physiker waren Beobachtungen, welche an Geisslerschen Röhren gemacht wurden. Hittorf fand bei stärkerer Luftverdünnung in denselben, dass von der Kathode Strahlen als schwach bläulicher Faden ausgehen. Crookes experimentierte später mit noch grösserer Luftverdünnung; wenn derselbe auch das Experiment in elegantere Form brachte, so hat Hittorf jedenfalls das Hauptverdienst, die Aufmerksamkeit der Physiker auf die folgenreiche Beobachtung gelenkt zu haben. Der letztgenannte Forscher wies vor allen Dingen nach, dass die Kathodenstrahlen sich nur geradlinig ausbreiten und dass, wenn sie etwa in einer gebogenen Geisslerschen Röhre erzeugt werden, sie nicht aus dem Knick heraustreten, sondern die Glaswand an letzterem lebhaft zur Phosphorescenz anregen. Plücker, Hittorf und Crookes fanden ferner, dass die Kathodenstrahlen durch den Magneten ablenkbar sind. Lenard nahm im vorigen Jahrzehnt diese Untersuchungen wieder auf. Derselbe setzte an die Stelle der Geisslerschen Röhre, welche durch die Kathodenstrahlen zum Phosphorescieren kam, ein sehr dünnes Aluminiumblatt als Fenster ein und sah zum ersten Mal die Kathodenstrahlen aus dem Geisslerschen Rohre in den freien Raum treten. Nun konnte Lenard auch nachweisen, dass die austretenden Strahlen sowohl Phosphorescenzerscheinungen auf einem Leuchtschirm, als auch photographische Wirkungen auf lichtempfindlichem Papier hervorrufen, indem sie letzteres schwärzen. Diese Entdeckungen blieben Gemeingut der Physiker, bis Röntgen mit seiner Entdeckung hervortrat und an sehr stark evakuierten Röhren nachwies, dass nun wirklich unsichtbare Strahlen durch das Glas in die Aussenwelt treten können und hier die bedeutenden photographischen Wirkungen hervorrufen, welche jetzt jedermann bekannt sind. Wir sehen an den Röntgenphotographieen die feinsten Strukturbilder, hervorgerufen durch Schattenbilder der mehr oder minder durchlässigen Teile des Objektes. Diese Schattenbilder zeigen, wie eine gewöhnliche Photographie, Lichter, Halbschatten und tiefe Schatten, und dieser Umstand bedingt gerade die vielseitige Verwendbarkeit

1) Vortrag, gehalten im Klub der Amateurphotographen zu München.

Figure 1.19. *Early work.*

Source: https://en.wikipedia.org/wiki/File:Unsichtbare_photographisch_wirksame_Strahlen.pdf.

Vascular contrast studies began using digital subtraction angiography (DSA) in the 1980s. Through digital processing and the subtraction of nonvascular anatomy, vascular structures are clearly displayed in DSA, which converts analog video signals from a TV camera to digital data. Rapid advancements in computer technology thereafter led to an expansion in the scope of diagnostic applications. Notable contributions to diagnostic and therapeutic medical physics were made by numerous prominent medical physicists working in the 20th century (Tables 1.1 and 1.2).

1.9.2. Radiography/Fluoroscopy

The process of attenuating an X-ray beam as it passes through a portion of the body and recording it for later medical interpretation of possible pathology (radiography) or showing it in real-time on a monitor for functional assessment (diagnostic fluoroscopy) or intervention (interventional radiology) is known as radiological imaging. The screen/film (S/F) combo in radiography and the image intensifiers and video cameras in fluoroscopy are gradually being replaced by new detectors of the computed radiography (CR) or digital radiology (DR) varieties.

S/F radiography uses luminescent intensifying screens as the primary X-ray absorber, whereas CR uses storage phosphor screens. In S/F, the film, the recording medium, can only receive the light that is emitted. The way images are processed in DR varies. Two categories of DR systems exist:

1. those that are based on charge-coupled devices (CCDs);
2. those that are based on amorphous silicon (a-Si:H) solid-state flat-panel detectors.

While indirect DR technologies need some intermediate steps, direct DR technologies transform the incident X-ray quanta into a measurable latent image signal. Direct detectors generate charge as a direct result of X-ray absorption in semiconductors (e.g., a-Se).

An X-ray scintillator or a thin-film transistor (TFT) photodiode array can convert light photons from an indirect detector into secondary signals, such as charge. Flat-panel detectors are a key element of image-guided radiotherapy and are revolutionizing fluoroscopic and radiographic imaging (Figure 1.20).

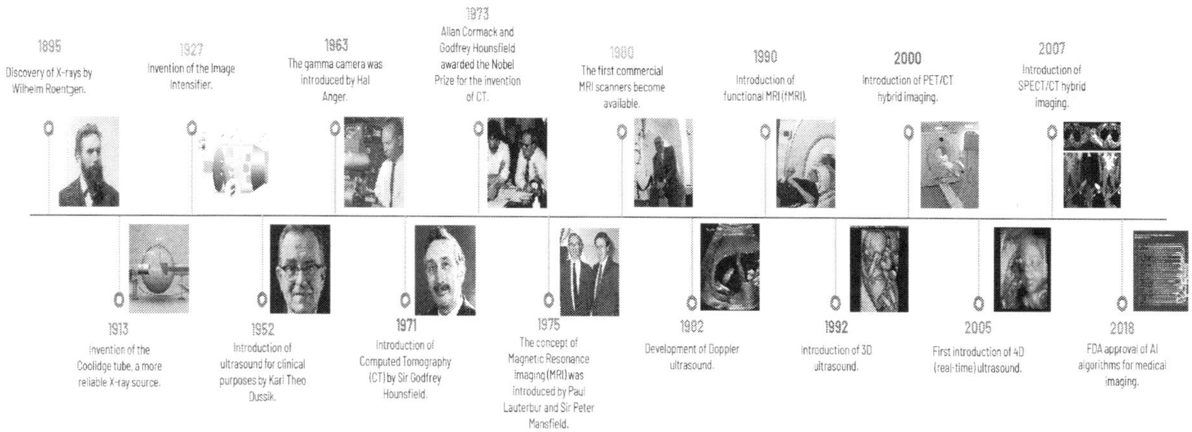

Figure 1.20. *A historical timeline of the key discoveries in medical imaging*

Source: *Najjar R. Redefining Radiology: A Review of Artificial Intelligence Integration in Medical Imaging. Diagnostics. 2023; 13(17):2760. https://doi.org/10.3390/diagnostics13172760.*

Other characteristics that affect image quality include contrast, contrast sensitivity (the ability to see differences in low-contrast objects), blurring and detail visibility (spatial resolution), visual noise, artifacts, and spatial attributes (magnification and distortion). The primary factor that influences X-ray image noise is the exposure level to the receptor. In traditional screen-film radiography, the receptor sensitivity is set at a specific value based on the film type, intensifying screens, and film processing quality. Due to the limited film latitude, exposures must fall within a specific range to avoid images being too light or too dark. The noise level in film radiographs is determined by the film and screen design, which dictates its sensitivity. In contrast, digital radiographic receptors can handle a wider range of exposure levels.

Since its beginnings, fluoroscopy has been and remains a vital imaging modality in the field of interventional radiology, which is concerned with using image guidance to perform minimally invasive procedures for both therapeutic and diagnostic purposes. A few of these procedures are embolization, angioplasty, pacemaker implantation, and angiography.

Because no other modality offers the same combination of high spatial and temporal resolution—which is crucial for the proper deployment of endovascular (from within the blood vessel) devices like stents or coils—X-ray fluoroscopy continues to be the predominant imaging modality in interventional radiology.

1.9.2.1. Radiography

By subjecting an anatomy of interest to X-rays and measuring the attenuation the radiation experiences as it passes through the object, radiography describes the process of producing two-dimensional projection images. It is a widely used type of X-ray imaging that is found in clinics all over the world. Examining fractures and alterations to the skeletal system is the primary application area. In this case, the high attenuation coefficient of the bones relative to the surrounding tissue provides a good contrast, facilitating the identification and categorization of fractures. Additionally, radiography can be used to identify changes in the density or consistency of a bone, e. g., if bone cancer or osteoporosis are present. Figure 1.21 shows two left-hand X-ray images of an arm with fractures in the radius and ulna bones. Additionally, two additional X-ray images of the treated arm, where metal plates have been used to fix the bones internally, are displayed in the figure along with a color image of the arm taken after intervention.

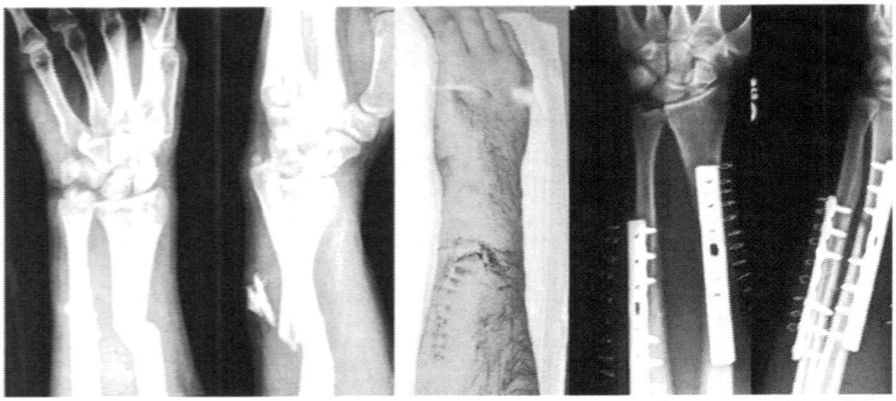

Figure 1.21. *Two left-hand X-ray images of an arm with fractures in the radius and ulna bones.*

Source: Berger, M., Yang, Q., & Maier, A. X-ray Imaging. 2018 Aug 3. In: Maier, A., Steidl, S., Christlein, V., et al., editors. Medical Imaging Systems: An Introductory Guide [Internet]. Cham (CH): Springer; 2018. Chapter 7. Available from: https://www.ncbi.nlm.nih.gov/books.

1.9.2.2. Fluoroscopy

Generally speaking, conventional radiography describes the taking of one or a few X-ray projection images for a particular view. On the other hand, fluoroscopy refers to a series of radiographic pictures that are taken on a regular basis at a specific frame rate. The X-ray source can either continuously expose the region of interest to radiation or it can be triggered for each frame. Image intensifiers and the more recent FPDs are potential sources of X-ray detection. The detection system's acquisition speed usually places a limit on the frame rate. It is determined by the final fluorescent screen's inertia for image intensifiers and by the speed of the electronic detector readout step for FPDs. Frame rates as high as 30 frames per second are feasible in practice. However, rates are frequently lowered for dosage-related reasons.

When performing minimally invasive procedures, fluoroscopy is especially crucial because it allows instruments such as catheters and endoscopes to be guided and used without making direct visual contact with the area being treated. As will be discussed in the next section, it is also the primary technology for using a contrast agent to visualize vessels, such as arteries or veins. An example image from a fluoroscopy sequence that illustrates the positioning of a heart pacemaker's two electrodes and wires is shown in Figure 1.22(a). Figure 1.22(b) depicts a typical clinical setup for a minimally invasive surgery, where a C-arm scanner that can be freely positioned around the patient serves as the X-ray imaging unit.

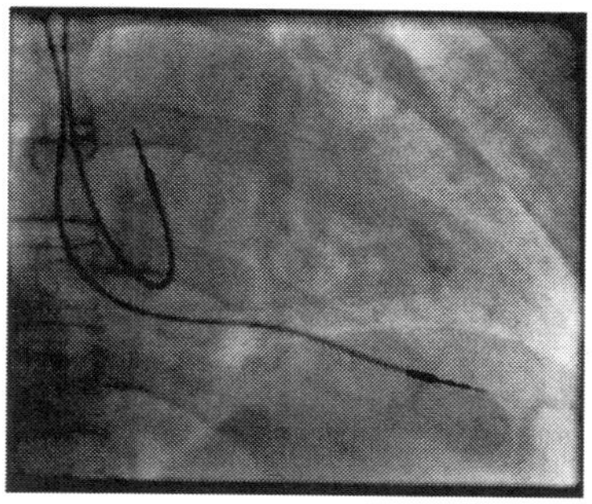

(a) Pacemaker Fluroscopy

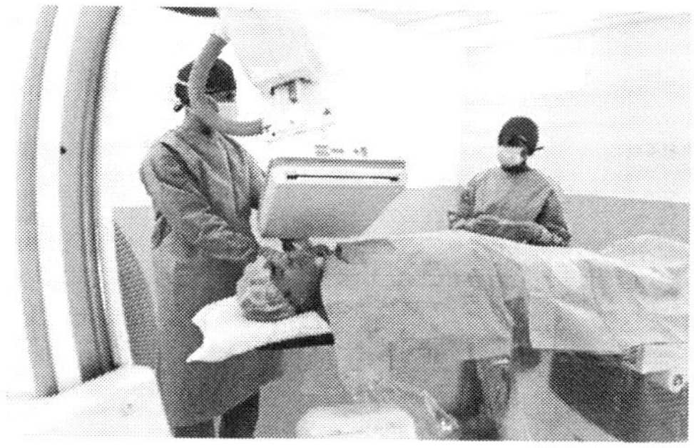

(b) Clinical Setup. Image courtesy of Siemens Healthineers AG

Figure 1.22. *Depicts a typical clinical setup for a minimally invasive surgery, where a C-arm scanner that can be freely positioned around the patient serves as the X-ray imaging unit*

Source: Berger, M., Yang, Q., & Maier, A. X-ray Imaging. 2018 Aug 3. In: Maier, A., Steidl, S., Christlein, V., et al., editors. Medical Imaging Systems: An Introductory Guide [Internet]. Cham (CH): Springer; 2018. Chapter 7. Available from: https://www.ncbi.nlm.nih.gov/books.

1.9.2.3. Digital Subtraction Angiography

Angiography is the term for the imaging of arteries (venography for veins) to analyze characteristics like lumen, size, shape, and flow rate. Because vessels' attenuation characteristics typically don't differ significantly from the surrounding tissue, X-ray-based imaging is difficult and produces poor contrast.

Contrast agent injections into the bloodstream are frequently used to improve contrast and image quality. A liquid that offers a higher attenuation coefficient than typical soft tissue is called a contrast agent. Iodine and barium are common contrast media; the former is used for intravascular procedures and the latter for gastrointestinal exams. Iodine is therefore injected into the bloodstream, whereas barium can be consumed to examine, for example, the stomach or colon.

A fluroscopic sequence of a fixed anatomy is obtained during DSA. Concurrently, the vessel system receives regular injections of contrast agent. Without a contrast agent, X-ray images of the scene are presumed to display background tissue, which is usually not of interest. We can measure the attenuation solely caused by the injected contrast agent if we now subtract the initially acquired background image from an X-ray image with contrast and assume that no patient motion has occurred. The result of such a subtraction will be a visualization of the vessels alone because the contrast agent is restricted to the vessel system in that it has been injected. A DSA acquisition example is shown in Figure 1.23. The contrast agent-free image comes first is obtained as illustrated in Figure 1.23(a), which is the mask image. Following the injection of contrast into the vascular system and some waiting, another image, i.e., the fill image, is obtained. The "angiogram," which solely displays the contrast agent's contributions and thus allows the vessels to be seen, is the difference between the two images.

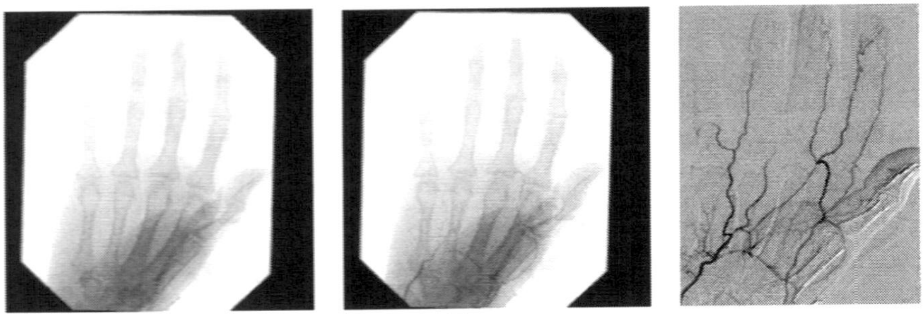

(a) Mask Image (b) Fill Image (c) Angiogram

Figure 1.23. *Creating the DSA.*

Source: Berger, M., Yang, Q., & Maier, A. X-ray Imaging. 2018 Aug 3. In: Maier, A., Steidl, S., Christlein, V., et al., editors. Medical Imaging Systems: An Introductory Guide [Internet]. Cham (CH): Springer; 2018. Chapter 7. Available from: https://www.ncbi.nlm.nih.gov/books.

1.9.3. Clinical Fluoroscopy Requirements for Interventional Radiology

The modern fluoroscope is made up of a large, C-shaped mount known as a C-arm, which includes an X-ray source at one end and an X-ray imager at the other. This setup allows for the acquisition of various projections of the patient's anatomy from different angles. In some cases, the C-arm is rotated around the patient while injecting a contrast dye to capture multiple projection images that can later be reconstructed into a detailed three-dimensional image of the vasculature. To ensure ease of positioning and patient access, the X-ray source and imager need to be compact and lightweight in design.

When using a fluoroscopic mode, an interventional physician inserts catheter-based devices, like stents or guide wires, into the lesion. The primary goal of this procedure is to track the device's position. Usually performed at relatively high imaging frame rates (7.5–30 image frames per second), this guidance—also known as a catheterization—allows the doctor to monitor the device's advancement toward the lesion while preventing complications from things like arterial tortuosity. To reduce patient radiation exposure, catheterization is frequently a lengthy procedure (ten minutes or more) that is carried out at very low X-ray exposures (mean exposure of 1 μR per frame at the imager). In fact, the X-ray exposures used are so low that the predominant type of noise in the fluoroscopic images produced with an XRII system is quantum noise, which is the stochastic variation in the spatial distribution of X-ray photons. Due to the high radioopacity of the interventional device under an image, these low exposures are frequently sufficient to obtain enough contrast to image the device. The cine mode records image sequences while an X-ray contrast agent is injected into the vasculature, usually using a catheter. These relatively quick (a few seconds) image acquisitions are made at higher exposures (~10 μR per frame) to produce better quality images (less quantum noise), which enhances the images' diagnostic value. When precise endovascular device deployment or positioning is required, this mode is also employed. Images are taken in the radiographic mode at even greater exposures (~100 μR per frame) for uses like digital subtraction angiography (DSA), which has been demonstrated to enhance the identification of specific lesions like thrombi or aneurysms.

High spatial resolution is crucial for cine and radiographic imaging in interventional procedures, as it can significantly impact the accuracy of diagnosis and treatment outcomes. Interventional devices like guide wires and stenos typically have wire diameters ranging from 50–200 μm. Despite the challenges posed by X-ray scattering, high-resolution imaging of individual stenos wires (struts) is achievable within a human head phantom, paving the way for novel asymmetrical stenos in specialized therapeutic neurovascular applications. In certain procedures such as coronary angiography, detecting small calcium deposits in coronary arteries, as small as tens of micrometers, is essential for evaluating atherosclerosis severity and predicting the success of angioplasty. To effectively capture fine details in interventional radiology, an imager should be capable of resolving 5 line pairs per millimeter, with a contrast ratio greater than 0.2 at a spatial frequency of 5 cycles per mm (MTF > 0.2).

From the discussion above, it follows that the key requirements for a clinical X-ray imager for interventional radiology - beyond a thin profile and providing unobstructed access to the patient - are:

1. quantum-noise limited (QNL) operation at the lowest clinical fluoroscopic x-ray exposures (in conformance with the ALARA principle);
2, capability for modes of operation that require significantly higher x-ray exposures and
3, capability of imaging fine features of interventional devices or lesions. The imager should also be able to operate at up to 30 frames per second.

1.9.4. X-ray Image Intensifiers

The XRII was, until recently, the most popular X-ray imaging system in interventional radiology. This electrooptical apparatus (Figure 1.24A) is housed in a vacuum enclosure and uses an input phosphor to transform X-rays into optical photons.

The phosphor is connected to a photocathode, which generates electrons when exposed to these optical photons. The latter strike an output phosphor screen after being accelerated in an electric field. For every photoelectron released from the photocathode, this process allows for the production of several thousand optical photons. A video camera or CCD is used in conjunction with an optical assembly to capture the final optical image. Because of the XRII's large internal gain, XRII/video systems offer excellent X-ray sensitivity—that is, the ability to detect small numbers of X-rays, ideally just one. However, the XRII also has significant limitations. These result in geometrical distortions (especially in the image periphery), spatial non-uniformities, and a reduction in imaging resolution. They are linked to the curvature of the input phosphor and the existence of multiple conversion stages. Moreover, the bulk and weight of these systems—they can weigh several hundred pounds—compromises image acquisition modes like cone-beam CT and rotational angiography as well as patient accessibility. Another important limitation of the XRII is its high sensitivity to magnetic fields (including the earth's magnetic field) which produces a distortion in the image that is shaped like an "S" and referred to as an S-distortion.

The availability of new solid-state technologies and these significant limitations have led to a progressive trend in recent years toward the replacement of XRII systems with flat-panel detectors.

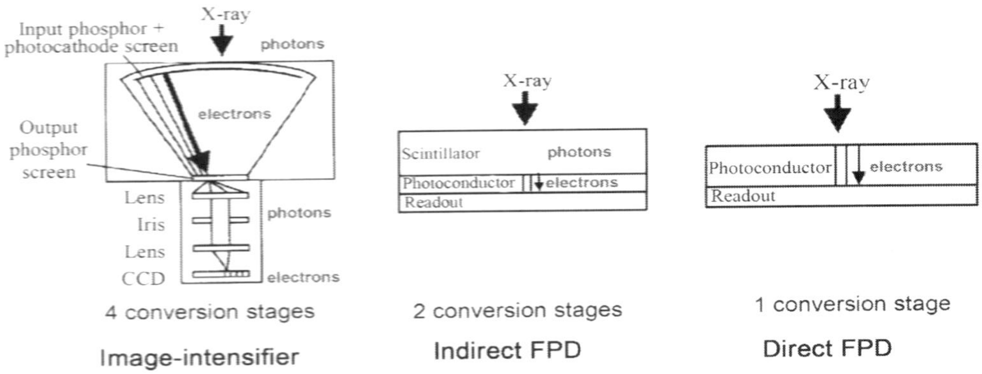

Figure 1.24. *This electrooptical apparatus is housed in a vacuum enclosure and uses an input phosphor to transform X-rays into optical photons.*

Source: *Mikla, V. I., Rusin, V. I., & Boldizhar, P. A. Advances in imaging from the first X-ray images. Journal of Optoelectronics and Advanced Materials. Vol. 14, No. 7–8, July–August 2012, pp. 559–570.*

1.9.5. A New Revolution in Optical Imaging

A new revolution in medical imaging did not start until the early 1970s, despite the fact that advancements in recording media significantly improved the quality and application of X-rays for medical purposes—fluoroscopy and nuclear imaging being the two most notable exceptions, which were developed decades later.

It wasn't until the 1970s that modern medical imaging became possible. An X-ray imaging device known as the "CAT" scanner, or Computerized Axial Tomograph device—long since renamed Computed Tomography, or CT—heralded in this modern era once more. This device made three major contributions to medical imaging that are still its cornerstone today: 1) the image was digital, created by a computer, and could be easily altered, analyzed, and displayed by computers; 2) the method provided sensitivity to differences in tissue density that could not have been achieved previously; and 3) the methodology provided cross-sectional views of the human body, eventually multiple cross-sectional views next to one another, providing a three-dimensional view of internal anatomic structures. Imaging adjacent thin body cross sections was a significant advancement in medicine's ability to more accurately see and understand the true nature of objects inside the body because the body is three-dimensional and the organs have different shapes, sizes, and positions relative to one another in three-dimensional space.

The 1970s saw the introduction of this scanner, which was followed quickly by the availability of 3D imaging and the quick development of additional modalities. The early 1980s saw the development of magnetic resonance imaging (MRI), which is noteworthy for its nearly revolutionary influence on soft tissue imaging. Functional imaging was first made possible by nuclear systems, most notably positron emission tomography (PET). High-speed CT (helical) and rapid magnetic resonance imaging (fMRI) came next. With notable advancements in imaging methodologies during the 1990s, interactive multi-dimensional, multimodality imaging was routinely used in large medical centers for better diagnosis, treatment, guidance, and therapy monitoring. The beginning of the

21st century saw the development of numerous image-guided interventions, which are frequently connected to minimally invasive surgery and are used for the planning, practice, and performance of a broad range of clinical and surgical procedures.

The following are the ongoing objectives for the development and acceptance of significant visualization display technology: (a) enhancing the display's dimensionality, quality, and speed; and (b) improving access to the data it represents by enabling interactive, user-friendly manipulation and measurement of the data it represents. Determining the quantitative information about the characteristics of anatomic tissues and how diseases relate to and impact them is one of these goals. With these developments, it will soon be feasible to deliver a number of significant clinical applications. Table 1.1 lists significant occurrences in diagnostic imaging.

These important developments have paved the way for an exciting future that will include real-time, multi-dimensional imaging, as well as extremely sensitive and specific imaging. Almost any number of orthogonal image variables can be fused and synchronized together to combine all the data collected and use it to help diagnose and treat diseases. Future medical practice will move toward genuinely synchronous, minimally invasive, highly specific, highly sensitive, and highly effective disease diagnosis and treatment as a result of the near future highly integrated capabilities for structural and functional information being demonstrated synchronously across space and time. The only process that can produce a gain big enough to meet the requirement (1) is avalanche multiplication of charge in a-Se, and the highly adjustable avalanche gain should also meet the requirement (2). Moreover, a-Se high intrinsic imaging resolution ought to satisfy the requirement (3).

Table 1.1. Major Events in Diagnostic Imaging Over the Last Five Decades

1950s	Utilization of an image-intensifier system for fluoroscopy Development of a gamma camera for radionuclide imaging
1960s	Development of a 90 s automated film processor Basic research on image quality, MTFs, Wiener spectra and quantum mottle
1970s	Development of rare-earth screen-film system, digital subtraction angiography (DSA), computed tomography (CT), ultrasound imaging with electronic scan Initial research on ROC analysis, MRI, PET, SPECT, PACS and electronic imaging
1980s	Development of computed radiography (CR), magnetic resonance imaging (MRI), color Doppler ultrasound imaging Initial research on computer-aided diagnosis (CAD)
1990s	Commercialization and clinical use of CAD system, flat-panel detector (FPD) systems, multi-detector computed tomography (MDCT), magnetic resonance angiography (MRA), harmonic/contrast imaging
2000s	Development and clinical use of real-time 3D ultrasound imaging, cone-beam CT, parallel MRI, PET/CT, full-field digital mammography (FFDM), MDCT with 256 detectors, molecular imaging and PACS

Source: Mikla, V. I., Rusin, V. I., & Boldizhar, P. A. Advances in imaging from the first X-ray images. Journal of Optoelectronics and Advanced Materials. Vol. 14, No. 7–8, July–August 2012, pp. 559–570.

1.10. Risk Factor

When X-ray exposure is high enough, cancer may result. X-rays were not initially suspected as the cause because this damage takes time to manifest. Clarence Dally, an assistant to Thomas Edison, was the first person to die as a result of radiation exposure from X-rays. Intense research was conducted into the effects of this radiation during the first half of the 20th century, and protective measures (like lead shielding) were developed to reduce exposure to it.

Predicting health issues early on is unquestionably crucial. Many imaging modalities, including computed tomography, magnetic resonance imaging, and X-rays, have been developed and used for several decades for both therapeutic and diagnostic medical care.

Nonetheless, doctors are now worried about the overuse of some diagnostic methods, especially those that expose patients to radiation, in the last few years. While a patient won't suffer any negative effects from infrequent use of computed tomography or X-ray scans, repeated radiation exposure over a brief period can seriously harm cells, raising the risk of cancer and other illnesses.

The negative impacts of ionizing radiation in fluoroscopy have been well-known for a long time, leading to the importance of keeping patient doses as low as possible during procedures. This guiding principle is commonly known as ALARA. Despite the risks, the use of X-ray radiation is deemed necessary when the potential benefits of the procedure outweigh the potential harm from the radiation.

Both direct and indirect effects are included in these biological effects.

- Ionizing radiation can have indirect effects on biological targets like DNA when electrons propelled by X-ray photons excite and ionize water molecules, resulting in the production of free radicals.
- DNA molecules are directly ionized by electrons in direct effects. Therefore, in some situations, like pediatric interventions, a particularly stringent adherence to ALARA is necessary because the cumulative stochastic effects of radiation exposure are more likely to impair tissue growth and development and raise the child's lifetime risk of developing cancer. Other imaging modalities are also associated with certain adverse effects. There is a known risk of heating from the electromagnetic radiofrequency pulses used in MRIs. This can be especially dangerous close to metallic implants or devices, like pacemakers or hearing aids. When exposed to ultrasonic waves, ultrasound contrast agents may also have potential bioeffects (i.e., rupturing of cell membranes) at the microcirculation level, though it's still unclear how useful these bioeffects would be in a clinical setting.

1.11. Medical Exposure Dosimetry

The International Commission on Radiological Protection (ICRP) uses the terms "equivalent dose" and "effective dose" to describe the stochastic effects of radiation protection. These terms are used in prospective dose assessments for planning and optimization in radiological protection, as well as to demonstrate regulatory compliance with dose limits for the public and occupationally exposed workers. They measure things in sieverts (Sv). "Effective dose is not recommended for epidemiological evaluations, nor should it be used for detailed specific retrospective investigations of individual exposure and risk." As indicated in table 6 from AAPM Report 96, effective dose in medical exposure can be used as a quality control tool to compare doses from various radiation modalities, but not to evaluate doses for specific patients. The International Commission on Radiation Units and Measurements (ICRU) states that "to assess the risk from stochastic and deterministic effects from medical x-ray imaging, it is necessary to know the organ or tissue doses, the dose distribution and the age and gender of the patients." The ICRU Report contains information on patient dose calculations and measurements, as well as amounts and units to be used in medical X-ray imaging. The gray is the unit (Gy).

In radiography and fluoroscopy, the patient doses can be calculated by measuring the airborne kerma for each radiation beam and multiplying the result by the technique factors that are utilized, which can be obtained manually or from the DICOM header. An additional option would be to fit an appropriately calibrated air-kerma-area-product meter (formerly known as a DAP meter) to every X-ray machine. CT doses may be calculated from "computed tomography air-kerma(dose) index"(CTDI) and "air-kerma (dose)-length product" (DLP) measurements. This is vital.

Table 1.2. Occupational Exposures for Various Job Categories

Workplace	Period	Monitored workers 10^3	Annual effective dose (mSv)
Uranium mining	2000–2002	12	1.9
Diagnostic radiology	2000–2002	6.670	0.5
Radiotherapy	2000–2002	264	0.5
Cyclotron			*WBD: 0.35–0.85 **WD: <7.95
Radiochemistry lab			*WBD: 0.60–1.80 **WD: <4.45

Source: Ali YF, Cucinotta FA, Ning-Ang L and Zhou G (2020) Cancer Risk of Low Dose Ionizing Radiation. Front. Phys. 8:234. doi: 10.3389/fphy.2020.00234.

As per the 2008 report by the United Nations Scientific Committee on the Effects of Atomic Radiation (UNSCEAR), the global annual number of diagnostic X-ray examinations performed is approximately 3.6 billion (3.1 for medical and 0.5 for dental). When comparing the annual examination frequency for this time period (1997–2007) to earlier UNSCEAR surveys, there has been a noticeable increase. The primary cause of this is population aging, as the majority of medical exposures involve elderly patients. In terms of dosage, the world annual dose from diagnostic medical exposures is 0.61 mSv, or 20% of the estimated global dose of 3.1 mSv (of which 79% is due to natural background). This percentage contribution is significantly different in developed nations like the United States, where an increase in medical uses between 1980 and 2006 raised the total annual effective dose from 3 to 5 mSv, making medical exposure equal to or greater than background exposure from natural sources. The number will rise if widespread CT screening methods—which are presently undergoing clinical trials—such as virtual colonoscopy, calcium scoring for atherosclerosis, coronary angiography, and lung cancer screening for smokers and ex-smokers, prove beneficial.

Assumingly, determining the necessity of the X-ray procedure is the first step towards radiological protection of diagnostic medical exposures, i.e., how will the study impact the care of patients.

When it comes to diagnostic medical exposures, the patient dose must be kept to the lowest amount required to meet the necessary diagnostic goal, while also taking into consideration pertinent reference levels for medical exposure and acceptable image quality standards set by relevant professional bodies. Thus, it is necessary to avoid exposures that result in doses higher than the minimal amounts that are clinically acceptable. It is crucial to realize that optimizing protection does not equate to lowering dosage, and that the determining factor should be diagnostic data rather than image quality. The patient's habits, the goal of the radiological examination, and the properties of the image receptor must all be taken into consideration when creating optimized images. Pregnant women and children should receive special attention.

Because noise and exposure have an inverse relationship, noise is the primary factor that restricts the amount of X-ray exposure and patient dose that can be decreased. This is true for all types of X-ray imaging, such as fluoroscopy and CT. In screen/film radiography, the film acts as the medium for acquisition, display, and storage, so the optimization process must be done during image acquisition. On the other hand, in digital radiography, the three processes are separate, allowing image optimization to be done through pre- and post-processing software. Various noise reduction methods have been documented, aside from increasing photon fluence (Buzug, 2008).

A Closer Look

Therapeutic Medical Physics

The employment of physicists in radiation therapy dates back to soon after X-rays were first used for treatment of diseases in the late 1890s and early 1900s. Physicists were needed because the early X-ray machines required constant nurturing to keep them running reliably and with some consistency in dose delivery. Many of the early developments in dose specification and measurement were made by physicists, culminating in the establishment of the first unit of "dose," the roentgen, in 1928. During this same period, a number of hospitals began to employ physicists to deal with the handling and dosimetry associated with radium and radon brachytherapy. Two pioneers in the United States whose names come to mind readily in this context were Giaoacchino Failla, DSc, and Edith Quimby, DSc, at the Memorial Hospital in New York City.

Medical physics has changed dramatically since 1895. There was a period of slow evolutionary change during the first 70 years after Roentgen's discovery of X-rays. With the advent of the computer, however, both diagnostic and therapeutic radiology have undergone rapid growth and changes. Technologic advances such as CT and MRI in diagnostic imaging and 3D treatment planning systems, stereotactic radiosurgery, and intensity-modulated radiation therapy in radiation oncology have resulted in substantial changes in medical physics. These advances have improved diagnostic imaging and radiation therapy while expanding the need for better educated and experienced medical physics staff.

Summary

- X-rays belong to the group of electromagnetic rays, hence, they follow the rules of electromagnetic radiation. Electromagnetic radiation transports energy, also called radiant energy, through space by waves and photons, just as radio waves, the visible light or microwaves. It can either be represented by photons or by a wave model.
- Rayleigh scattering is a coherent process and is the predominant kind of scattering at low X-ray energies. It is caused by an interaction of the incident wave with several, usually outer shell electrons.
- X-ray imaging is a process that uses electromagnetic waves to create images of the inside of the body. X-rays pass through the body, and different parts of the body absorb them differently.
- X-rays are electromagnetic radiations having wavelengths roughly within the range from 0.05 to 100 Angstroms. Their similarities to light led to the tests of established wave optics: polarization, diffraction, reflection and refraction.
- X-rays are also used extensively in industry as a nondestructive testing method that examines the volume of a specimen. Radiographs of a specimen showed any changes in thickness, internal and external defects, and assembly details invisible to the naked eye.
- Radiological imaging is a process by which the attenuation of an X-ray beam traversing a part of a human body is either recorded in a medium for later medical interpretation of potential pathology (radiography) or displayed in real time on a monitor for functional assessment (diagnostic fluoroscopy) or intervention (interventional radiology).
- Angiography refers to the imaging of arteries (venography for veins) to analyze properties such as shape, size, lumen, or flow rate. Usually, the attenuation properties of vessels do not substantially differ from that of the surrounding tissue which makes X-ray-based imaging hard and yields poor contrast.

References

1. Buzug, T. M. (2008). *Computed Tomography: From Photon Statistics to Modern Cone-Beam CT*. Berlin, Germany: Springer. DOI:10.1118/1.3176026.
2. Kasap, S. O., Frey, J. B., Belev, G., Tousignant, O., Mani, H., Greenspam, J., Laperriere, L., Bubon, O., Reznik, A., DeCrescenzo, G., Karim, K. S., & Rowlands, J. (2011). Amorphous and polycrystalline photoconductors for direct conversion flat panel image sensors. *Sensors, 11*, 5112.
3. Lorch, B., Maier, A., Hofmann, H. G., & Fahrig, R. (2015). Projection and reconstruction-based noise filtering methods in cone beam CT. In H. Handels (Ed.), *Bildverarbeitung für die Medizin 2015* (pp. 59–64). Lübeck, Germany: Springer.
4. Maier, A., & Fahrig, R. (2015). GPU denoising for computed tomography. In X. Jia & S. Jiang (Eds.), *Graphics Processing Unit-Based High Performance Computing in Radiation Therapy* (1st ed., Vol. 1). Boca Raton, FL: CRC Press. https://doi.org/10.1201/b18968-9.

5. Maier, A., Steidl, S., Christner, F., Wigström, L., Hofmann, H. G., & Fahrig, R. (2011). Three-dimensional anisotropic adaptive filtering of projection data for noise reduction in cone beam CT. *Medical Physics, 38*(11), 5896–5909. https://doi.org/10.1118/1.3633901.

6. Rowlands, J. A. (2002). The physics of computed radiography. *Physics in Medicine & Biology, 47*, R123.

7. Schmahl, W. W., & Steurer, W. (2012). Laue centennial. *Acta Crystallographica Section A: Foundations and Advances, 68*(1), 1.

8. Wang, J., & Blackburn, T. J. (2000). The AAPM/RSNA physics tutorial for residents. *RadioGraphics, 20*(5), 1471–1477.

Chapter

COMPUTED TOMOGRAPHY

2

Contents

Introduction

The term CT scan is commonly used to refer to computed tomography. A CT scan is a diagnostic imaging technique that creates images of the inside of the body by combining computer technology and X-rays. Any part of the body, including the bones, muscles, fat, organs, and blood vessels, can be seen in detail.

Compared to regular X-rays, CT scans provide more details. An energy beam is directed towards the body part under examination in standard X-rays. Following its passage through skin, bone, muscle, and other tissue, the energy beam's variations are captured by a plate located behind the affected body part. A standard X-ray can reveal a lot of information, but it does not provide much detail regarding internal organs or other structures.

The X-ray beam in a CT scan circles the patient's body. This offers far more detail and numerous perspectives of the same organ or structure. The X-ray data is sent to a computer, which decodes it and projects it onto a monitor in two dimensions. Computer software and newer technology enable the creation of three-dimensional images. CT scans can be used to look for internal injuries or damage, look into internal bleeding, or assist in the diagnosis of tumors. Tissue or fluid biopsies can also be performed with CT (Calabrese, 2011).

Orientation and Directional Terms

Term	Definition	Illustration
Spiral CT	Spiral CT is a vast improvement over conventional CT scans. The patient lies on an exam table that passes through a doughnut-shaped scanner, while an X-ray tube rotates around the table. This movement results in a spiral shaped continuous data set without any gaps. With the helical CT, there is less likelihood to miss small tumors or abnormalities, and spiral CT is about 8 to 10 times faster than a traditional CT. This procedure is especially beneficial to the elderly, very young patients and acutely injured patients who are sensitive to longer exam times.	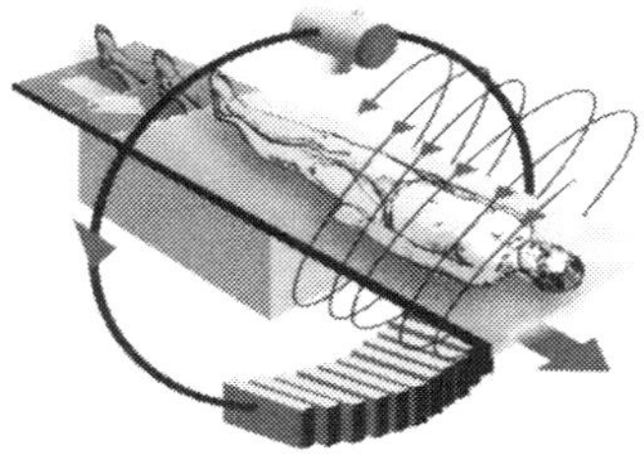
Angiography	Angiography is a type of X-ray used to check blood vessels. Blood vessels do not show clearly on a normal X-ray, so a special dye called a contrast agent needs to be injected into your blood first. This highlights your blood vessels, allowing your doctor to see any problems.	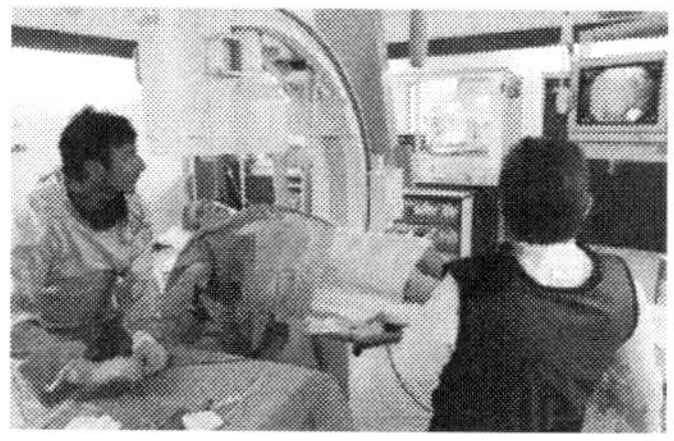
Multiplanar reconstruction (MPR)	Multiplanar reconstruction (MPR) involves the process of converting data from an imaging modality acquired in a certain plane, usually axial, into another plane. It is most commonly performed with thin-slice data from volumetric CT in the axial plane, but it may be accomplished with scanning in any plane and whichever modality capable of cross-sectional imaging, including magnetic resonance imaging (MRI), PET and SPECT.	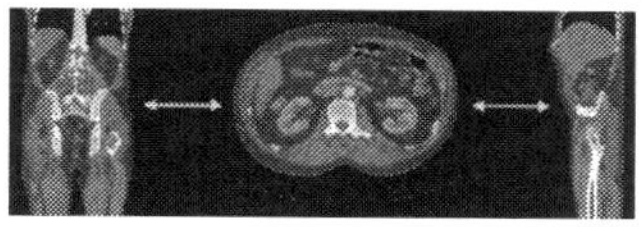
Maximum intensity projection	Maximum intensity projection (MIP) is a method for 3D data that projects in the visualization plane the voxels with maximum intensity that fall in the way of parallel rays traced from the viewpoint to the plane of projection. This implies that two MIP renderings from opposite viewpoints are symmetrical images if they are rendered using orthographic projection.	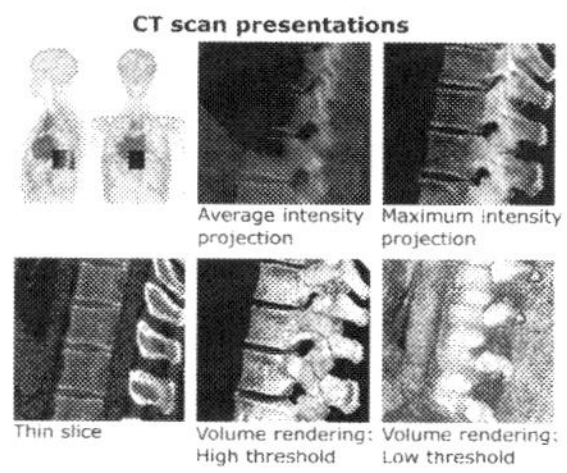
Windowing	Windowing is the process in which the CT image grayscale component of an image is manipulated via the CT numbers; doing this will change the appearance of the picture to highlight particular structures. The brightness of the image is adjusted via the window level. The contrast is adjusted via the window width.	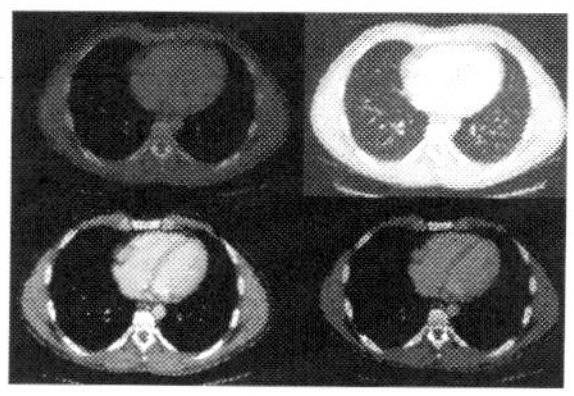

2.1. Advents Of Computed Tomography

One significant scientific advance has been the identification of X-ray radiation. This has been credited to Wilhelm Conrad Röentgen, a German scientist who, on November 8, 1895, carried out the first cathode tube experiments (Crookes tube). This radiation penetrates opaque objects, sensitizes the film, and exhibits fluorescence. This radiation was called "X-ray radiation" by Röentgen. Three-dimensional objects are penetrated by X-rays that are irradiated. X-rays that pass-through objects are captured as two-dimensional images on film or detectors. Radiography is the term commonly used to describe this. Overlap causes information to vanish, it is difficult to distinguish between tissues with small absorption coefficients, and scattering X-rays negatively affect the formation of images.

The terms "computed" and "tomography" are derived from the Greek words "tomo" (which means "to cut" or "section") and "graphy" (which means "to describe"). The term "computed" in CT (computed tomography) denotes calculated or reconstructed. X-rays are the foundation for CT scanner operations. Generally speaking, general CT uses energy between 100 and 150 kV.

The mathematical underpinnings of the Radon transformation (also known as the Radon theorem), which was published in 1917 by Austrian mathematician Johann Radon—who also supplied the formula for the inverse transform—are the basis for the CT image reconstruction algorithms. According to the Radon theorem, it is possible to reconstruct an image from projections; specifically, an infinite set of the image's projections obtained through rotational scanning can be used to obtain the image distribution function.

The mathematical computation technique that allowed cross-sectional images of internal distributions to be calculated from projection of attenuation data due to X-rays that penetrated the body at different angles based on the rotation of the X-ray source and electronic detector around a three-dimensional object was published in the early 1960s by Allan M. Cormack, an American physicist of South African descent. The British engineer Godfrey N. invented the CT scanner, which uses X-rays, in 1972. Hounsfield. Hounsfield and Allan M. Cormack were jointly awarded the 1979 Nobel Prize in Physiology and Medicine for the invention of CT. Two of the earliest clinical CT scanners were a head scanner installed in 1972 at the Atkinson Morley Hospital in London, UK, and a whole-body scanner installed in 1976 at Georgetown University Medical Center in the United States.

2.2. Basic Physical Principles of Computed Tomography

2.2.1. X-ray Attenuation through an Object

The X-rays propagate through the sample wherein some of the X-ray photons are absorbed, and others are transmitted to the detector. The general form of X-ray attenuation is $I_x = I_0 \cdot \exp^{-\mu x}$, where I_0 is the X-ray intensity before the object is reached, I_x is the X-ray intensity after they penetrate through the object with a thickness x (where exp=e=the exponential coefficient=2.7182818...), μ is the X-ray linear attenuation coefficient, and x is the thickness of the absorbing material in chosen distance units, e.g., in mm. If X-rays pass through multiple objects with a total thickness x, as shown in Figure 2.1, the penetrated X-ray intensity can be expressed according to $I = I_0 \cdot e^{-\mu 1x} \times e^{-\mu 2x} \times e^{-\mu 3x} \times e^{-\mu 4x} = I_0 \cdot e^{-(\mu 1+\mu 2+\mu 3+\mu 4)x}$, known as the Beer-Lambert ssslaw. Therefore, the total linear attenuation coefficient can be written as the sum of contributions of $\mu_{tot} = \mu_1 + \mu_2 + \mu_3 + \mu_4$ shown in Figure 2.1. Thus, the intensity of the X-rays measured on a position of the detector is proportional to the integral of the two-dimensional (2D) transparency of the object, and is exactly equal to the sum of the linear attenuation coefficient along their passage.

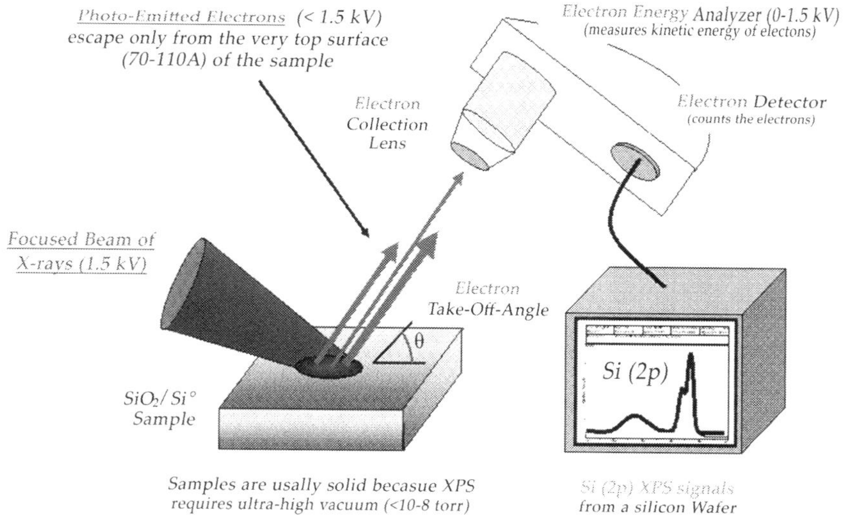

Figure 2.1. *X-ray beam.*

Source: By Bvcrist (talk); transferred to Commons by Lauro Chieza de Carvalho (Carvalho, Lauro Chieza de) – System2.gif in english Wikipedia (log), Public Domain, https://commons.wikimedia.org/w/index.php?curid=7333849.

2.2.2. Computed Tomography Image Data Acquisition

An object is placed on a table in order to obtain a CT image. The object is rotated around by an X-ray source (located within a CT scanner gantry), and any X-rays that pass through it are detected on the other side. The data acquisition system receives the detections obtained at various angles (DAS). These provide projection data to form tomographic images. The basic requirements of CT image acquisition include: a) One tomographic image is reconstructed from X-ray projection data of the object acquired at different angles for general 360° (or 180°) rotations; and b) objects must be still and included in every projection dataset during the scan. These are the fundamental requirements for acquiring CT images.

2.2.3. Computed Tomography Image Reconstruction

In computed tomography (CT) image reconstruction, the 2D cross-sectional attenuation distribution function [f(x,y)] is derived from a sequence of one-dimensional (1D) X-ray projections [P(r,θ)s] obtained as the line integrals at numerous angles around the three-dimensional (3D) object. The attenuated set of parallel X-rays (or isotropic X-rays emitted from a point source) passing through a 2D object of interest forms a projection, [P(r,θ)]. A sinogram is a group of projections made at various angles during one rotation of the X-ray source-detection system. This is essentially a linear transformation of the object's cross-sectional image. All of the various projections for any slices stacked together are simply displayed on sinograms. In actuality, we are able to measure the intensity I of the detected X-ray beam and know the intensity I_0 of the incident X-ray beam. Therefore, what we are interested in learning is the distributions of the object's individual X-ray attenuation coefficients. These specific coefficients in the object's internal structure must be calculated to reconstruct images in CT. An example is given below:

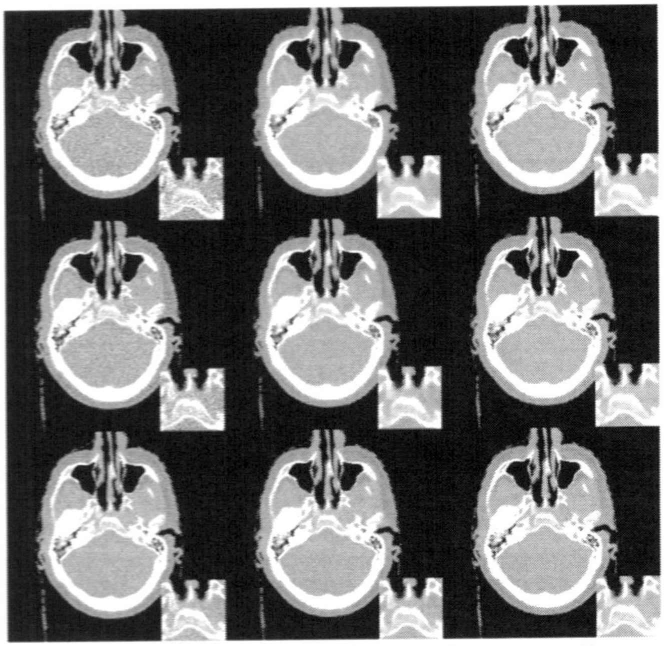

Figure 2.2. *Computed tomography: an example study of image reconstruction methods.*

Source: *Wu, J., Wang, X., Mou, X., Chen, Y., & Liu, S. Low dose CT image reconstruction based on structure tensor total variation using accelerated fast iterative shrinkage thresholding algorithm. Sensors. 2020; 20(6), 1647. https://doi.org/10.3390/s20061647.*

Matrix inversion, iterative, backprojection, analytical, 2D Fourier transformation, and filtered backprojection methods in conventional CT; and 3D Radon transform, 3D filtered backprojection methods in spiral CT or conical beam CT (CBCT), and nutating slice are among the numerous techniques that can be used for CT image reconstruction. To bring the rays close to the image plane, algorithms for reconstructing tilted image planes are adjusted to the spiral path. A single ray in a given projection is simply the sum of all the pixels the ray passes through on its way through the object. The iterative reconstruction (IR) method is an algebraic reconstruction technique that starts with an image assumption and adjusts its value based on the difference between estimated and measured values until the two are in agreement. The initial reconstruction algorithm used when CT was developed in the 1970s was the IR, which required about 45 minutes to reconstruct a single slice. A faster filtered backprojection (FBP) algorithm was subsequently developed and has been employed in CT imaging for over thirty years. However, the relatively high noise levels cause issues for the FBP. For each projection, the backprojection technique "smears back" the projection inversely across the image plane at the measurement angle. FBP was developed with filtering to change (or modify) the projections with a reconstruction Kernel prior to applying standard backprojection in order to improve the blurring issue that arises in backprojection. The theorem that connects the Fourier transform—currently the most widely used reconstruction technique in the field of medical imaging—and the Radon is called the central slice theorem (CST), sometimes referred to as the projection slice theorem or Fourier slice theorem.

The objective is to deduce from the P(r, θ) function of the projections (sinogram) in polar coordinates the function f(x, y) of the attenuation coefficient map of the object in the x-y rectangular coordinate system. Understanding the relationships between different operations in the f(x, y) space and those in the Fourier F(u, v) space is always useful. The relationship between the object's Radon transform and the 2D Fourier transform of the sinogram P(r, θ) is defined by the CST. Consequently, the radial slice obtained through the object's 2D Fourier domain at an angle θ is equal to the 1D Fourier transform of the projection measured at that same angle. As indicated in Figure 2.2, the computed coefficient distributions of F(u,v) in the frequency domain are then subjected to an inverse Fourier transform to yield the f(x, y) attenuation coefficient distributions.

2.2.4. Computed Tomography Numbers/Hounsfield Units

A CT scanner's image is a digital image. It is composed of a square matrix of picture elements, or pixels, each of which represents a voxel, or volume element, of the object's (the patient's) internal structure. Each pixel in a CT section actually represents a small volume element, or voxel (pixel area × slice thickness), because a CT section has a finite thickness. This voxel's dimensions are determined by the thickness of the section, the chosen field-of-view (FOV), and the matrix size. The numerical pixel matrix corresponding to a spatial location in the image is transformed into an image based on the allocation/transformation of the pixel values to a corresponding grayscale value. These pixel values are the average linear attenuation coefficients of the interior tissue corresponding to the spatial locations of these pixels.

With an image depth of 12 bits (4,096 gray levels) and a square matrix of 512 by 512 pixels, a typical CT image is created. However, in recent years, matrices made of 1,024 by 1,024 or 2,046 by 2,048 (ultrahigh-resolution CT) pixels have become more common. CT numbers (Hounsfield units [HU]) are defined as the attenuation values of the imaged tissues normalized to that of water:

$$CT\ number\left(HU\right)=1{,}000\times\frac{\mu_{pixel}-\mu_{water}}{\mu_{water}}$$

where μ_{pixel} denotes the linear attenuation coefficient of a specific pixel and μ_{water} denotes the linear attenuation coefficient of water. The definition of CT number (HU) states that the range of CT numbers for water and air are 0 and −1,000, respectively.

2.2.5. General Classifications of Computed Tomography Scanners

The fan-beam X-ray source is primarily used for diagnostic purposes, and the CT scanner is categorized as spiral (helical) and traditional (axial) CT depending on the data acquisition method. Furthermore, radiation therapy is the primary use of the conical beam X-ray source in CBCT scanners. Using a fan-shaped X-ray beam, the conventional (traditional) CT scanner acquires one slice image per scan before moving on to the next slice scan position. The fan-shaped X-ray beam and detector (or multidetector) in the spiral (helical) CT scanner move in a helical path with respect to the object using a DAS. Actually, as the gantry rotates, the scanned object on the CT couch is moved to the scanner's bore.

With just one rotation around the object being scanned, the conical beam X-ray used by the CBCT scanner can cover a sizable volume. On the other hand, the linear array of detector elements (in a single slice CT) found in spiral and conventional CT scanners is replaced by a 2D array of detector elements in the multidetector CT (MDCT). The acquisition of multiple slices (or sections) of large volume simultaneously during CT scanning is made possible by the 2D detector array, which also significantly speeds up the process of acquiring CT images.

2.2.6. Components of Computed Tomography Scanner

The basic components of a modern CT scanner consist of a gantry that is outfitted with an X-ray tube, high-voltage generator, filters, collimators, detector arrays, DAS, couch (patient table), operating console, and computer for image reconstruction. The current CT X-ray tube must maintain 60–80 kW on a focal spot as small as 1 point 3 by 10 mm for up to 20 seconds. The X-ray tube receives high voltages (usually between 120 and 140 kV) from a very stable three-phase generator. The range exposure parameters, including the X-ray characteristics of kV and mA, are determined by the generator's power capacity, which is expressed in kW.

Low-energy X-rays that increase patient dose rather than aid in image formation are removed by the filter positioned between the patient and the X-ray tube. The patient and the filter are separated by the collimator. Its function is to limit the scattered X-rays from the outer regions of the relevant slice and to lower the radiation dose. Numerous varieties of CT detectors were created, such as solid-state scintillation detectors, gas-filled detectors, and others. A gas-filled detector is made up of distinct subdetectors and a single vessel that is filled with high-pressure gases (about 25 atm) of high-atomic-number elements (Krypton, Xenon, or Krypton and Xenon). Sodium iodide scintillation crystals (NaI) combined with a photomultiplier tube were used in early CT scanners. The X-rays are transformed into visible light photons by the majority of solid-state detectors, which then use photodiodes to convert the photons into electrical signals. Because solid-state detectors use crystals that fluoresce when X-ray photons interact with them, they are also known as scintillation detectors. The scintillation lights are converted to electrical signals by a photodiode.

Because carbon fibers have a low photon absorption rate, they don't interfere with X-rays, which is why patient couches and tables are made of them. To establish the scanning position and regulate the patient's movements following position settlement during the examination, patients lie on the couch and are moved through the gantry aperture. For a CT couch to support weights up to 204 kg, it must be sturdy and rigid. While diagnostic CT uses a rounded table top for patient comfort, radiation therapy tables are flat to reconstruct the patient's image in the same condition as a treatment machine. In radiation therapy simulations, the gantry's bore size is larger to account for scenarios where immobilization devices result in a large overall diameter of the imaging volume. Furthermore, for better results from treatments, specific patient postures are frequently required (85 cm for radiation treatment vs. 70 cm to aid in diagnosis). The control center of the CT scan is the operating console. It is made up of computers, several monitors, and a keyboard that are used to control the scanner, get data from the DAS, and recreate the CT image.

2.2.7. Developments of Computed Tomography Scanner

The way that CT scanners worked in the past was as follows. A single detector measured the X-ray pencil beam, and the X-ray tube and detector moved in tandem (translation movement). Then, for a single slice, these steps were repeated while the X-ray and detector rotated simultaneously at a different angle. After that, the detector and X-ray moved in unison to a new slice, and the procedure was repeated. With the exception of using a row of up to 30 detectors simultaneously that were integrated with narrow fan X-ray beams, the second generation of CT scanners was operated similarly to the first-generation scanners. The scanning time for each slice using this method was between 5 and 90 seconds. A row of detectors on the third generation CT scanner was sufficiently wide to image the entire slice at a single angle orientation. As a result, the translation movement was abandoned. This procedure was repeated until a single slice was scanned before acquisitions were made for a different slice (axial scanning). The X-ray and detector rotated together at different angles. These days, this technique is most frequently employed. It takes about 0.3 seconds to image a single slice. A fixed full ring of detectors was adopted by the fourth generation CT. As a result, the X-ray tube only moved to a new slice after rotating around the previous one. These days, this approach is not very popular. The fifth generation of CT electron beam scanners does away with mechanically moving parts, such as the television tube case, by using a stationary X-ray tube and a stationary detector ring. The patient is surrounded by a fixed array of tungsten anode targets that receive an electron beam that is magnetically deflected toward them. By sweeping the electron beam over the target, the magnetic deflection produces an X-ray source that essentially rotates around the patient. The lack of mechanically moving parts allows for the completion of a sweep in as little as 50–250 ms.

The sixth generation CT, helical (spiral) CT, was developed by Willi A. Kalender (German medical physicist) in 1989. The third and fourth CT generations' concepts were combined with slip-ring technology to create the helical CT. A continuously rotating X-ray beam and gantry detector system moved the patient in the direction of the gantry. In terms of cutting down on scanning time, spiral CT is far more effective. The scanning time was significantly reduced by combining continuous data acquisition with continuous table translation and slip-ring-based volumetric data transmission. The X-ray tube and detector array system installed in the gantry, using slip-ring technology, can rotate at different speeds ranging from 0.25 to 3 seconds per rotation. In the late 1990s and early 2000s, MDCT, the seventh generation of CT scanners, was unveiled. It featured a 2D multiple detector array that could scan multiple slices simultaneously in a single rotation. High-speed image acquisition that is proportionate to the number of detector rows has been made possible by the development of MDCT. One row of detectors was present in the first single-slice CT scanner. All CT scanners nowadays, however, have multislice detector arrays with 8–320 rows of detectors. Unlike single-detector row CT, which has multiple detectors along the gantry but only one row, multidetector row (also known as multislice) CT uses multiple rows of CT detectors instead of just one. It simply recreates one slice in the z-direction. Because more body parts are contained in each gantry turn, MDCT has the advantage of faster scanning. With MDCT, the multiple rows of detectors reconstruct multiple slices per projection. The MDCT pitch is computed by dividing the movement of the table by the total beam width. Similar numbers to the single-slice version are obtained in this way: contiguous helices correspond to a pitch of 1.

As seen in Figure 2.3, modern, cutting-edge novel CT technologies have brought dual-energy CT (DECT) and detector-based spectral CT to the market. Compared to a standard single energy helical CT, DECT, also referred to as spectral CT, uses two distinct X-ray energy tubes, typically rated at 80 kVp and 140 kVp. This allows the image enhancement of substances through the application of subtraction imaging techniques, which exhibit distinct attenuation behaviors at different energies. Attenuation varies depending on the material when the tube's rated voltage is changed. DECT takes advantage of the following effects: two datasets with varying attenuation levels are acquired by two X-ray sources operating concurrently at different energies. The material-specific difference in attenuation in the resulting images makes it possible to classify the scanned tissue's basic chemical composition with ease. Furthermore, a fused image is offered for preliminary diagnosis. To distinguish materials like iodine, calcium, and uric acid from soft tissues, DECT techniques may be helpful. Using traditional helical CT protocols, detector-based spectral computed tomography uses two layers of detectors to simultaneously gather low- and high-energy data from a single X-ray tube in all patients. Based on the material densities or atomic numbers of the different components in the body, this spectral information can show the different shades of gray or even colors in the final image to differentiate the X-ray attenuation differences of those elements. Better tissue discrimination can already be facilitated by DECT, which makes it simpler to distinguish between materials. For example, tissues containing calcium and iodine can appear similar on conventional, monochromatic CT techniques. In a variety of clinical settings, including the improvement of conspicuity and identification of smaller vessels connected to subsegmental pulmonary emboli, it may also raise diagnostic accuracy.

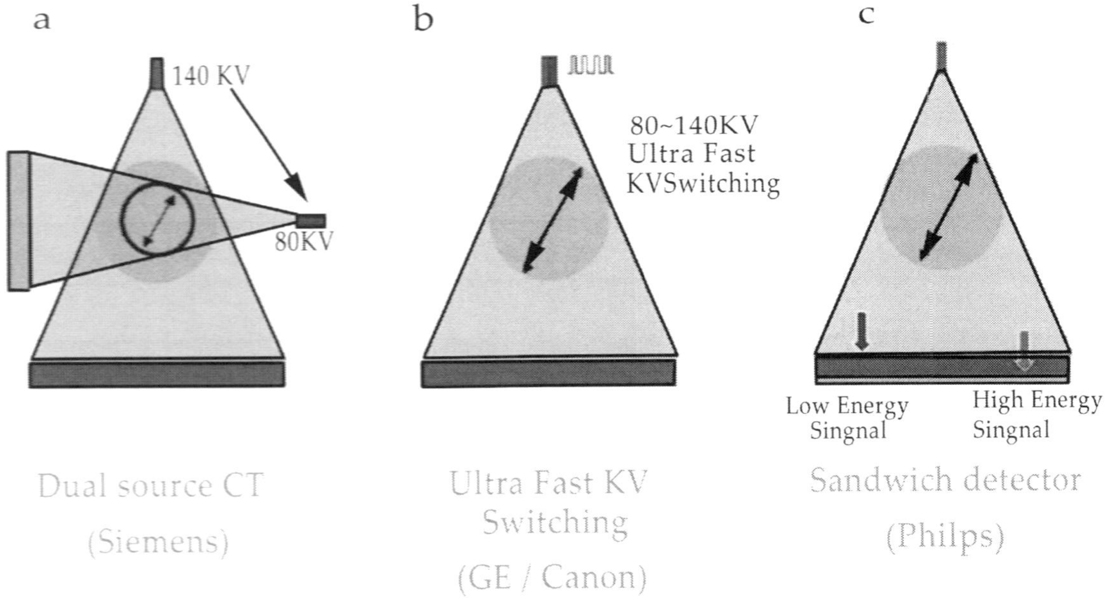

Figure 2.3. *Dual-energy computed tomography (CT). This is a schematic showing (**a**) a dual-source CT in which X-rays of different tube voltages are simultaneously irradiated from two bulbs with 90° orientation differences, (**b**) a single-source CT system in which the tube voltage is switched to a fast switching mode (Fast kV switching) of 0.5 ms or less, and (**c**) a single-tube voltage X-ray irradiated with a stacked detector.*

Source: *Tsurusaki M, Sofue K, Hori M, Sasaki K, Ishii K, Murakami T, Kudo M. Dual-Energy Computed Tomography of the Liver: Uses in Clinical Practices and Applications. Diagnostics. 2021; 11(2):161. https://doi.org/10.3390/diagnostics11020161.*

2.3. Types of Computed Tomography

There are many different kinds of scanners on the market, each based on how images are acquired and processed.

2.3.1. Sequential CT

The CT table moves stepwise in a sequential CT scan, commonly referred to as step-and-shoot CT. The rotation of the X-ray tube and the acquisition of a slice occur after the table advances to a specific point and stops. After that, the table increases once more, and another slice is taken. When taking slices, the table must come to an end. This causes the scanning time to increase.

2.3.2. Spiral CT

An entire X-ray tube is spun around the central axis of the area being scanned in a spinning tube scan, also known as spiral CT or helical CT. These scanners are the most common kind available because they are less expensive to produce and buy, and they have been around for a longer time. The primary constraint on this kind of CT scan is the weight and inertia of the apparatus (the detector array and X-ray tube assembly on the other side of the circle), which sets a maximum spin speed limit. To increase temporal resolution, certain designs make use of two X-ray sources and detector arrays that are angled.

2.3.3. Electron Beam Tomography

A particular type of CT called electron beam tomography (EBT) involves building a sufficiently large X-ray tube so that deflection coils are only used to spin the path of the electrons as they travel between the cathode and anode of the tube. This type has a significant advantage over others because of its ability to achieve much faster sweep speeds, which reduces blurry imaging of moving structures like the heart and arteries. Compared to spinning tube types, fewer scanners of this design have been manufactured, primarily because of the higher construction costs of a much larger X-ray tube and detector array as well as the limited anatomical coverage.

2.3.4. Dual Energy CT

A development of computed tomography, dual-energy CT, also called spectral CT, uses two energies to produce two sets of data. To obtain two distinct sets of data, a dual-energy CT can use a single source with a dual detector layer, a single source with energy switching, or a dual source.

- A dual-source CT scanner uses two X-ray tubes for detection, as opposed to the single tubes used in traditional single-tube systems. The two detector systems are positioned at a 90-degree angle in the same plane on a single gantry. Because they can acquire an entire CT slice in just half a rotation, Dual Source CT scanners enable faster scanning with higher temporal resolution. Rapid imaging can potentially shorten the breath-hold duration by reducing motion blurring at high heart rates. This is especially helpful for sick patients who can't take medicine to lower their heart rate or who have trouble holding their breath.

- Another Dual energy CT mode is a Single Source with Energy switching, where a single tube is operated at two different energies by frequently switching the energies.

2.3.5. CT Perfusion Imaging

A particular type of CT used to measure blood vessel flow while administering a contrast agent is called CT perfusion imaging. It is possible to compute blood flow, blood transit time, and organ blood volume with a respectable level of specificity and sensitivity. Although its sensitivity and specificity for identifying anomalies are still lower than those of other CT types, this kind of scan can be applied to the heart. This can also be applied to the brain, where a CT perfusion scan can frequently identify inadequate brain perfusion long before a traditional spiral CT scan does. When diagnosing strokes, this is superior to other types of CT.

2.3.6. PET CT

The hybrid CT modality known as positron emission tomography–computed tomography (PET–CT) combines an X-ray computed tomography (CT) scanner and a positron emission tomography (PET) scanner on a single gantry. Sequential images are obtained from both devices during the same session and combined into a single superposed (co-registered) image. Functional imaging from PET scans, which show the body's metabolic or biochemical activity distribution spatially, can therefore be more precisely aligned or correlated with anatomic imaging from CT scans.

PET-CT is useful in identifying various cancer types and provides anatomical and functional details of an organ under examination (Rosen et al, 2003; Mettler et al, 2008).

2.4. Medical Use

Ever since its debut in the 1970s, computed tomography (CT) has grown in importance as an adjunct to traditional X-ray imaging and medical ultrasonography. In more recent times, it has been applied to preventive medicine and disease screening; examples include full-motion heart scans for individuals at high risk of heart disease and CT colonography for those with a high risk of colon cancer. Due to the radiation dose involved, many institutions offer full-body scans to the general public, although this practice is against the official position of many professional organizations in the field.

In many nations, the use of CT scans has skyrocketed in the past 20 years. In the US, there were over 80 million scans in 2015 compared to an estimated 72 million in 2007.

- **Head:** Usually, infarction (stroke), tumors, calcifications, hemorrhage, and bone trauma are found via CT scanning of the head. Among the aforementioned, hyperdense (bright) structures suggest calcifications and hemorrhage, hypodense (dark) structures can suggest edema and infarction, and bone trauma can be observed as a disjunction in bone windows. Tumors can be identified by surrounding edema or by the swelling and anatomical distortion they produce. Using a tool called the N-localizer, CT scanning of the head is also utilized in radiosurgery and CT-guided stereotactic surgery to treat intracranial tumors, arteriovenous malformations, and other surgically treatable conditions.
- **Neck:** When it comes to adult neck masses, contrast CT is typically the first investigation of choice. Thyroid computed tomography (CT)

is a valuable diagnostic tool for thyroid cancer. The most common method of investigation for thyroid abnormalities is a CT scan, which also frequently uncovers thyroid abnormalities by coincidence.

- **Lungs:** The lung tissue, or lung parenchyma, can undergo both acute and chronic changes that can be found with a CT scan. This is especially important because typical two-dimensional X-rays don't display these kinds of flaws. Various methods are employed, based on the suspected anomaly. Thin sections with high spatial frequency reconstructions are used to assess chronic interstitial processes like fibrosis and emphysema; frequently, scans are done during both inspiration and expiration. High-resolution CT is a specialized method that creates lung samples rather than continuous images.

  On lung CT scans, bronchial wall thickening is visible and typically (though not always) indicates bronchial inflammation.
- **Angiography:** When a nodule is discovered by accident and there are no symptoms, it's called an incidentaloma. This can cause worry because it could be a benign or malignant tumor. To perform surveillance on the nodules, patients and physicians occasionally consent to an intensive schedule of CT scans, sometimes up to every three months and beyond the advised guidelines. This may be the result of fear. According to established guidelines, patients who do not have a history of cancer and whose solid nodules have not grown over the course of two years are not likely to be suffering from malignant cancer. Patients shouldn't undergo CT screening beyond what is advised by established guidelines due to these reasons, the lack of evidence in favor of intensive surveillance producing better results, and the risks involved with the procedure.
- **Cardiac Anatomy:** To learn more about the anatomy of the heart or coronaries, a CT scan of the heart is done. Traditionally, coronary artery disease has been identified, diagnosed, or monitored using cardiac CT scans. In the rapidly developing field of transcatheter structural heart interventions, particularly in the transcatheter repair and replacement of heart valves, CT has recently assumed a pivotal role.

The main forms of cardiac CT scanning are:

- **Coronary CT angiography (CCTA):** Coronary CT angiography (CCTA) is the process of evaluating the heart's coronary arteries with CT scans. After the patient gets an intravenous injection of radiocontrast, a high-speed CT scanner scans the heart, enabling radiologists to determine the degree of coronary artery occlusion and, typically, make a diagnosis of coronary artery disease.
- **Coronary CT Calcium:** Another tool for determining the severity of coronary artery disease is the coronary CT calcium scan. It searches the coronary arteries specifically for calcium deposits,

which can narrow the arteries and raise the risk of a heart attack. A standard coronary CT calcium scan is performed without radiocontrast, though it might also be performed using contrast-enhanced images.

Post-processing of the images is common to improve the anatomy's visualization. Volume rendering and multiplanar reconstructions (MPR) are the most popular. To obtain a deeper understanding of more intricate anatomy and procedures, like heart valve interventions, a true 3D reconstruction or a 3D print is made using these CT images.

- **Abdomen and Pelvis:** CT is a reliable method for identifying diseases of the abdomen, such as Crohn's disease, GIT hemorrhage, cancer diagnosis and staging, and post-treatment follow-up to evaluate response. It is frequently employed to look into sudden stomach pain.

  These days, the gold standard for diagnosing urinary stones is non-enhanced computed tomography. To assist clinicians in directing additional treatment, the size, volume, and density of stones can be estimated; size plays a particularly significant role in predicting the spontaneous passage of a stone.
- **Axial Skeleton and Extremities:** Because CT can reconstruct the area of interest in multiple planes, it is frequently used to image complex fractures, particularly those around joints, in the axial skeleton, and extremities. With a 0.2 mm resolution, fractures, ligamentous injuries, and dislocations are easily identifiable. Modern dual-energy CT scanners have opened up new applications, like helping with gout diagnosis.

2.5. Interpretation of Results

Understanding the visual representations of the body's internal structures that the computed tomography (CT) scan captures is necessary for interpreting the results.

2.5.1. Presentation

The result of a CT scan is a volume of voxels, which may be presented to a human observer by various methods, which broadly fit into the following categories:

- Slices (of varying thickness): A thin slice is typically defined as a thickness of less than 3 mm, while a thick slice is usually considered to be between 3 mm and 5 mm in thickness.
- Projection, including maximum intensity projection and average intensity projection
- Volume rendering (VR)

The difference between projections and volume renderings is a little hazy because, technically, all volume renderings turn into projections when viewed on a two-dimensional display. The best volume rendering models combine various techniques, like shading and coloring, to produce observable and realistic images.

Conventionally, two-dimensional CT images are displayed as though the patient is standing on the image and looking up at it. Thus, the image's left side corresponds to the patient's right side and vice versa; likewise, the image's anterior side corresponds to the patient's anterior side and vice versa. This left-right exchange reflects the typical perspective that doctors have when they are in front of patients.

- **Grayscale:** Relative radiodensity is the metric used to display pixels in a CT scan image. On a scale from +3,071 (most attenuating) to −1,024 (least attenuating) on the Hounsfield scale, the pixel itself is displayed based on the mean attenuation of the tissue(s) that it corresponds to. A pixel is a two-dimensional representation of the field of view and matrix size. A voxel is a three-dimensional unit that is used when the thickness of the CT slice is also taken into consideration. Air has an attenuation of −1,000 HU, cancellous bone is usually +400 HU and cranial bone can reach 2,000 HU. Water has an attenuation of 0 HU. The attenuation of metallic implants is dependent on the element's atomic number: iron steel can totally block the X-ray and is therefore responsible for the well-known line-artifacts in computed tomograms. Titanium, on the other hand, typically has an amount of +1000 HU. Abrupt transitions between low- and high-density materials produce artifacts because they cause data values to exceed the processing electronics' dynamic range.
- **Windowing:** The high dynamic range of CT data sets needs to be decreased to be displayed or printed. Usually, "windowing" is used to accomplish this, mapping a range of pixel values to a grayscale ramp. For example, a window spanning from 0 HU to 80 HU is typically used to view CT images of the brain. Values inside the window are shown as a gray intensity proportional to position within the window; values of 0 and below are displayed as black, and values of 80 and above are displayed as white. To maximize the visible detail, the display window must match the X-ray density of the object of interest. A scan's windowing can be adjusted using the window width and window level parameters.
- **Multiplanar Reconstruction and Projections:** The process of transforming data from one anatomical plane—typically transverse—to other planes is known as multiplanar reconstruction or MPR. It can be applied to projections as well as thin slices. With the nearly isotropic resolution that current CT scanners offer, multiplanar reconstruction is feasible.

Almost all scans employ MPR. It is commonly used to examine the spine. Only one vertebral bone can be seen at a time in an axial plane image of the spine, and its relationship to other vertebral bones is not shown. The sagittal and coronal planes can be used to visualize the relative position by reformatting the data in different planes.

Organs that are not in orthogonal planes can be seen thanks to new software that reconstructs data in non-orthogonal (oblique) planes. As the bronchi do not lie orthogonal to the scan direction, it is more appropriate for visualizing their anatomical structure.

Curved-plane reconstruction (or curved planar reformation = CPR) is performed mainly for the evaluation of vessels. By straightening a vessel's bends, this kind of reconstruction makes it easier to see the entire vessel in a single image or a series of images. Measurements like cross-sectional area and length can be taken of a straightened vessel. This is useful for evaluating a surgical procedure before it is performed.

- **Volume Rendering:** The operator sets a threshold value for radiodensity (e.g., a level that corresponds to bone). The original data can be used to create a 3D model that is shown on screen using edge detection image processing algorithms. Different colors can be applied to each anatomical component, such as muscle, bone, and cartilage, to enable differentiation based on a variety of thresholds. This mode of operation, however, is unable to display internal structures.

  Surface rendering is a limited technique because it only shows surfaces that face the viewer and match a specific threshold density. Nonetheless, volume rendering uses colors, shading, and transparency to make it simple to display a volume in a single image. Pelvic bones, for instance, might be shown as semi-transparent so that, even when viewed from an oblique angle, one portion of the image does not obscure another.

2.5.2. Image Quality

2.5.2.1. Dose versus Image Quality

How to lower the radiation dose during CT exams without sacrificing image quality is a major concern in radiology today. Higher radiation doses typically produce images with greater resolution, whereas lower doses tend to produce images with more noise and less sharpness. The risk of radiation-induced cancer is one of the negative side effects that increase with dosage; a four-phase abdominal CT scan exposes the patient to the same amount of radiation as 300 chest X-rays. There are many ways to lower the amount of ionizing radiation that is exposed to during a CT scan.

- The required radiation dose can be greatly decreased with the use of new software technology. Super-resolution may be possible with new iterative tomographic reconstruction algorithms (such as iterative Sparse Asymptotic Minimum Variance) without needing a greater radiation dosage.
- Consider the body type and the organ under examination when customizing the examination and adjusting the radiation dosage. The amounts of radiation required for different body types and organs vary.
- In certain situations, such as when detecting small pulmonary masses, a higher resolution is not necessary (Rosen et al, 2000; Rosen et al, 2003).

2.6. Adverse Effects

Computed tomography (CT) scans are useful medical instruments for diagnosing conditions, but they do have some risks and side effects, just like any radiation-related procedure.

2.6.1. Cancer

CT scans use radiation that can harm body cells and DNA, potentially causing cancer. The amount of radiation received from CT scans varies, with doses 100 to 1,000 times higher than traditional X-rays. However, a lumbar spine X-ray and a head CT have similar levels of radiation. Media reports often inflate the risks of CT scans by comparing them to lower-dose X-rays. Overall, a routine abdominal CT scan has a radiation dose equivalent to three years of average background radiation.

Numerous large-scale population-based studies have repeatedly shown that low-dose radiation from CT scans affects the incidence of various types of cancer. For instance, it was discovered that radiation from CT scans may be the cause of up to 4% of brain cancers in a sizable population-based cohort. According to some experts, medical imaging will eventually be the cause of three to five% of all cancer cases. According to an Australian study involving 10.9 million people, irradiation was primarily responsible for the cohort's higher incidence of cancer following CT scan exposure. In this cohort, an excess cancer was detected after one out of every 1,800 CT scans. After a CT scan, the absolute risk increases to 40.05% if the lifetime risk of developing cancer is 40%. Patients who will be getting CT scans again in a short time—between one and five years—need to be particularly aware of the risks associated with these scans.

Some experts note that CT scans are known to be "overused," and "there is distressingly little evidence of better health outcomes associated with the current high rate of scans." However, a recent study that examined patient data from those who received high cumulative doses revealed a high level of appropriate use. This raises significant concern about these patients' cancer risk. Additionally, a highly significant finding that was not previously publicized is that some patients received CT scan doses of more than 100 mSv in a single day, refuting previous criticisms by some investigators regarding the relative benefits of acute versus prolonged exposure.

There are opposing viewpoints, and discussion is still going on. Several studies have demonstrated that publications suggesting a higher risk of cancer from standard body CT scan dosages are beset by severe methodological flaws and several wildly unlikely findings, leading them to conclude that there is no proof that these low doses have any long-term negative effects. According to one study, CT scans may have contributed as much as 0.4% of cancer cases in the US, and based on the percentage of CT scans performed in 2007, this may have increased to as much as 1.5 to 2%. Some disagree with this estimate because it is not universally agreed upon that the low radiation levels used in CT scans result in harm. In many situations, lower radiation doses are employed, as in the study of renal colic.

The age of an individual is a major factor in their subsequent risk of developing cancer. An abdominal CT scan of a one-year-old is estimated to carry a lifetime cancer mortality risk of 0 point 1%, or 1 in 1000 scans. Twenty-year-olds have a risk that is half that of forty-year-olds, with a significantly lower risk in the elderly. A 2012 review found no correlation between medical radiation exposure and cancer risk in children, noting the limitations in the evidence upon which the review is based. CT scans can be performed with different settings for lower exposure in children, with most manufacturers of CT scans as of 2007 having this function built in. The International Commission on Radiological Protection estimates that the risk to a fetus being exposed to 10 mGy (a unit of radiation exposure) increases the rate of cancer before 20 years of age from 0.03% to 0.04%.

Moreover, kids may need to undergo several CT scans due to specific conditions.

As of right now, patients should be made aware of the risks associated with CT scanning. Yet, imaging center staff members typically don't discuss these risks with patients unless they specifically ask.

2.6.2. Contrast Reactions

In contrast, CTs with intravenous injections of radiocontrast agents account for half of all CT scans performed in the US. These drugs typically cause mild side effects, such as nausea, vomiting, and itchy rashes. Rarely, severe reactions that pose a threat to life may happen. Overall, responses happen in 1–3% of individuals using nonionic contrast and 4–12% of those using ionic contrast. Rashes on the skin can develop in up to 3% of cases in just one week.

The newer, low-osmolar radiocontrast agents cause reactions in 0.01–0.04% of cases, compared to 1% of cases with the older agents causing anaphylaxis. About 2 to 30 people die for every 1,000,000 administrations of the drug; newer agents are safer. Individuals who are female, elderly, or in poor health are more likely to die, usually as a result of either acute kidney injury or anaphylaxis.

Nephropathy brought on by the contrast agent is a possibility. This happens in 2–7% of patients receiving these agents; individuals with reduced intravascular volume, diabetes, or kidney failure prior to treatment are more at risk. It is typically recommended that individuals with mild renal impairment make sure they are fully hydrated for several hours prior to and following the injection. Iodinated contrast should not be used for moderate kidney failure; this may require switching from CT to another method. Less stringent precautions are necessary for those with severe kidney failure who need dialysis because the kidneys' remaining function is so low that any additional damage would be undetectable and the dialysis will remove the contrast agent; nevertheless, scheduling dialysis as soon as possible after contrast administration is usually advised to minimize any negative effects of the contrast.

When examining the abdomen, oral contrast agents are frequently used in addition to intravenous contrast. Just diluted to about 10% of the concentration, these are often identical to the intravenous contrast agents. Oral substitutes for iodinated contrast do, however, exist. One such substitute is a very diluted suspension of barium sulfate (0.5–1% w/v). While diluted barium sulfate has the benefit of not causing allergic reactions or kidney failure, it cannot be administered to patients who may have a suspected bowel injury or perforation because it can leak into the bloodstream and cause fatal peritonitis.

Patients with kidney disease may experience adverse effects from intravenous contrast agents during certain CT scans, although this risk is now thought to be lower than previously believed (Mettler et al, 2008; Schauer and Linton, 2009).

2.7. Effective Dose (Radiation)

In the radiological protection system of the International Commission on Radiological Protection (ICRP), an effective dose is a dose quantity.

It represents the stochastic health risk to the entire body, which is the likelihood of ionizing radiation-induced cancer and genetic effects, and is the tissue-weighted sum of the equivalent doses in all designated human tissues and organs. It accounts for the type of radiation and the characteristics of each organ or tissue that is being exposed to radiation, allowing for the summation of organ doses resulting from varying levels and types of radiation, both internal and external, to produce an overall calculated effective dose.

The sievert (Sv), which denotes a 5% chance of developing cancer, is the SI unit for an effective dose. The amount absorbed dose determines the severity of acute tissue damage that is guaranteed to occur; the effective dose is not meant to be a measure of these deterministic health effects.

Wolfgang Jacobi developed the concept of effective dose, which was published in 1975. The ICRP included this concept as "effective dose equivalent" in their 1977 general recommendations because it was so compelling. In 1991, the term "effective dose" took the place of "effective dose equivalent." It has served as the primary dose limitation quantity in the international community's radiological protection system (ICRP) since 1977.

2.7.1. Uses

The prospective dose assessment for planning and optimization in radiological protection, as well as the demonstration of dose limit compliance for regulatory purposes, are the primary applications of effective dose, according to the ICRP. For regulatory purposes, the effective dose is therefore a central dose quantity.

According to the ICRP, effective dose has also played a major role in radiological protection by allowing doses from radionuclide intake and whole and partial body exposure to various forms of external radiation to be added up.

- **Usage for External Dose:** When the human body is partially or non-uniformly exposed to radiation, the effective dose must be calculated because the equivalent dose only takes the radiation type into account without taking the affected tissue into account. Because different body tissues react differently to ionizing radiation, the ICRP has given specific tissues and organs sensitivity factors so that, if the irradiated regions are known, the effect of partial irradiation can be calculated. There will be less danger from a radiation field that only exposes a section of the body than from a field that exposes the entire body. This is taken into consideration when calculating and adding the effective doses to the various body parts that have been exposed to radiation. This becomes the dose quantity that is effective for the entire body. It is a "protection dose" quantity that can be computed but not actually measured.

  Regardless of the application site, an effective dose carries the same effective risk to the entire body as an equivalent dose applied uniformly in the same amount to the entire body.
- **Usage for Internal Dose:** The internal dose from breathing, consuming, or injecting radioactive materials can be used to compute the effective dose.

The dose quantity used is:

The committed effective dose, denoted as E(t), is the product of the committed organ or tissue equivalent doses and the relevant tissue weighting factors WT. The integration time, measured in years after the intake, is represented by the variable t. For adults, the commitment period is 50 years, and for children, it is 70 years.

2.7.2. Calculation of Effective Dose

The material being irradiated absorbs energy from ionizing radiation. The absorbed dose, a physical dose quantity that depends on the incident radiation level and the irradiated object's absorption characteristics, is the unit used to express this. The International Commission on Radiation Units and Measurements (ICRU) and the International Council on Radiological Protection (ICRP) developed the dose quantities equivalent dose and effective dose to calculate the biological effect of an absorbed dose because the absorbed dose is a physical quantity and is not a satisfactory indicator of biological effect. This allows consideration of the stochastic radiological risk.

A weighted average of the equivalent dose quantity (HT) received in irradiated body tissues is obtained by first correcting the calculated absorbed organ dose (D_T) for the radiation type using factor WR. This produces an effective dose quantity E. The result is then further corrected for the tissues or organs being irradiated using factor WT.

The effective dosage for the entire body is the total of the effective doses given to all of the body's tissues and organs. The effective dose is only determined for the areas of the body that have received radiation. The tissue weighting factors add up to 1.0, meaning that the effective dose and the equivalent dose for a whole body exposed to uniformly penetrating external radiation are the same.

- **Use of Tissue Weighting Factor $W_{T:}$** The accompanying table contains the ICRP tissue weighting factors as well as the equations needed to calculate from either the equivalent dose or the absorbed dose.

Certain tissues, such as bone marrow, exhibit high sensitivity to radiation and are assigned a weighting factor that is substantially larger than their proportion of body mass. Conversely, tissues like the hard bone surface are relatively resistant to radiation and therefore receive a disproportionately low weighting factor.

Calculating from the equivalent dose:

$$E = \sum_T W_T \cdot H_T = \sum_T W_T \sum_R W_R \cdot \bar{D}_{T,R}$$

$$E = \sum_T W_T \sum_R W_R \cdot \frac{\int_T D_R(x,y,z)\rho(x,y,z)dV}{\int_T \rho(x,y,z)dV}$$

where; E is the effective dose to the entire organism; H_T is the equivalent dose absorbed by tissue T; W_T is the tissue weighting factor defined by regulation; W_R is the radiation weighting factor defined by regulation; $\bar{D}_{T,R}$ is the mass-averaged absorbed dose in tissue T by radiation type R; D_R (x,y,z)} is the absorbed dose from radiation type R as a function of location; ρ (x,y,z)} is the density as a function of location; V is volume; and T is the tissue or organ of interest.

The fraction of biological effects or health risks that can be attributed to the specified tissue is represented by the ICRP tissue weighting factors.

Table 2.1. Effective Dose by Medical Imaging Type

Target Organs	Exam Type	Effective Dose in Adults	Equivalent Time of Background Radiation
CT of the head	Single series	2 mSv	8 months
	With + without radiocontrast	4 mSv	16 months
Chest	CT of the chest	7 mSv	2 years
	CT of the chest, lung cancer screening protocol	1.5 mSv	6 months
	Chest X-ray	0.1 mSv	10 days
Heart	Coronary CT angiography	12 mSv	4 years
	Coronary CT calcium scan	3 mSv	1 year
Abdominal	CT of abdomen and pelvis	10 mSv	3 years
	CT of abdomen and pelvis, low dose protocol	3 mSv	1 year
	CT of abdomen and pelvis, with + without radiocontrast	20 mSv	7 years
	CT Colonography	6 mSv	2 years
	Intravenous pyelogram	3 mSv	1 year
	Upper gastrointestinal series	6 mSv	2 years
	Lower gastrointestinal series	8 mSv	3 years
Spine	Spine X-ray	1.5 mSv	6 months
	CT of the spine	6 mSv	2 years
Extremities	X-ray of extremity	0.001 mSv	3 hours
	Lower extremity CT angiography	0.3 – 1.6 mSv	5 weeks – 6 months
Dental X-ray		0.005 mSv	1 day
DEXA (bone density)		0.001 mSv	3 hours
PET-CT combination		25 mSv	8 years
Mammography		0.4 mSv	7 weeks

Source: https://en.wikipedia.org/wiki/Template:Effective_dose_by_medical_imaging_type.

2.7.3. Dose Reduction Strategies

Even though the precise carcinogenic potential of ionizing radiation is unknown, the medical community has an intrinsic duty to maintain radiation doses "as low as reasonably achievable (ALARA)." Every imaging procedure must be optimized and justified, and in every clinical situation, the goal should always be to obtain a diagnostic CT scan with the least amount of radiation possible. Considerable progress has already been made in reducing radiation doses thanks to improved technology. Since the 1980s, a variety of technological advancements have resulted in a two- to three-fold decrease in the dosage obtained from a combined CT study of the abdomen and pelvis. Nevertheless, depending on variable parameters, radiation exposure has been demonstrated to vary over a tenfold range in clinical practice for the same investigation, even with these technological advancements and emphasis on the ALARA principle. With significant variations in the reported average dosage, this kind of variation can occur both within and between different institutions. There is currently no legal requirement for routine monitoring of cumulative effective radiation dose that patients may be exposed to during the diagnostic process, even though standards and limits exist for healthcare workers and those who regularly undergo occupational radiation exposure.

Integration of hospital PACS systems at both national and international levels would facilitate the tracking of cumulative radiation exposure for each patient. The scanning industry is currently working on developing this type of database. These platforms also provide optimization tools that can help radiographers and radiologists minimize radiation exposure while maximizing clinical information obtained from each scan and avoiding duplication of scans that have already been performed at other facilities. Specific exposure limits can be set for each type of scan, and the technology will alert physicians if these limits are exceeded. This system would also allow departments to review and improve their practices. Additionally, the online collection of radiation dose data associated with imaging procedures would alert departments to instances of high radiation exposure, enabling immediate action to prevent large numbers of patients from experiencing very high radiation levels from diagnostic imaging. It is possible to optimize scanning techniques to try and obtain a usable image at a lower exposure level (Thibault et al, 2007; Smith-Bindman et al, 2012) (Table 2.2).

Table 2.2. Data Acquisition Protocols Used for Dose Optimization in Default Clinical Brain Protocols of the Neusoft NeuViz 128 CT Scanner

Parameters	**Default (Optimized Protocol)**
kVp	120 (80, 100, 140)
mAs	300 (100, 200, 400)
Rotation time	1.0 s
Pitch	0.5
Slice thickness	5 mm
SNR level	1.0 (0.3, 0.7, 1.3, 1.7)
FOV	250 mm
Kernel	F20
IR	50% (20%, 30%, 40%, 60%) Clearview
Matrix	512 × 12

Source: *Prabsattroo, T., Wachirasirikul, K., Tansangworn, P., Punikhom, P., & Sudchai, W. The dose optimization and evaluation of image quality in the adult brain protocols of multi-slice computed tomography: A phantom study. Journal of Imaging. 2023; 9(12), 264. https://doi.org/10.3390/jimaging9120264.*

Depending on their size, patients will need varying radiation dosages. The most fundamental aspect that can be adjusted for each patient is the tube current. For instance, the amperage used in pediatric scanning ought to be substantially less than that used in adult scanning (and ought to be higher in patients who are obese). The total attenuation of the anatomic region under evaluation should be taken into account when adjusting the tube current. Other methods, like current modulation based on the electrocardiogram, can assist in lowering the dose during cardiac CT. A relatively new method called automatic exposure control adjusts the tube current during each scan following the various anatomical regions' attenuations. Delivering the ideal dosage to produce the ideal diagnostic image is an additional benefit of this. Radiologists can help with the challenging task of balancing image quality and radiation exposure by defining the amount of noise that is appropriate for specific clinical scenarios before the scan.

It has been shown that there are published strategies to design an optimal tube potential for different diagnostic tasks and patient sizes, which can reduce doses by 40% for the abdomen and by 70% for the chest. With regard to cardiac CT, dose reductions ranging from 30% to 90% are possible thanks to electrocardiographic-based tube current modulation. Increases in efficiency with a dual-source CT system allow for dose reductions of up to 10–12 times.

- **Iterative Reconstruction:** Iterative reconstruction is a major advancement in CT scanning technology, particularly for reducing radiation dosage. By using this technique alongside or instead of filtered back projection, images can have better noise and spatial characteristics. This results in higher-quality images being produced with lower radiation exposure. With ongoing advancements in technology and software, it is expected that iterative reconstruction algorithms will continue to improve.
- **Noise Reduction Filters:** This method has been shown to significantly lower radiation dose and has the potential to optimize the quality of the acquired image by removing noise.
- **Low Dose Protocols:** It has been demonstrated that low dose techniques for abdominal CT scanning in kids and teens are comparable to standard dose CT in terms of the likelihood of a negative appendectomy. Up to four times as little radiation can be used with these low-dose techniques as compared to the standard dose protocol.
- **Spacing of CT Slices:** The radiation dose to the patient may increase significantly if a large number of thin adjacent CT slices are used. Because of scan overlap, placing the CT scanner closer to the patient, and increased scatter radiation, multi-slice CT scanners also provide a significantly higher radiation dose. Thus, choosing a slice that is both large enough to guarantee an acceptable radiation dose and small enough to produce the best possible diagnostic image requires careful consideration.
- **Maintaining the Limits of the Radiation Field Within the Anatomy of Interest:** The region being scanned in a CT scan frequently contains additional images that are not in the original field of interest. According to one study, extra images above

the diaphragm were obtained in 97% of cases, and images below the symphysis pubis were obtained in 94% of patients when evaluating the use of abdomino-pelvic CT scans. This translated to an additional 1280 images in 106 patients. Although the images increased each patient's radiation exposure, most of these cases had little additional diagnostic data. Restricting the field of view to the region of interest may enable reduced cumulative dosage and possibly better pictures through targeted imaging.

- **Decision Support at the Time of Ordering a Scan:** Utilizing automated prompts and advice in online radiology ordering systems can significantly decrease the number of low utility examinations conducted, as shown by a study that found that this system reduced such examinations by three times.
- **Split Bolus Techniques for Urological Studies:** Multiple image acquisitions have been necessary for standard CT urography protocols in order to obtain the unenhanced, contrast-enhanced nephrographic, and contrast-enhanced excretory phase images. A considerable radiation burden is necessary for this multiple image acquisition method (cited between 15–35 mSv). Split bolus protocols, on the other hand, can greatly lessen this burden and expose the patient to doses comparable to those found in routine abdomino-pelvic CT scans that are neither enhanced by contrast nor enhanced by it.
- Virtual Non-contrast CT from Dual Energy CT
  - **Rational Scanning:** The aforementioned strategies have the potential to significantly reduce the dosage that is given to the patient during different scanning procedures. The best approach to reducing dosage, though, is to refrain from unnecessary scanning. Regretfully, research indicates that a significant number of scans are performed annually without a reliable clinical indication. In fact, it's been estimated that if scan decisions were made under the guidelines that are currently available, maybe 20–40% of all CT scans could be avoided. It has been demonstrated that in the pediatric population, one-third of all CT scans could be performed using alternative techniques or not at all. In the same population, concerns have also been raised about the routine use of CT for appendicitis diagnosis, despite CT's remarkable ability to lower the rate of negative appendectomy. Other diagnostic modalities may be preferred over CT in terms of replacement or reduction. Both magnetic resonance imaging (MRI) and ultrasound offer the advantage of not subjecting the patient to ionizing radiation; however, their usefulness is limited by their accessibility [for MRI], and image quality [for ultrasound]. When compared to CT, MRI does not

always provide the same level of diagnostic information in clinical settings.

Although they are challenging to create, decision support software programs that assess a CT scan's appropriateness as a doctor orders it have demonstrated remarkably large decreases in the number of CT scans performed. The introduction of these initiatives to encourage physicians to reevaluate the clinical necessity for each scan is encouraging, as evidence-based guidelines indicate that 20–40% of CT scan orders are incorrect. The American College of Radiologists has acknowledged the need for comprehensive guidelines to help doctors determine which scans to use and when. A word of caution regarding the use of these kinds of decision support is that, somewhat surprisingly, the implementation of a no-denial policy on radiological imaging did not lead to a rise in the use of imaging modalities.

Naturally, the benefit-risk ratio is almost always significantly in favor of imaging when it is clinically indicated. But far too frequently, time restraints, medicolegal issues, or patient preferences drive the decision to image. The onus of determining the risk-benefit ratio for radiological investigations rests with the referring physician and radiologist; no study has attempted to do so to date. Guidelines must therefore be the foundation for optimizing clinical decision-making when it comes to imaging, as this can potentially lessen the impact of convenience factors on their own.

Every patient has a unique risk/benefit ratio. The radiation-induced cancer risk is influenced by the following factors.

- **Genetic Considerations:** Some groups of people may be more radiosensitive than others, and they may be more likely to develop cancer after radiation exposure. For instance, it has been demonstrated that certain patient groups with a genetic defect that predisposes them to cancer are more vulnerable to the effects of radiation.
- **Age at Exposure:** The BEIR VII report illustrated the correlation between the age at exposure and the lifetime attributable risk of cancer incidence, indicating that the earlier a patient was exposed to high radiation doses, the higher their risk of developing cancer. Most medical imaging is performed on older patients, but shorter life expectancy lowers the risk of radiation-induced cancers. Imaging standards for these patients shouldn't always be the same as those for younger patients with treatable conditions. Recent population-based studies from Australia and the United Kingdom have confirmed that there is more opportunity for malignancy to arise in the pediatric population due to their longer post-radiation life expectancy.
- **Sex:** Even with comparable radiation exposures, there seems to be a trend toward a higher incidence of cancer in women than in men after radiation exposure.
- **Illness:** Numerous patients receiving

treatment for illnesses that are likely to shorten life expectancy will undergo repeated imaging. It is unlikely that this imaging radiation will have carcinogenic effects.

- **Fractionation and Protraction of Exposure:** Due to the impact of DNA damage repair, it is generally thought that there is a higher risk associated with high radiation doses administered quickly compared to the same (or lower) doses administered over an extended period of time. Surprisingly, though, it has been suggested that the cumulative dose given over a longer time has little effect.

2.8. Clinical Applications of Computed Tomography

2.8.1. Computed Tomography Scanning Parameters

The characteristics and abilities of X-ray CT scanners are determined by a number of closely related parameters. The type of examination and the CT scanner's performance specifications are the main factors influencing the CT scanning time. Short scan times are necessary to minimize the artifacts related to the patient's physiological movements, such as peristaltic, respiratory, and digestive tract motions. The time needed for the X-ray tube and detector to circle the object one full rotation (360°) is known as the gantry rotation time for a helical CT scan.

The gantry rotation time has been reduced by technological advancements to as little as 0.3 seconds. A scan length of 240 mm is needed for the head and 400 mm for the chest or abdomen during a standard CT examination. For a standard head CT scan, the CT slice thickness (also known as slice collimation) is usually 5 mm. For blood vessel and thin-section facial bone CT, or 3D image processing, it varies between 0.625 and 1.25 mm. The ability to process scans is indicated by the CT patient throughput, which is correlated with the number of exams performed each hour.

2.8.2. Causes and Types of Computed Tomography Image Artifacts

Fundamentally, spatial resolution, image contrast, image noise, and artifacts—all of which are closely related to one another—are used to characterize image quality in CT and all other medical imaging modalities. The imaging system's technical parameters, the user—a radiology technologist or radiologist during image acquisition and evaluation—and the patient—the patient's size and movement—all have an impact on the quality of CT images. Features that show up on CT scans that weren't present in the original clinic are known as artifacts. This main cause is linked to CT's primary limitation as well as its own malfunction and improper adjustment.

Artifacts can arise from a variety of sources, including motion, metal, partial volume, beam hardening, technical flaws, or operator error. Motion artifacts are patient-specific characteristics that arise from the patient's breathing, twitching, or other movements during a scan. Patients may experience motion artifacts if they move. Thus, in order to avoid these, patient movements should be kept to a minimum. Using a motion artifact correction algorithm in conjunction with breathing control during image acquisition can help reduce motion artifact. Furthermore, the motion correction algorithm has the ability to compensate for motion artifacts. When tissues in complex bone structures with significantly different X-ray absorption characteristics are included in the same CT slice, partial volume artifacts result. As a result, there is a beam attenuation that varies proportionally to the mean of each slice. This is because high-contrast errors are caused by the extremely dense structures (bones), which are only partially included in the slice. When there are significant structural variations in the direction of the slice thickness, these are explained by the partial volume effect. It is advised to use a thin-slice thickness to lessen the partial volume artifacts. The phenomenon known as "beam hardening" happens when an X-ray beam with varying energies goes through a dense material and causes lower energy photons to selectively attenuate. In theory, the beam hardening effect works similarly to a high-pass filter in that it keeps only photons with higher energies in the beam. As a result, the mean beam energy gets "hardened" or increased. The streaking (dark band) artifacts caused by the beam hardening effect are multiple streaking bands situated between two dense tissues or cupping artifacts, which make an object's edges appear brighter than its center. By using a metal filter before the CT scan, the X-ray spectrum can minimize lower energy photons and thereby lessen the beam hardening effect. In this regard, metal artifact reduction algorithms are a feature of CT scanners. Many factors, such as beam hardening, scatter, Poisson's noise, motion, and edge effects in the scanned objects—such as hair pins, clips, and metals inside the patient—can result in metal streak artifacts. Metals absorb X-rays almost entirely, such as gold-implanted objects within human bodies. This results in "radiation shadows," which cause distinct streaks of light and dark across the entire reconstructed image. The only way to prevent this is to tilt the gantry so that the unsettling metallic objects are not in the slice plane. In a CT scanner, ring artifacts can be caused by miscalibration or technical malfunction of one or more detector elements. This can also be brought on by a contrast medium on the detector cover becoming contaminated or by insufficient X-ray intensity. They typically appear on multiple slices and occur near the scan's isocenter.

2.8.3. Computed Tomography Image Noise

There are numerous components to image quality, and numerous technical factors influence it. Low-contrast objects are less visible in CT because noise introduces undesired pixel value changes into a homogeneous image. The amount of noise influencing contrast resolution varies depending on various factors such as operating mode, patient size, reconstruction algorithm, mAs, kVp, and slice thickness.

CT image noise levels affect image reconstruction algorithms. Although it generates a good edge definition, an edge-enhancing (HighRes) algorithm has high noise levels. Although HighRes algorithms produce more noise, they offer superior spatial resolution. Although a smoothing algorithm reduces noise, it also results in a worse definition of edges. Soft algorithms offer reduced noise and improved contrast detectability. Generally, a standard algorithm is advised for routine studies.

The standard deviation of the beam thickness has an inverse relationship with image noise. Although there is more image noise with thinner slices, it is easier to see small lesions. For soft tissues, thicker slices improve contrast detectability by producing less noise. For bony structures, thinner slices produce better spatial resolution. Consequently, as a function of slice thickness, a compromise between contrast detectability and the spatial resolution for the diagnostic content should be taken into account.

According to generally accepted guidelines, for larger patient body sizes, the noise level doubles every 10 cm increase in patient diameter for abdominal scans and every 13 cm increase for lung scans. A two-squared (or one-point-four) reduction in the noise level results from doubling the dose (in milliampere-hours). It is especially crucial to use higher mAs in soft tissue studies to minimize noise. It is easier to identify structures with minute variations in density at lower noise levels. Higher mAs are not required, though, for studies on the lungs or bones.

2.8.4. Computed Tomography Image Reformatting

Cross-sectional (axial) images are the most widely used application of X-ray CT. These images are used in many different medical fields for both diagnostic and therapeutic purposes. The techniques of multiplanar reconstruction (MPR), maximum intensity projection (MIP), minimum intensity projection (MinIP), cine (movie) mode, shaded surface display (SSD, also known as surface rendering), 3D volume rendering, and virtual endoscopy (VE), such as angioscopy, bronchoscopy, and colonoscopy, are among the many reformatted images that can be navigated and visualized using the modern CT workstations.

Using a variety of software and a workstation, the MPR technique entails the image processing tasks required to convert thin-slice data from volumetric CT in the axial plane from another plane (such as coronal, sagittal, or oblique) to control the window level (WW) and center the image to view whichever structures are needed. The MPR display can be used to generate interactive slices in Cartesian planes (axial, sagittal, and coronal) or even in oblique planes based on the 3D reconstruction of a series of tomographic images. This implies that, in comparison to the images from the original sequence, the doctor can obtain views of the patient's internal structures that offer more clarity. To identify all of the hyperdense structures (bone or contrast material-filled structures) in a volume, the MIP technique uses 3D data and projects the voxels with the highest intensity (highest Hounsfield number) that get in the way of parallel rays traced from the viewpoint to the plane of projection in the 2D viewing plane. A 2D visualization technique called MinIP makes it possible to identify low-density structures within a given volume. The MinIP images are multiplanar slab images created by displaying only the lowest attenuation value encountered along a ray cast through an object toward the viewing plane. These images are primarily used to diagnose lung diseases. Using edge detection image processing algorithms, the surface-shaded display is an established visualization technique for 3D imaging of sectional image data. By choosing attenuation thresholds, an SSD offers a realistic three-dimensional representation of the surface of a structure of interest within the designated volume. Using specialized software, volume rendering is a type of data visualization technique that converts 3D imaging of sectional image data into a 2D projection. Transparency, color, and shading are used in volume rendering to improve the volume's visual representation in a single image. The main purposes of volume rendering are improved human anatomy visualization, surgical treatment planning, and medical education. VE is a noninvasive method that provides accurate spatial relationships between pathological regions and their surrounding structures by combining the features of cross-sectional volumetric imaging and endoscopic viewing to explore internal structures. The colon, bronchi, stomach, blood vessels, bladder, kidney, esophagus, and other organs have all been assessed using VE within the human anatomy.

The CINE mode is a dynamic movie display format on a monitor that consists of a sequence of quickly captured images captured at sequential time cycles. In CINE mode, four-dimensional (4D) helical CT is used to acquire

CINE CT images. In planar geometry, a stationary volume scanning mode is continuously scanned in time and in space in succession. The realization of high-speed image reconstruction has made real-time continuous observations possible during scans such as X-ray fluoroscopy. The CINE CT images are sequentially shown as continuous slice images like a movie on a display device that uses 3D data. Because these images are constantly being reviewed, it is simple to identify differences between each image in the stack and to observe the shapes of organs and the operation of blood vessels.

2.8.5. Computed Tomography Image Windowing

By changing the WL and window width (WW), T images can be shown with any brightness and contrast. The brightness is determined by the position of the scale's center or WL. The contrast is set by selecting a range of CT numbers for grayscale amplification, or WW. CT density values span from -1,000 to +3,000, although the human eye can only detect a maximum of 30–40 grayscale levels. As a result, the window settings need to match the structures that are to be seen.

A narrow window width (WW) suggests that the change from black to white will happen much more quickly, giving the impression of a high-contrast image. However, structures outside of that window range might not be properly represented or might be missed. Tissue types with comparable tissue densities, like the liver or brain, can be effectively displayed using narrow WWs, which are defined as the range between 50 and 350 HUs. A wide WW, which is the 400–2,000 HU range, means that the grayscale is wider and that areas with small density variations, like the lungs or cortical tissue, appear homogeneous.

2.8.6. Clinical Challenges of Computed Tomography Scanner Technology

In order to increase the signal intensity from arteries, veins, and tissues throughout the body, a special contrast medium (dye) is injected during a CT angiography (CTA) examination. The heart, aorta, and other major blood vessels, as well as the lungs, kidneys, head, neck, arms, and legs, can all be seen with CTA. It is possible to 3D reconstruct CTA images to view and rotate the cerebral vessels along with any associated pathology from any angle. Structures that are normally invisible or only dimly visible can be imaged using contrast media. Intravenous contrast agents are used to make blood vessels and organs more visible. To see the digestive tract, oral contrast agents are utilized. Through an intravenous line in the hand or arm, the contrast media for a CT scan is administered. CT contrast media is typically an iodine compound that is transparent and colorless, meaning that it is impervious to X-rays. A CT contrast injector is used to inject between 100 and 150 mL into a vein at a speed of 2–3 mL/s during a single CT exam. Uncommon allergic reactions, bronchospasm, kidney damage, nausea, vomiting, and/or hives, as well as brief unconsciousness, can all result from the contrast media. Radiation oncologists plan to ascertain the type of cancer, its precise location, its size and shape, its staging, the vital structures that are closely related to the cancer, the radiation dose required for the cancer treatment, and the patient's general health and medical history before beginning an external beam radiotherapy treatment.

With only minor additions, CT simulators (CTSim) used for radiotherapy are derived from standard diagnostic CT scanners. A flat tabletop to mimic the radiotherapy treatment unit couch, a larger bore size to accommodate patient immobilization devices, a laser positioning and marking system as a reference for patient positioning, and a virtual simulation software workstation are all common features of CTSim. A variety of information is provided by the CTsim 3D imaging data of the patient's anatomy to enable a more precise delineation of the tumor and the surrounding normal tissues. Furthermore, the associated tissue density data that is needed to calculate radiation dose distributions is already included in the pixel HU values by default. This is essential for 3D radiotherapy treatment planning for X-ray radiation treatments. A phantom calibration is used to complete the conversion, and yearly checks are necessary. Cutting-edge CTSim can also gather data from 4D imaging. The internal organs impacted by respiratory motion can use the 4D CT simulations. These sophisticated CT imaging simulation methods enable precise tumor localization, visualization of the course of treatment, and administration of that course of care.

MicroCT is comparable to standard diagnostic CTs in terms of imaging acquisition principles, but it has substantially higher spatial resolution, a much smaller applied slice thickness, and a much smaller bore-size scale. Common microCT scanners are capable of imaging objects with pixel sizes in the micrometer range, up to 20 cm in diameter. Without having to section the samples, the microCT scanner can be used to examine the internal structure of biological and material samples for materials science and small animal imaging, including mice, rats, and occasionally rabbits. This preserves the samples or specimens for use in future research. Microfossils, food, biomedical samples, tiny animals (in vivo scanners), and other investigations requiring minute detail are commonly performed using standard microCT scanners. They have an enclosed microfocus X-ray source and a charge-coupled device (CCD) camera with a detection system. These are operated on a table top with high-accelerating voltages ranging from 70 to 225 kV with specific beam currents, aluminum filters, radiation doses less than a few μSv/h at 10 cm from the instrument's surface, long scanning times varying from a few minutes to 10 hours depending on the region of interest's size, and a few minutes for image reconstruction.

Planning radiation therapy, specialized breast imaging, implant dentistry diagnosis, and industrial applications as a nondestructive testing tool have all seen an increase in the use of CBCT. The primary distinction between CBCT and traditional helical CT is that the former uses a narrow, collimated, fan-shaped X-ray beam and a linear group of detectors, while the latter uses a divergent cone-shaped X-ray beam and a large area flat panel detector. Using 3D volume reconstruction algorithms, CBCT uses a single rotation around a stationary object to capture the entire image volume. The growing adoption of kV systems installed on the current generation of linear accelerators has led to a rise in the use of CBCT in radiotherapy. Gantry-mounted kV CBCT is primarily used in image-guided radiotherapy to confirm patient positioning and setup, locate tumors, and monitor tumor changes over treatment. However, since HU values can be measured and calibrated for use in treatment planning, it also creates the possibility of re-optimizing adaptive radiotherapy treatment plans in real-time. When conical-shaped beams are used in radiotherapy, the use of CBCT results in poor image quality of the moving object within all slices and acquisition times ranging from 40 seconds to two minutes per gantry rotation. Furthermore, compared to fan-beam helical CT, cone beam geometry covers a larger FOV in a single rotation, which increases the scattered radiation component. For clinical applications, however, the use of CBCT necessitates an additional radiation dose and length of treatment time. Due to the lack of offline viewing, these have an adverse effect on doctors and residents who must be present during the CBCT acquisition. Because CBCT imaging doses are small and infrequent compared to the therapeutic dose used to treat patients, they have historically been disregarded in radiation therapy. CBCT raises the dosage that is given to both the healthy tissues and the tumor. Depending on the treatments given to the patients, the additional dose may range from 2 to 8 cGy.

Another type of clinical CT is portable or mobile CT. Its primary feature is its ability to transform any hospital room—such as the operating room, intensive care unit (ICU), radiation oncology suites, and emergency department—into an advanced imaging suite. This is particularly useful for situations where patients require flexible, real-time portable imaging at their bedsides. When patients are in the intensive care unit, clinic, operating room, or emergency room, these portable CTs are designed specifically for them to enhance the standard of care and lessen the challenges related to getting them to a traditional CT imaging scanner. ENTs use portable CT scanning primarily for neuroradiological head and neck imaging in the intensive care unit (ICU), trauma, orthopedic, and vascular imaging during surgery, and interoperative imaging of the bone and sinuses.

Currently, most modern MDCT scanners offer special image acquisition protocols with a significantly lower radiation dose that can be used to find treatable cases of lung cancer. Low-dose CT (LDCT) examinations are used for lung cancer screenings to detect lung nodules that may represent lung cancer. The tube current, low-tube potentials, which vary from 80 to 100 kV, and the innovative low-dose reconstruction algorithm are the most crucial scan parameters for maximizing the radiation dose from LDCT. This technique can reduce radiation exposure in an LDCT scan by up to five times compared to a standard CT scan. It is well known that LDCT screening is a far more efficient method than standard chest X-ray radiography. Since there is typically too much margin of error when dealing with individuals who do not exhibit any symptoms of the disease, LDCT scans are typically reserved for adults between the ages of 55 and 80 who have a history of smoking and who have either stopped smoking in the last 15 years or who are already patients with lung cancer. This often leads to more standard tests being performed than is necessary.

2.8.7. Radiation Dose of Computed Tomography

The amount of radiation exposure from CT scans varies depending on the type of scanner, the body part being examined, and the imaging parameters used. For example, an abdominal scan using specific settings may result in a radiation dose of 21 mGy at the center of the body and 35 mGy at the edges. Overall, the effective dose from CT scans typically ranges from 1 to 10 mSv.

2.8.8. Quality Control and Imaging Phantom of Computed Tomography

Maintaining optimal image quality, appropriate radiation doses to patients, and appropriate electromechanical component performance all depend on periodic quality control, or quality assurance, of CT scans. The roles and responsibilities of radiologists, radiologic technologists, and medical physicists, as well as the regular test cycle consisting of weekly (some perform daily), monthly, semi-annual, and annual tests, are categorized as the CT QC program. The ACR recommended minimum QC test frequencies in the CT QC manual, including the annual tests of qualified medical physicist surveys, which include the following: scout prescription and alignment light accuracy, table travel accuracy, radiation beam width, low-contrast performance, spatial resolution, CT number accuracy, artifact evaluation, CT number uniformity, dosimetry, calibration of the CT scanner display, artifact evaluation (daily), visual checklist (monthly), dry laser printer QC (monthly), and gray level performance of CT scanner acquisition display monitors (monthly) (Cardis et al, 2007; O'Sullivan et al, 2010).

A Closer Look

Electron Beam Computed Tomographic Scanning in Preventive Medicine

Most electron beam computed tomography (EBCT) scans are done in a population that is mainly asymptomatic to evaluate and fine-tune cardiac risk. More than 200 articles and editorials have been published since the first EBCT scans for the measurement of coronary artery calcification were obtained in 1988, demonstrating the usefulness of this method for the evaluation of coronary atherosclerosis. 10% or so of asymptomatic patients will have scan results that indicate they are at risk enough to warrant additional testing for diagnosis. Physicians can use the majority of scans, however, to determine which patients will benefit and who won't from risk factor modification, including medication intervention.

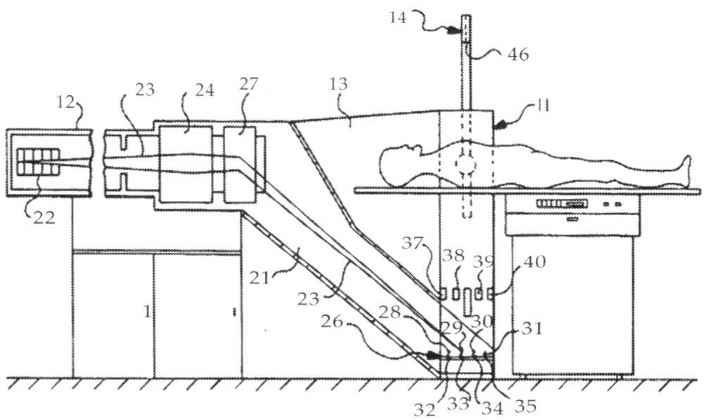

Figure: 2 from U.S. patent 4,672,649, Public Domain, https://en.wikipedia.org/w/index.php?curid=1507649.

A July 2000 expert consensus document on EBCT from the American College of Cardiology/American Heart Association (ACC/AHA) cites a high false-positive rate for the detection of obstructive disease and criticizes the use of EBCT for the "diagnosis and prognosis of coronary artery disease." The data have been misinterpreted by the committee's experts, only one of whom was an expert in EBCT. It's possible that a positive scan for coronary artery calcification won't be followed by the 75% narrowing required for an angiographic or stress test result to be consistently positive. This does not negate the EBCT test; on the contrary, the test's sensitivity to early atherosclerosis allows for inexpensive, practical lifestyle modifications that can halt the advancement of obstructive disease. There is no evidence, in opposition to the writing committee chairman's belief, that the early detection of subclinical disease—whether through EBCT or another technique—requires "further expensive and unnecessary testing to rule out a diagnosis of coronary artery disease." Actually, there is strong evidence supporting the cost-effectiveness of employing this extremely delicate procedure in all cases to save the most vulnerable. Coronary angiography alone may be appropriate for these individuals, who are typically those with typical angina, as the final test before a scheduled intervention.

Current Status of EBCT Scanning

- **Subclinical Disease Assessment in Asymptomatic Subjects:** The ACC/AHA statement has a generally negative tone, but the committee acknowledges that EBCT has a role to play in determining whether people who are assumed to be at high risk may actually be at much lower risk if there is no calcification. Either way, shifting the course of treatment would probably enable funding for medical care to be directed toward the people who would gain the most. The committee confirmed the conclusions of a 1996 AHA statement:
    1. A negative EBCT test makes the presence of atherosclerotic plaque, including unstable plaque, very unlikely.
    2. A negative test is highly unlikely in the presence of significant luminal obstructive disease.
    3. Negative tests occur in the majority of patients who have angiographically normal coronary arteries.
    4. A negative test may be consistent with a low risk of a cardiovascular event in the next 2–5 years.
    5. A positive EBCT confirms the presence of a coronary atherosclerotic plaque.
    6. The greater the amount of calcium, the greater the likelihood of occlusive coronary artery disease, but there is not a 1-to-1 relationship, and findings may not be site-specific.
    7. The total amount of calcium correlates best with the total amount of atherosclerotic plaque, although the true "plaque burden" is underestimated.
    8. A high calcium score may be consistent with a moderate to high risk of a cardiovascular event within the next 2–5 years.

The document seems to lay the groundwork for EBCT to be widely used by any prevention expert who already believes that standard risk factor assessment is inadequate, by allowing its use in asymptomatic patients only after "the more standard cardiac risk assessment by the physician is considered insufficient to direct further therapy plans." According to published research, risk ratios for "abnormal" cholesterol as a predictor of cardiac events or stenosis are typically about 2, whereas risk ratios for EBCT can range from 5 to 20. Most scanning centers perform a thorough questionnaire and document risk factors in addition to EBCT, which gives the referring physician quick access to a set of data that is exceptional in its accuracy.

Incidental findings from every EBCT data set are also noteworthy. These include various spinal abnormalities that appear in these high-resolution EBCT studies, enlarged lymph nodes, masses in the superior part of the liver, and small pulmonary nodules, which may be a sign of lung cancer.

- **Assessment of Progression or Regression of Coronary Calcific**ation: The use of EBCT to measure the progression, stabilization, and even regression of coronary disease was published by Callister et al. in 1998. Since then, findings from two additional independent studies have confirmed that EBCT has a new use in calculating the rate at which calcification volume changes over periods of 12 months or longer. Subjects receiving statin therapy reported significantly lower rates of progression—on average, 61%. Furthermore, one year later, 98% of individuals who had zero calcium scores at baseline still had zero.

Summary

- Computerised tomography, CT, is an ideal form of tomography yielding sequence images of thin consecutive slices of the patient and providing the opportunity to localize in three dimensions.
- To acquire a CT image, an object is placed on a table. An X-ray source (within the gantry of a CT scanner) rotates around the object, and X-rays that pass through the object are detected on the opposite side.
- The image of a CT scanner is a digital image. It consists of a square matrix of pixels (picture elements), each of which represents a voxel (volume element) of the interior structure of the object (patient).
- The CT scanner according to the data acquisition method is classified as traditional (axial) and spiral (helical) CT with the fan-beam X-ray source used mainly for diagnostic purposes.
- Sequential CT also known as step-and-shoot CT is a type of scanning method in which the CT table moves stepwise.
- Spinning tube, commonly called spiral CT, or helical CT, is an imaging technique in which an entire X-ray tube is spun around the central axis of the area being scanned.
- Electron beam tomography (EBT) is a specific form of CT in which a large enough X-ray tube is constructed so that only the path of the electrons, traveling between the cathode and anode of the X-ray tube, are spun using deflection coils.
- CT perfusion imaging is a specific form of CT to assess flow through blood vessels whilst injecting a contrast agent.
- A CT scan of the heart is performed to gain knowledge about cardiac or coronary anatomy.
- CT is an accurate technique for diagnosis of abdominal diseases like Crohn's disease, GIT bleeding, and diagnosis and staging of cancer, as well as follow-up after cancer treatment to assess response.
- An important issue within radiology today is how to reduce the radiation dose during CT examinations without compromising the image quality. In general, higher radiation doses result in higher-resolution images, while lower doses lead to increased image noise and unsharp images.
- The radiation used in CT scans can damage body cells, including DNA molecules, which can lead to radiation-induced cancer.3

References

1. Bernstein, C. N., Blanchard, J. F., Kliewer, E., & Wajda, A. (2001). Cancer risk in patients with inflammatory bowel disease: A population-based study. *Cancer, 91*(4), 854–862.
2. Berrington de González, A., & Darby, S. (2004). Risk of cancer from diagnostic X-rays: Estimates for the UK and 14 other countries. *Lancet, 363*(9406), 345–351.
3. Berrington de González, A., Mahesh, M., Kim, K. P., Bhargavan, M., Lewis, R., Mettler, F., &

Land, C. (2009). Projected cancer risks from computed tomographic scans performed in the United States in 2007. *Archives of Internal Medicine, 169*(22), 2071–2077.

4. Brenner, D. J., & Hall, E. J. (2007). Computed tomography—An increasing source of radiation exposure. *New England Journal of Medicine, 357*(22), 2277–2284.
5. Calabrese, E. J. (2011). Muller's Nobel lecture on dose-response for ionizing radiation: Ideology or science? *Archives of Toxicology, 85*(12), 1495–1498.
6. Cardis, E., Vrijheid, M., Blettner, M., Gilbert, E., Hakama, M., Hill, C., Howe, G., Kaldor, J., Muirhead, C. R., Schubauer-Berigan, M., et al. (2007). The 15-country collaborative study of cancer risk among radiation workers in the nuclear industry: Estimates of radiation-related cancer risks. *Radiation Research, 167*(4), 396–416.
7. Desmond, A. N., O'Regan, K., Curran, C., McWilliams, S., Fitzgerald, T., Maher, M. M., & Shanahan, F. (2008). Crohn's disease: Factors associated with exposure to high levels of diagnostic radiation. *Gut, 57*(11), 1524–1529.
8. Doss, M. (2014). Linear no-threshold model may not be appropriate for estimating cancer risk from CT. *Radiology, 270*(1), 307–308.
9. Esses, D., Birnbaum, A., Bijur, P., Shah, S., Gleyzer, A., & Gallagher, E. J. (2004). Ability of CT to alter decision making in elderly patients with acute abdominal pain. *American Journal of Emergency Medicine, 22*(3), 270–272.
10. Fazel, R., Krumholz, H. M., Wang, Y., Ross, J. S., Chen, J., Ting, H. H., Shah, N. D., Nasir, K., Einstein, A. J., & Nallamothu, B. K. (2009). Exposure to low-dose ionizing radiation from medical imaging procedures. *New England Journal of Medicine, 361*(9), 849–857.
11. Hatch, M., Ron, E., Bouville, A., Zablotska, L., & Howe, G. (2005). The Chernobyl disaster: Cancer following the accident at the Chernobyl nuclear power plant. *Epidemiologic Reviews, 27*(1), 56–66.
12. Heiken, J. P., Peterson, C. M., & Menias, C. O. (2005). Virtual colonoscopy for colorectal cancer screening: Current status. *Cancer Imaging, 5*(Spec No A), S133–S139.
13. Hendee, W. R., & O'Connor, M. K. (2012). Radiation risks of medical imaging: Separating fact from fantasy. *Radiology, 264*(2), 312–321.
14. Henschke, C. I., Yankelevitz, D. F., Libby, D. M., Pasmantier, M. W., Smith, J. P., & Miettinen, O. S. (2006). Survival of patients with stage I lung cancer detected on CT screening. *New England Journal of Medicine, 355*(17), 1763–1771.
15. Hidajat, N., Mäurer, J., Schröder, R. J., Wolf, M., Vogl, T., & Felix, R. (1999). Radiation exposure in spiral computed tomography: Dose distribution and dose reduction. *Investigative Radiology, 34*(1), 51–57.
16. Hricak, H., Brenner, D. J., Adelstein, S. J., Frush, D. P., Hall, E. J., Howell, R. W., McCollough, C. H., Mettler, F. A., Pearce, M. S., Suleiman, O. H., et al. (2011). Managing radiation use in medical imaging: A multifaceted challenge. *Radiology, 258*(3), 889–905.
17. Kinsella, S. M., Coyle, J. P., Long, E. B., McWilliams, S. R., Maher, M. M., Clarkson, M. R., & Eustace, J. A. (2010). Maintenance hemodialysis patients have high cumulative radiation exposure. *Kidney International, 78*(8), 789–793.
18. Mettler, F. A., Bhargavan, M., Faulkner, K., Gilley, D. B., Gray, J. E., Ibbott, G. S., Lipoti, J. A., Mahesh, M., McCrohan, J. L., Stabin, M. G., et al. (2009). Radiologic and nuclear medicine

studies in the United States and worldwide: Frequency, radiation dose, and comparison with other radiation sources—1950–2007. *Radiology, 253*(2), 520–531.

19. Mettler, F. A., Bhargavan, M., Thomadsen, B. R., Gilley, D. B., Lipoti, J. A., Mahesh, M., McCrohan, J., & Yoshizumi, T. T. (2008). Nuclear medicine exposure in the United States, 2005-2007: Preliminary results. *Seminars in Nuclear Medicine, 38*(5), 384–391.
20. Mettler, F. A., Huda, W., Yoshizumi, T. T., & Mahesh, M. (2008). Effective doses in radiology and diagnostic nuclear medicine: A catalog. *Radiology, 248*(1), 254–263.
21. Mettler, F. A., Thomadsen, B. R., Bhargavan, M., Gilley, D. B., Gray, J. E., Lipoti, J. A., McCrohan, J., Yoshizumi, T. T., & Mahesh, M. (2008). Medical radiation exposure in the U.S. in 2006: Preliminary results. *Health Physics, 95*(5), 502–507.
22. Mettler, F. A., Wiest, P. W., Locken, J. A., & Kelsey, C. A. (2000). CT scanning: Patterns of use and dose. *Journal of Radiological Protection, 20*(4), 353–359.
23. O'Sullivan, J., O'Connor, O. J., O'Regan, K., Clarke, B., Burgoyne, L. N., Ryan, M. F., & Maher, M. M. (2010). An assessment of medical students' awareness of radiation exposures associated with diagnostic imaging investigations. *Insights into Imaging, 1*(2), 86–92.
24. Preston, D. L., Ron, E., Tokuoka, S., Funamoto, S., Nishi, N., Soda, M., Mabuchi, K., & Kodama, K. (2007). Solid cancer incidence in atomic bomb survivors: 1958–1998. *Radiation Research, 168*(1), 1–64.
25. Rosen, M. P., Sands, D. Z., Longmaid, H. E., Reynolds, K. F., Wagner, M., & Raptopoulos, V. (2000). Impact of abdominal CT on the management of patients presenting to the emergency department with acute abdominal pain. *AJR American Journal of Roentgenology, 174*(5), 1391–1396.
26. Rosen, M. P., Siewert, B., Sands, D. Z., Bromberg, R., Edlow, J., & Raptopoulos, V. (2003). Value of abdominal CT in the emergency department for patients with abdominal pain. *European Radiology, 13*(2), 418–424.
27. Schauer, D. A., & Linton, O. W. (2009). National Council on Radiation Protection and Measurements report shows substantial medical exposure increase. *Radiology, 253*(2), 293–296.
28. Scott, B. R. (2008). Low-dose radiation risk extrapolation fallacy associated with the linear-no-threshold model. *Human & Experimental Toxicology, 27*(2), 163–168.
29. Smith-Bindman, R., Miglioretti, D. L., Johnson, E., Lee, C., Feigelson, H. S., Flynn, M., Greenlee, R. T., Kruger, R. L., Hornbrook, M. C., Roblin, D., et al. (2012). Use of diagnostic imaging studies and associated radiation exposure for patients enrolled in large integrated healthcare systems, 1996–2010. *JAMA, 307*(22), 2400–2409.
30. Thibault, J. B., Sauer, K. D., Bouman, C. A., & Hsieh, J. (2007). A three-dimensional statistical approach to improved image quality for multislice helical CT. *Medical Physics, 34*(11), 4526–4544.
31. Tsapaki, V., Ahmed, N. A., AlSuwaidi, J. S., Beganovic, A., Benider, A., BenOmrane, L., Borisova, R., Economides, S., El-Nachef, L., Faj, D., et al. (2009). Radiation exposure to patients during interventional procedures in 20 countries: Initial IAEA project results. *AJR American Journal of Roentgenology, 193*(2), 559–569.
32. Tubiana, M. (2005). Dose-effect relationship and estimation of the carcinogenic effects of low doses of ionizing radiation: The joint report of the Académie des Sciences (Paris) and

of the Académie Nationale de Médecine. *International Journal of Radiation Oncology Biology Physics, 63*(2), 317–319.

33. Tubiana, M., Feinendegen, L. E., Yang, C., & Kaminski, J. M. (2009). The linear no-threshold relationship is inconsistent with radiation biologic and experimental data. *Radiology, 251*(1), 13–22.

34. van Randen, A., Bipat, S., Zwinderman, A. H., Ubbink, D. T., Stoker, J., & Boermeester, M. A. (2008). Acute appendicitis: Meta-analysis of diagnostic performance of CT and graded compression US related to prevalence of disease. *Radiology, 249*(1), 97–106.

Chapter 3

MAGNETIC RESONANCE IMAGING

Contents

Introduction

A non-invasive imaging method that creates three-dimensional, finely detailed anatomical images is called magnetic resonance imaging (MRI). It is frequently employed in the diagnosis, monitoring, and detection of diseases. It is based on advanced technology that rotates protons in the water that makes up living tissues, excites them, and detects when their direction changes.

Protons in the body are forced to align with the strong magnetic field created by the powerful magnets used in MRIs. The protons are then stimulated and spin out of equilibrium when a radiofrequency current is pulsed through the patient, pushing against the magnetic field's pull. The energy released as the protons realign with the magnetic field is detectable by the MRI sensors when the radiofrequency field is switched off. The environment and the chemical makeup of the molecules affect how long it takes the protons to realign with the magnetic field and how much energy is released. These magnetic characteristics allow doctors to distinguish between different kinds of tissues.

A patient is put inside a big magnet to get an MRI, and they have to stay motionless the entire time to avoid blurring the picture. To accelerate the rate at which protons realign with the magnetic field, a patient may receive intravenous contrast agents—which frequently contain the element gadolinium—before or during the magnetic resonance imaging (MRI). The image gets brighter the faster the protons realign.

MRI scanners are especially useful for imaging the body's soft tissues and non-bony parts. They are different from computed tomography (CT) in that they don't utilize X-rays' harmful ionizing radiation. Because MRI provides a much clearer image of the brain, spinal cord, and nerves than standard X-rays and CT do, it is frequently used to image injuries to the knee and shoulder.

In the brain, MRI can differentiate between white matter and gray matter and can also be used to diagnose aneurysms and tumors. When repeated imaging is needed for diagnosis or treatment, especially in the brain, magnetic resonance imaging (MRI) is the preferred imaging modality since it doesn't involve radiation or X-rays. MRIs cost more than CT scans or X-ray imaging, though.

Functional Magnetic Resonance Imaging (fMRI) is a type of specialized MRI scan. Through the observation of brain structures, it is possible to ascertain which regions of the brain "activate"—that is, use more oxygen—during different types of cognitive tasks. It contributes to the growing body of knowledge regarding the structure of the brain and may establish a new benchmark for evaluating neurological health and neurosurgical risk.

Orientation and Directional Terms

Term	Definition	Illustration
Magnetic resonance spectroscopy	Magnetic resonance spectroscopy (MRS) provides a non-invasive 'window' on biochemical processes within the body.	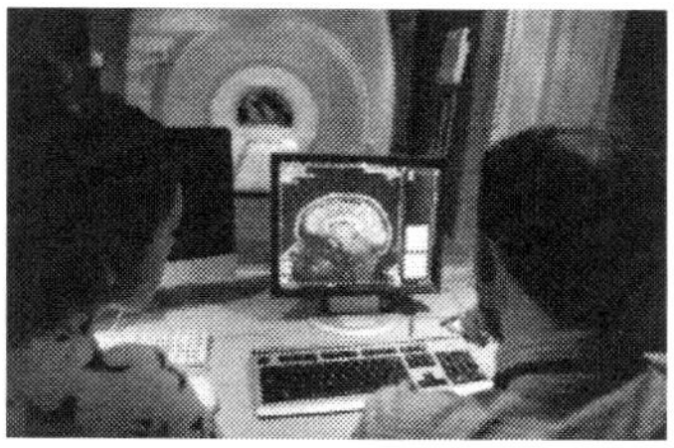
Real-time MRI	Real-time magnetic resonance imaging (RT-MRI) refers to the continuous monitoring ("filming") of moving objects in real-time.	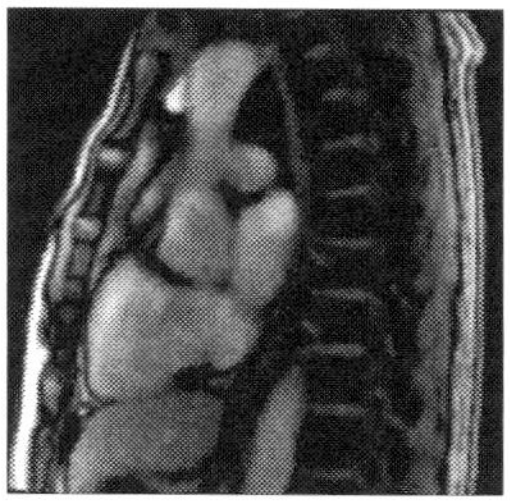
Interventional MRI	Interventional magnetic resonance imaging, also interventional MRI or IMRI, is the use of magnetic resonance imaging (MRI) to do interventional radiology procedures.	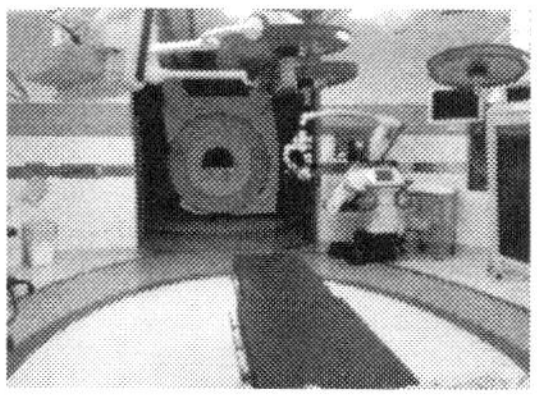
Magnetic resonance guided focused ultrasound	Magnetic resonance guided focused ultrasound surgery (MRgFUS) is a non-invasive way to treat benign and malignant tumors.	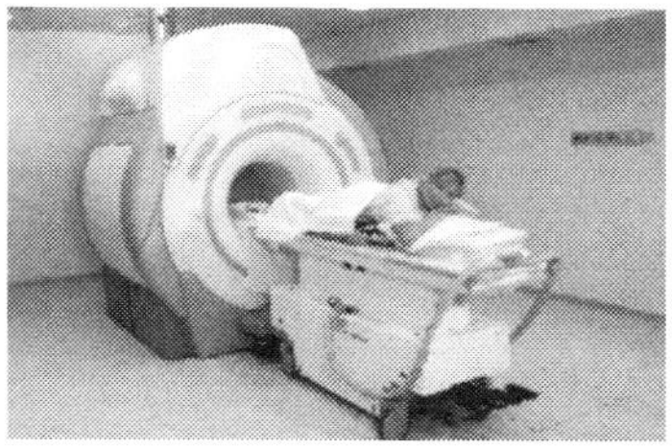
Quantitative MRI	Quantitative magnetic resonance imaging (qMRI) goes beyond conventional MRI, which aims primarily at local image contrast.	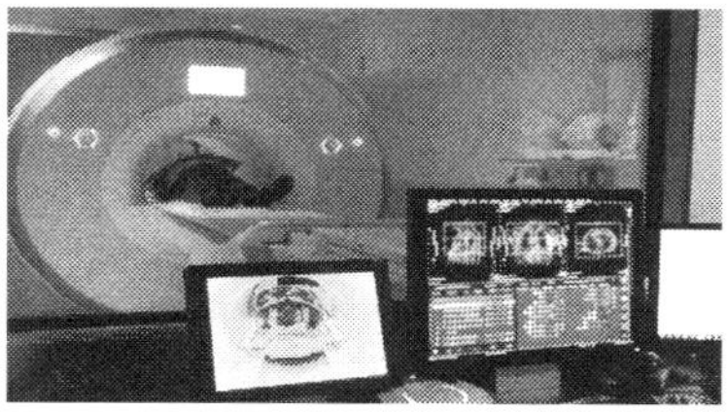

3.1. History of NMR and MRI

When radio frequency is added to a magnetic field, nuclei's spin orientation shifts, as Isidor Rabi's research on the nature of the force binding protons to atomic nuclei in the 1930s eventually revealed. This was the first study done by humans on the relationship between radio frequency, magnetic field, and atomic nuclei. As a result, he was given the 1944 Nobel Prize in Physics for this outstanding contribution.

A decade later, in 1946, Harvard University's Purcel and F. Magnetic nuclei in a magnetic field absorb electromagnetic radiation and reemit it, as was independently discovered by Block of Stanford University. They were awarded the Nobel Prize in Physics in 1952 for their discovery of nuclear magnetic resonance and subsequent advancements in this field.

As soon as the phenomenon of nuclear magnetic resonance was discovered, researchers began using this technique to study the structure and properties of nuclei, including measuring their nuclear magnetic moments, among other useful studies. According to the effects of molecular structure on the surrounding magnetic field of hydrogen, chemists developed NMR spectroscopy. From one-dimensional 1H spectroscopy to two-dimensional, 13-carbon, and other sophisticated techniques, NMR spectroscopy emerges as a dominant method for determining molecular structure. This method was even used on proteins by scientists in the 1990s, enabling precise molecular structure determination of liquid phase proteins. Molecular structure and composition analysis, medical diagnosis, and many other fields of chemistry, biology, and research now make extensive use of nuclear magnetic resonance technology.

NMR can distinguish between tumor and normal tissue in vivo because, as discovered by R. Damadian in 1971, both the longitudinal relaxation time (T1) and transverse relaxation time (T2) in tumors are longer than those in normal tissue. This work offered a fantastic opportunity to introduce the NMR technique into medical research. Paul Lauterbur first used magnetic resonance imaging on tiny test tube samples in 1973, and the first cross-sectional image of a live mouse was released in January 1974. The Fourier Transform, which forms the basis of modern MRI techniques, and phase and frequency encoding were proposed by Richard Ernst in 1975 for use in magnetic resonance imaging. Richard Ernst received the 1991 Chemistry Nobel Prize in recognition of his contributions to pulsed Fourier Transform NMR and MRI, while Paul C. In 2003, Sir Peter Mansfield of the University of Nottingham and Lauterbur of the University of Illinois were granted the Nobel Prize in Medicine for their research on magnetic resonance imaging. MRI is still a commonly used diagnostic and tumor detection tool (Kuperman, 2000; Peter, Jezzard, Matthews Paul M, and Smith Stephen M, 2001; Edelman, 2006; Schröder, Leif, and Cornelius Faber, 2011).

3.2. Nuclear Magnetism

Subatomic particles exhibit the quantum mechanical phenomenon known as spin. Nuclei like ^{1}H, ^{2}H, ^{3}He, ^{23}Na, and ^{31}P possess a non-zero spin, resulting in a magnetic moment. Spin-1/2 nuclei, such as 1H, have two distinct spin states, often termed as up and down. Nuclei like 12C have no net spin due to no unpaired neutrons or protons, while isotope ^{13}C does. When these spins are exposed to a strong external magnetic field, they rotate around an axis in alignment with the field. Protons align in two energy states (known as the Zeeman effect): one low-energy and one high-energy, separated by a small energy difference.

3.2.1. Resonance and Relaxation

A single proton's behavior can only be accurately modeled using quantum mechanics. However, the behavior of an ensemble of protons can be adequately described by classical mechanics. When the spin of a single proton is measured, it can only produce one of two outcomes, known as parallel or anti-parallel, just like with other spin 1/2 particles. The wave function of a proton, which is a linear combination of its parallel and anti-parallel states, is what we mean when we talk about the state of a proton or protons.

The protons will appear to precess at the Larmor frequency in the presence of the magnetic field, B_0, which is determined by the gyromagnetic ratio of the particle and the strength of the field. Precession, which is equivalent to an radiofrequency (RF) photon, is caused by the static fields that are most frequently used in MRIs. Due to a small excess of protons in the lower energy state, thermodynamic equilibrium results in net longitudinal magnetization. As a result, the net polarization is parallel to the outside field. An RF pulse applied can cause this net polarization vector to tip sideways (with, i.e., aso-called90°pulse), or even go the other way (using a "180° pulse"). The RF pulse and the protons will bring each other into phase.

Longitudinal, or T_1 relaxation, is the exponential process that results in the recovery of longitudinal magnetization with a time constant T_1. Transverse or T_2 relaxation is the term used to describe the loss of phase coherence in the transverse plane. The enthalpy of the spin system, or the proportion of nuclei with parallel versus anti-parallel spin, is thus linked to T_1. The number of nuclei in phase, or the system's entropy, is related to T_2, on the other hand.

The transverse vector component creates an oscillating magnetic field that causes a small current to be induced in the receiver coil when the radio frequency pulse is turned off. The free induction decay (FID) is the name given to this signal. The FID in an idealized nuclear magnetic resonance experiment decays with a time constant T2 in an approximately exponential fashion. Nevertheless, in real-world MRI, the Larmor frequency varies throughout the body due to minute variations in the static magnetic field at various spatial locations, or "inhomogeneities." Destructive interference results from this, shortening the FID. The T^*_2 relaxation time, which is always less than T_2, is the time constant for the FID's observed decay. Simultaneously, the longitudinal magnetization begins its exponential recovery, with a time constant T_1 significantly larger than T_2.

A field gradient coil is used in MRI to increase the static magnetic field and vary it throughout the scanned region, assigning distinct precession frequencies to different spatial locations. Excitation will only occur in areas where the field is such that the precession frequencies coincide with the RF frequency. The almost limitless range of RF and gradient pulse sequences that make MRI so versatile are how these field gradients, which are typically modulated to sweep across the region to be scanned, are used. The responding FID signal is spread in the frequency domain by a change of field gradient; however, this can be recovered and measured by a digital post-processing of the spread signal, a refocusing gradient (to create a so-called "gradient echo"), or a radio frequency pulse (to create a so-called "spin-echo"). Once some T_1-relaxation has taken place and the spins' thermal equilibrium has been roughly restored, the entire procedure can be repeated. The interval of time between two consecutive excitations of the same slice is known as the repetition time (TR).

Soft tissues typically have T_1 times less than a second and T_2 and T^* times less than a few tens of milliseconds. These values, however, can differ significantly between tissues and between various external magnetic fields. One of the things that gives MRIs such amazing soft tissue contrast is this behavior. Gadolinium(III)-containing MRI contrast agents, for example, function by changing (shortening) the relaxation parameters, particularly T_1 (Kuperman, 2000; Peter, Jezzard, Matthews Paul M, and Smith Stephen M, 2001; Edelman, 2006; Schröder, Leif, and Cornelius Faber, 2011).

3.2.2. T_1 and T_2

Two distinct processes are identified as responsible for the decay of RF-induced NMR spin polarization, each having a unique time constant. After pulse excitation, a process known as T_1 is in charge of the resonance intensity being lost. The width or broadness of resonances is characterized by the other process, T_2. Formally speaking, T_1 is the time constant for the physical processes that lead to the relaxation of the nuclear spin magnetization vector M's constituent parts parallel to the external magnetic field, B_0 (commonly referred to as the z-axis). The coherent components of M perpendicular to B_0 are impacted by T_2 relaxation. T_1 controls the maximum time an NMR spectrum can be obtained and sets a limit on the pulse repetition rate in conventional NMR spectroscopy. T_1 values vary from milliseconds to several seconds, contingent upon the molecule's size, solution viscosity, sample temperature, and potential presence of paramagnetic species (e.g., O_2 or ions of metal).

3.2.2.1. T_1

The longitudinal (or spin-lattice) relaxation time T_1 is the decay constant for the recovery of the z component of the nuclear spin magnetization, M_z, towards its thermal equilibrium value, $M_{z,eq}$. In general;

$$M_z(t) = M_{z,\text{eq}} - [M_{z,\text{eq}} - M_z(0)]e^{-t/T_1}$$

In specific cases:

- $M_z(0)=0$ indicates that M has been tilted into the xy plane, and the recovery is straightforward.

  $$M_z(t) = M_{z,\text{eq}}\left(1 - e^{-t/T_1}\right)$$

  i.e., after one time constant T1, the magnetization returns to 63% of its equilibrium value.
- The initial magnetization is inverted in the inversion recovery experiment, $M_z(0) = -M_{z,eq}$, which is frequently used to measure T_1 values. As a result, the recovery occurs.

  $$M_z(t) = M_{z,\text{eq}}\left(1 - 2e^{-t/T_1}\right)$$

To achieve the thermal equilibrium distribution, T_1 relaxation entails redistributing the populations of the nuclear spin states. This is not energy-saving by definition. Furthermore, at NMR frequencies, spontaneous emission is incredibly slow. Therefore, nuclear spins that are truly isolated would exhibit very low T_1 relaxation rates. Nonetheless, nuclear spins can exchange energy with the lattice, their surroundings, through a variety of relaxation mechanisms, which enables the spin populations to equilibrate. The alternative description, spin-lattice relaxation, originates from the fact that T_1 relaxation involves an interaction with the environment.

Take notice that T_1 relaxation rates (i.e., $1/T_1$) typically fluctuate significantly with magnetic field strength B and are heavily reliant on the NMR frequency. A sample's relaxation rate is greatly accelerated by minute concentrations of paramagnetic materials. Liquid samples easily achieve T_1/T_2 values of ten seconds or more through degassing, which eliminates dissolved oxygen.

Spin Saturation Transfer

Spin Saturation Transfer (SST) technique provides information on chemical exchange reactions, particularly for molecules exhibiting slowly relaxing (T_1) signals. The technique works well with fluxional molecules. If rates surpass 1/ T_1, this magnetization transfer technique yields data.

3.2.2.2. T_2

An illustration of a proton's spin in a magnetic field B_0 that is always present. The relaxation times for T_1 and T_2 are visualized. For the component of M perpendicular to B_0, denoted M_{xy}, M_T, or $M_\perp$, the decay constant is the transverse (or spin-spin) relaxation time T_2.

$$M_{xy}(t) = M_{xy}(0)e^{-t/T_2}$$

i.e., the transverse magnetization vector decreases with one-time constant T_2 to 37% of its initial magnitude.

Although T_2 relaxation is a multifaceted phenomenon, at its most basic level, it is associated with a transverse nuclear spin magnetization decoherence. Random variations in the instantaneous NMR precession frequency of various spins are caused by fluctuations in the local magnetic field. Consequently, the original phase coherence of nuclear spins is lost, leading to the phases' eventual disorder and the absence of net xy magnetization. T_2 relaxation is frequently referred to as "spin-spin" relaxation since it only takes into account the phases of other nuclear spins.

Compared to T_1 values, T_2 values typically depend much less on field strength, B. The T_2 time can be determined using the Hahn echo decay experiment, as the animation below illustrates. The echo's size is measured at various intervals between the two applied pulses. This displays the decoherence that the 180° pulse does not refocus. In basic scenarios, the T_2 time describes an exponential decay that is measured.

- **T_2*and Magnetic Field Inhomogeneity:** In an ideal system, all nuclei within a specific chemical environment will precess in a magnetic field at the same frequency. However, real systems exhibit slight variations in chemical environments, leading to a distribution of resonance frequencies. This distribution can cause a dispersion of magnetic spin vectors and result in signal loss (free induction decay). In magnetic resonance experiments, this "relaxation" process typically dominates, leading to dephasing.

Nevertheless, decoherence resulting from the inhomogeneity of the magnetic field is not a genuine "relaxation" process; rather, it is contingent upon the molecule's position within the magnet. In the case of stationary molecules, a spin echo experiment can be used to recover the signal since the departure from ideal relaxation is constant over time. Therefore, T_2^*, which is typically substantially smaller than T_2, is the corresponding transverse relaxation time constant. In contrast to T_2, T_2^* is affected by irregularities in the magnetic field gradient. For water samples in imaging magnets, the T_2^* relaxation time is usually milliseconds and is always less than the T_2 relaxation time. The following relation is absolutely true in NMR systems: $T_2 \leq 2T_1$. Generally speaking (though not always), T_1 is larger than T_2. While uncommon, $2T_1 > T_2 > T_1$ cases are not unheard of.

3.2.3. Bloch Equations

When relaxation times T_1 and T_2 are present, the nuclear magnetization $M = (M_x, M_y, M_z)$ as a function of time is determined using Bloch equations. Felix Bloch introduced the concept of phenomenological equations, or Bloch equations, in 1946.

$$\frac{\partial M_x(t)}{\partial t} = \gamma(\mathbf{M}(t) \times \mathbf{B}(t))_x - \frac{M_x(t)}{T_2}$$
$$\frac{\partial M_y(t)}{\partial t} = \gamma(\mathbf{M}(t) \times \mathbf{B}(t))_y - \frac{M_y(t)}{T_2}$$
$$\frac{\partial M_z(t)}{\partial t} = \gamma(\mathbf{M}(t) \times \mathbf{B}(t))_z - \frac{M_z(t) - M_0}{T_1}$$

Where × is the cross-product, γ is the gyromagnetic ratio and $\mathbf{B}(t) = (B_x(t), B_y(t), B_0 + B_z(t))$ is the magnetic flux density experienced by the nuclei. Typically, the z component of the magnetic flux density B consists of two terms: $B_z(t)$, which depends on time, and B_0, which is constant in time. It is a component of magnetic resonance imaging and aids in the NMR signal's spatial decoding. The Bloch equations correspond to the equations mentioned above in the section on T_1 and T_2 relaxation (Kuperman, 2000; Peter, Jezzard, Matthews Paul M, and Smith Stephen M, 2001; Edelman, 2006; Schröder, Leif, and Cornelius Faber, 2011).

3.3. Diagnostics

MRI is commonly used in medical diagnosis with over 25,000 scanners in use globally.

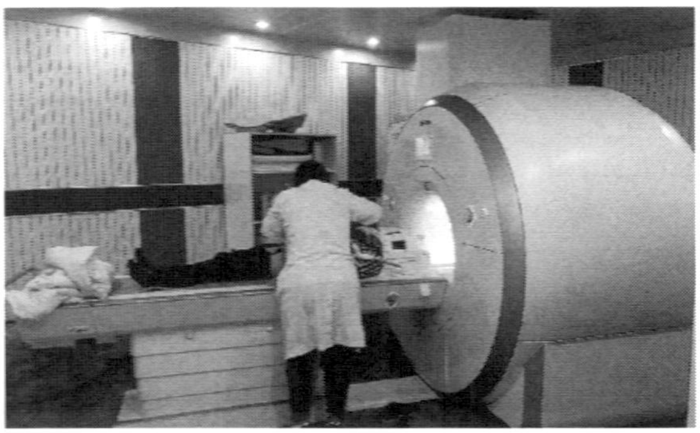

Figure 3.1. *A patient being positioned for MRI of the head and abdomen.*

Source: By Ptrump16-Ownwork, CCBY-SA4.0, https://commons.wikimedia.org/w/index.php?curid=64157788.

Its impact on health outcomes varies across specialties, but it is particularly useful in preoperative staging for rectal and prostate cancer. Additionally, MRI plays a crucial role in diagnosing, staging, and monitoring various tumors, as well as identifying tissue samples for biobanking (Figure 3.1).

3.3.1. Neuroimaging

Ionizing radiation (X-rays) or radioactive tracers are not needed for magnetic resonance imaging (MRI), which creates high-quality two- or three-dimensional images of the brain, brainstem, and cerebellum.

3.3.1.1. History

Under the direction of Ian Robert Young and Hugh Clow, two research groups at EMI Laboratories produced the first magnetic resonance images of a human brain in 1978. 1986 saw Charles L. Denis Le Bihan acquired the first images and subsequently patented diffusion MRI, while Dumoulin and Howard R. Hart at General Electric developed MR angiography. Arno Villringer and team proved in 1988 that susceptibility contrast agents could be used in perfusion magnetic resonance imaging. Seiji Ogawa at AT&T Bell Laboratories discovered the method underlying Functional Magnetic Resonance Imaging (fMRI) in 1990 when he noticed that blood with depleted hemoglobin (dHb) was drawn to a magnetic field.

Diffusion tensor imaging (DTI) was created in the early 1990s by NIH employees Peter Basser and Le Bihan, as well as Aaron Filler, Franklyn Howe, and associates. In 1992, Graeme Bydder, Young, and Joseph Hajnal reported using the FLAIR pulse sequence to show high signal regions in normal white matter. John Detre, Alan P., et al in the same year. Arterial spin labeling was developed by Koretsky and associates. In 1997, Reichenbach, Jürgen R., E. Mark Haacke at Washington University in St.

Louis with colleagues. Susceptibility weighted imaging was created by Louis.

Both in 1994 at 3.0 T and in 1998 at 8 T, the first studies of the human brain at these temperatures were published. Researchers have studied the human brain at 9.4 T (2006) and as high as 10.5 T (2019). As a result of their research on MRI, Paul Lauterbur and Sir Peter Mansfield were granted the 2003 Nobel Prize in Physiology or Medicine (Figure 3.2).

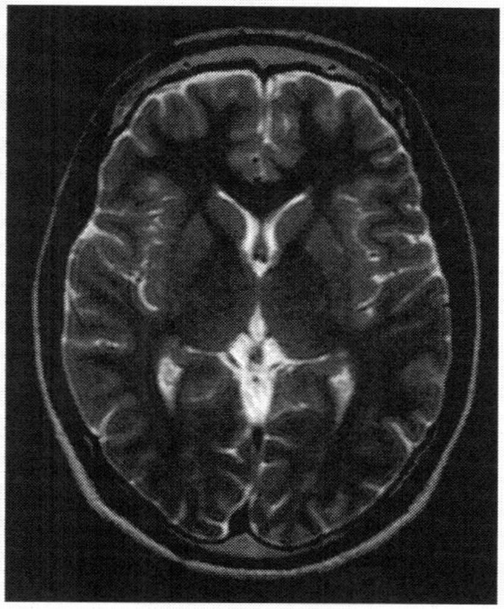

Figure 3.2. *This axial T2-weighted (CSFwhite) MRI scan shows a normal brain at the level of the lateral ventricles.*

Source: ByNovaksean-Ownwork, CCBY-SA4.0, https://commons.wikimedia.org/w/index.php?curid=44348140.

100 microns is the record for the highest spatial resolution of a postmortem, whole intact brain from Massachusetts General Hospital. On October 30, 2019, the information was published in Scientific Data.

3.3.1.2. Applications

Better tissue contrast and fewer artifacts are two benefits of magnetic resonance imaging (MRI) over computed tomography (CT) when viewing the brainstem. Additionally, MRI works better for pituitary imaging. It might, however, be less successful in detecting cerebritis early on. An MRI should not be performed after a concussion unless there are focal neurological findings, progressive neurological symptoms, or a concern about a skull fracture during the examination. Measurements of global connectivity, cerebral blood flow, mean diffusivity, fractional anisotropy, and other factors can be used in the analysis of a concussion to see how the pathophysiological mechanisms develop during the healing process. MRI gives more information about gyration than ultrasound when analyzing the fetal brain. Brain abscesses can be detected with high sensitivity using MRI.

Many different imaging modalities or sequences can be used with imaging the nervous system:

- T_1-weighted (T1W) images: Dark fluid surrounds the brain. Normal anatomy can be seen with T1-weighted images.
- T_2-weighted (T2W) images: Compared to T_1, CSF is lighter, but fat (and hence white matter) is darker. T2-weighted images can help visualize pathology.
- Diffusion-weighted images (DWI): DWI produces contrast in MR images by utilizing the diffusion of water molecules.
- Proton density (PD) images: Because of its comparatively high proton content, CSF appears bright. Compared to white matter, gray matter is brighter.
- Fluid attenuation inversion recovery (FLAIR): iiis beneficial for assessing white matter plaques in the vicinity of the ventricles. It helps to recognize demyelination.

3.3.1.3. Diagnostic Usage

A brain or head MRI can be used for a variety of diagnostic purposes, such as the detection of tumors, aneurysms, strokes, and other brain injuries. When differentially diagnosing other diseases, magnetic resonance imaging (MRI) is helpful in many cases, including Parkinson's and Alzheimer's. Regarding diagnosis, brain tumors have been identified through the use of deep learning networks and MRI data.

3.3.2. Cardiovascular

Cardiovascular magnetic resonance imaging, or cardiac magnetic resonance imaging (cardiac MRI, CMR), is a non-invasive magnetic resonance imaging (MRI) technique used to evaluate the structure and function of the cardiovascular system. Congenital heart disease, cardiomyopathies, valvular heart disease, aortic diseases such as dissection, aneurysm, and coarctation, and coronary heart disease are among the conditions under which it is carried out. It is also useful for examining pulmonary veins. You can find patient information here.

It is not recommended if you have claustrophobia or have any metal or electronic implants, such as intracerebral clips. To find out if these are MRI conditional, you can look them up. Nearly all patients with pacemakers or defibrillators can be scanned, but specific procedures are required. ECG gating and high temporal resolution protocols are used to modify standard MRI sequences for cardiac imaging. Research on the development of cardiac MRI is ongoing, and new and cutting-edge methods are being developed at a rapid pace.

3.3.2.1. Uses

When combined with other imaging modalities like nuclear medicine, cardiac CT, and echocardiography, cardiovascular MRI is a useful tool. In the evidence-based diagnosis and treatment of cardiovascular disease, the technique plays a crucial role. Myocardial ischemia and viability assessment, cardiomyopathies, myocarditis, iron overload, vascular diseases, and congenital heart disease are among the conditions for which it is used. It serves as the benchmark for evaluating the structure and function of the heart and is helpful in the diagnosis and surgical planning of complex congenital heart disease.

It plays a role in identifying and characterizing myocardial ischemia caused by diseases affecting the microvasculature and epicardial vessels when combined with vasodilator stress. To characterize cardiomyopathy and determine viability, infarction and fibrosis can be identified using late gadolinium enhancement (LGE) and T_1 mapping. To evaluate congenital or acquired anomalies of the coronary arteries and great vessels, magnetic resonance angiography can be done with or without a contrast agent.

Limited access to scanners, a shortage of technologists and qualified clinicians, comparatively high costs, and competing diagnostic modalities are some of the barriers preventing its broader application. To enable more clinics to implement CMR into their operations, some organizations are working on ways to lessen these barriers. These solutions are frequently software platforms that enhance procedure efficiency and offer clinical decision support.

3.3.2.2. Risks

Comparing cardiac MRI to other imaging indications, there are no particular risks involved. When used in CT scans, gadolinium-based contrast medium—which is primarily used in patients with renal disease—has been linked to nephrogenic systemic fibrosis. Gadolinium has been found to deposit intracranially more recently; however, no neurological side effects have been noted. Although cardiac MRI has been shown to have genotoxic effects both in vivo and in vitro, more recent research has not confirmed these results, and it is unlikely that cardiac MRI will cause the intricate DNA damage linked to ionizing radiation.

3.3.2.3. Physics

The fundamental ideas of CMR and other MRI methods are the same. Cardiovascular imaging is typically carried out with cardiac gating, which is a modification of traditional ECG methods. Balanced steady state free precession, or bSSFP, provides intrinsic image contrast and good temporal resolution for acquiring cardiac cine sequences. T_1-weighted sequences are employed to identify intra-myocardial fat and to visualize anatomy. Another technique for measuring diffuse myocardial fibrosis is T_1 mapping. Myocardial edema, which can arise in cases of acute myocarditis or infarction, is primarily detected by T_2-weighted imaging. Phase-contrast imaging is used to quantify shunts and evaluate valve disease by using bipolar gradients to encode velocity in a specific direction.

3.3.2.4. Techniques

A CMR study usually consists of a series of steps in a protocol that are customized to the particular exam indication. Localizers are used in the study to help with image planning, and a series of retrospectively-gated cine sequences are used to evaluate biventricular function in conventional orientations. Intravenous contrast medium is used to measure LGE and myocardial perfusion. Phase contrast imaging can be used to calculate the shunt volume and valvular regurgitant fraction. MR angiography and T_1 and T_2-weighted imaging are possible additional sequences. Here are some examples:

- **Heart Function using Cine Imaging:** Cine sequences of bSSFP are used to obtain structural and functional information. Because of the blood's comparatively high T_2:T_1 ratio in comparison to the myocardium, these are typically retrospectively-gated and have intrinsically high contrast in cardiac imaging. To achieve the standard cardiac planes used for assessment, images are usually planned sequentially. Dephasing and signal loss brought on by turbulent flow enable a qualitative understanding of valvular disease. Acquired from base to apex, the left ventricular short axis cines are used to measure myocardial mass and end-diastolic and end-systolic volumes. Strain can be measured by using tagging sequences to activate a grid pattern that changes with cardiac contraction.
- **Late Gadolinium Enhancement:** For the best contrast between the normal and infarcted myocardium, intravenous gadolinium-based contrast agents are given, and delayed imaging is carried out at least ten minutes later. Using an inversion recovery (IR) sequence, the signal from a healthy myocardium is eliminated. Transmural enhancement can be used to measure the viability of the heart. Non-ischemic LGE patterns can also be characteristic of inflammatory, infiltrative, and cardiomyopathic diseases.
- **Perfusion:** By acting as a vasodilator through the A_{2A} receptor, adenosine can increase the perfusion difference between myocardial territories supplied by coronary arteries that are normal and stenosed. A bolus of

contrast medium is given while obtaining saturation recovery images of the heart with a high temporal resolution readout, following a few minutes of continuous intravenous infusion until there are hemodynamic signs of vasodilatation. An inducible myocardial perfusion defect clearly shows promise. Its use is frequently limited to patients with intermediate pre-test probability due to cost and availability, but research has shown that, when compared to guidelines-directed care, it reduces unnecessary angiography.

- **4D flow CMR:** By applying flow-sensitive gradients in three orthogonal planes within a three-dimensional volume throughout the cardiac cycle, conventional phase contrast imaging can be extended. By encoding the blood flow rate at every voxel in the volume, 4D imaging makes it possible to visualize fluid dynamics through specialized software. Due to the difficulty of post-processing and the comparatively lengthy acquisition times, it is not routinely used in clinical practice. However, applications include complex congenital heart disease and research into cardiovascular flow characteristics.

3.3.2.5. Children and Congenital Heart Disease

The most common major birth defect is congenital heart defects. It is crucial to accurately diagnose these defects to create effective treatment plans. Cardiac magnetic resonance imaging, or CMR, can provide detailed information about the nature of congenital heart defects safely without the use of X-rays or invasive procedures. However, it is not typically the primary or only diagnostic test used for congenital heart disease.

Instead, it is usually combined with other diagnostic methods. Generally speaking, there are four main clinical reasons for a CMR examination: (1) when cardiac ultrasound, or echocardiography, is unable to provide enough diagnostic information; (2) as a risk-free substitute for diagnostic cardiac catheterization, which involves radiation exposure from X-rays; (3) to obtain specific diagnostic information for which CMR offers special benefits, such as blood flow measurement or the identification of cardiac masses; and (4) when clinical assessment and other diagnostic tests are inconsistent. Tetralogy of Fallot, transposition of the great arteries, coarctation of the aorta, single ventricle heart disease, anomalies of the pulmonary veins, atrial septal defect, connective tissue diseases like Marfan syndrome, vascular rings, anomalous origins of the coronary arteries, and cardiac tumors are a few conditions for which CMR is frequently used.

In children, CMR exams usually take 15 to 60 minutes. Throughout the examination, the child needs to stay extremely still to prevent blurry images. While pediatric CMR protocols vary amongst institutions, most children 7 years of age and older can cooperate well enough for a high-quality examination. A successful study is more likely if the child is given an age-appropriate explanation of the process beforehand. Parents may be permitted entry into the MRI scanner room to assist their child in finishing the exam following the appropriate safety screening. To lessen anxiety and increase cooperation, some centers let kids watch movies or listen to music on a special audiovisual system that is compatible with MRI scans. However, any form of entertainment or distraction that doesn't involve sedation usually yields better results in terms of pediatric cooperation than the presence of a composed, supportive, and encouraging parent. General anesthesia or sedation with intravenous medication may be required if the child is not cooperative enough. It might be possible to examine very young infants while they are sleeping naturally. Modern image capture methods like 4D flow necessitate a shorter scan time and may result in less sedation being required.

3.3.2.6. Different Cardiac-capable Magnet Types

Most CMR is carried out at 1.5T or 3T using traditional superconducting MRI equipment. A greater signal-to-noise ratio can be obtained by imaging at 3T field strength in exchange for better temporal or spatial resolution, which is most useful for first-pass perfusion studies. However, many studies are routinely conducted at 1.5T due to higher capital costs and the effects of off-resonance artifact on image quality. Research on imaging at 7T field strength is expanding, although the technology is still relatively new. MRI scanners with cardiac capabilities are currently made by Philips, Siemens, Hitachi, Toshiba, and GE.

3.3.3. Musculoskeletal

Soft tissue tumors, joint disease assessment, and spinal imaging are among the musculoskeletal system's applications. Additionally, systemic muscle diseases, including genetic muscle diseases, can be diagnosed with MRI techniques. Motion artifact over the imaged spine can result from swallowing movement of the throat and esophagus. Thus, this artifact can be avoided by applying a saturation pulse over the throat and esophagus. By timing the MRI pulse following heart cycles, motion artifacts resulting from the heart's pumping can be minimized. Applying saturation pulses above and below the region of interest can help minimize blood vessel flow artifacts. A variation of the fMRI technique designed for use in the brain is spinal fMRI or functional magnetic resonance imaging of the spinal cord. While the fundamental principles of the methods remain the same, spinal fMRI necessitates several specific modifications to account for the periodic motion of the spinal cord, its small cross-sectional dimensions (approximately 8 mm × 15 mm at the largest region) and length (~45cminadulthumans). Additionally, the magnetic field used for MRI varies depending on the position of the spinal cord due to differences in magnetic susceptibility between bone and tissues. Neuronal activity at most levels of the spinal cord in response to a variety of stimuli, including touch, vibration, and temperature changes, as well as when performing motor tasks, has been mapped using spinal fMRI. To date, studies of normal sensory and motor function as well as investigations into the effects of multiple sclerosis and trauma on the spinal cord have been conducted using spinal fMRI.

Two distinct techniques for acquiring the data have been used: one is based on the well-established BOLD (blood-oxygen-level dependent) functional magnetic resonance imaging (fMRI) methods used in the brain, and the other is based on the contrast of SEEP (signal enhancement by extravascular water protons) with proton-density weighted spin-echo imaging. The SEEP contrast method is the foundation for most of the studies that have been published to date. Using a heartbeat recording to account for the related time course of spinal cord motion, acquiring image data with relatively high (~1–2 mm) spatial resolution to detect fine structural details, and acquiring images in thin contiguous sagittal slices to span a large extent of the spinal cord are some of the methods that have been demonstrated to overcome the challenges mentioned above. In order to lessen the effects of spatial magnetic field distortions, BOLD contrast-based methods have used imaging slices transverse to the spinal cord and parallel imaging techniques to speed up data acquisition. SEEP contrast techniques were specifically developed because of their low sensitivity to distortions in the magnetic field and their sensitivity to changes in neuronal activity.

3.3.4. Liver and Gastrointestinal

The liver, pancreas, and bile duct lesions can be found and identified using hepatobiliary magnetic resonance imaging. Dynamic contrast enhancement sequences and diffusion-weighted, opposed-phase imaging can be used to assess focal or diffuse liver disorders. Modern hepatobiliary contrast agents also offer the possibility of performing functional biliary imaging, although extracellular contrast agents are still commonly used in liver MRIs. In magnetic resonance cholangiopancreatography (MRCP), a heavily T2-weighted sequence is used to achieve anatomic imaging of the bile ducts. The pancreas is imaged functionally after secretin has been administered. MR enterography offers a non-invasive method for evaluating small bowel tumors and inflammatory bowel disease. Large polyps in patients at higher risk of colorectal cancer may be found with MR-colonography.

3.3.5. Angiography

A collection of methods based on magnetic resonance imaging (MRI) for blood vessel imaging is known as magnetic resonance angiography (MRA). To assess arteries (and less frequently veins) for anomalies such as stenosis (abnormal narrowing), occlusions, aneurysms (dilatations in the vessel wall that are susceptible to rupture), or other conditions, magnetic resonance angiography is used to create images of the arteries. MRA is frequently used to assess the renal arteries, the arteries in the legs (the latter exam is often called a "run-off"), the arteries in the neck and brain, and the thoracic and abdominal aorta.

3.3.5.1. Acquisition

A range of methods based on flow effects or contrast (natural or pharmacologically produced) can be applied to produce images of blood vessels, including arteries and veins. The most widely used MRA techniques include the use of intravenous contrast agents, especially those that contain gadolinium to shorten blood's T1 to approximately 250 ms, which is shorter than the T_1 of all other tissues (apart from fat). The blood appears brightly in short-TR sequence images. Nonetheless, there are numerous additional methods for carrying out MRA that fall into two broad categories: "flow-dependent" and "flow-independent" methods.

- **Flow-Dependent Angiography:** Blood flow is the basis for one class of MRA techniques. These techniques are known as flow-dependent MRA. They use the blood flowing through the vessels as a distinguishing factor between the vessels and other static tissue. In this manner, pictures of the vasculature can be generated. There are two types of flow-dependent MRA: phase-contrast MRA (PC-MRA), which uses phase differences to separate blood from static tissue, and time-of-flight MRA (TOF MRA), which takes advantage of the fact that moving blood spins receive fewer excitation pulses than static tissue, e.g., when picturing a slender slice.

  Flow compensation and a brief echo time are used in time-of-flight (TOF) or inflow angiography to make flowing blood appear significantly brighter than stationary tissue. Since flowing blood has not yet reached saturation due to a limited amount of excitation pulses, it exhibits a significantly higher signal than the saturated stationary tissue. Due to the reliance of this technique on blood flow, regions with sluggish blood flow (like massive aneurysms) or blood flow that is in the image plane might not be clearly visible. This produces finely detailed, high-resolution images and is most frequently used in the head and neck. Additionally, it is the method most frequently employed for routine angiographic assessment of the intracranial circulation in ischemic stroke patients.

- **Phase-contrast MRA:** A phase shift proportional to the spins' velocities occurs when spins are traveling in the same direction as a magnetic field gradient. Phase-contrast angiography is based on this principle. Bipolar gradients, or two gradients with the same magnitude but opposite directions, are used to encode the spin velocities in the most basic phase-contrast pulse sequence. The application of the two gradients results in no net phase change for stationary spins. Due to their differing spatial positions, moving spins will perceive the second gradient at a different magnitude than the first. A net phase shift is the outcome of this. The spins' velocities can be ascertained directly from this data. An angiogram can also be obtained by subtracting the image from one that was acquired without the velocity encoding gradients.
- **Flow-independent Angiography:** Non-contrast enhanced flow-independent methods exist in MRA, although the majority of techniques rely on contrast agents or flow into the blood to generate contrast (Contrast Enhanced techniques). As the name implies, these techniques rely on the variations in T_1, T_2, and chemical shift of the various tissues within the voxel rather than flow. One of the key benefits of these techniques is that they make it easier to image the areas of slow flow that are frequently present in vascular disease patients. Furthermore, the use of additional contrast agents—which have recently been connected to nephrogenic systemic fibrosis in patients with chronic kidney disease and kidney failure—is not necessary with non-contrast enhanced methods.

MRI contrast agents are injected during contrast-enhanced magnetic resonance angiography (CEA), which is currently the most widely used MRA technique. After injecting the contrast agent into a vein, pictures are taken before and after the agent's initial passage through the arteries. In post-processing, an image is produced by subtracting these two acquisitions, which, in theory, only displays blood vessels and not the surrounding tissue. If the timing is right, this could produce very high-quality images. An alternative is to use a contrast agent known as a "blood-pool agent," which stays in the bloodstream for up to an hour instead of exiting the vascular system like most agents do after a few minutes. Higher-resolution imaging is feasible because there is more time available for image acquisition. The simultaneous enhancement of veins and arteries, however, presents a challenge if higher-resolution images are needed.

Contrast-enhanced magnetic resonance angiography without subtraction: Thanks to advancements in MRA technology, high-quality contrast-enhanced MRA images can now be produced without subtracting a non-contrast-enhanced mask image. Because it avoids both the motion subtraction artifacts and the rise in image background noise, which are both direct consequences of image subtraction, this method has been demonstrated to improve diagnostic quality. Excellent body fat suppression over sizable image regions is a prerequisite for this strategy, which can be met by utilizing mDIXON acquisition techniques. Conventional MRA suppresses body fat-related signals during the actual image acquisition process. However, because this method is sensitive to even minute variations in the magnetic and electromagnetic fields, it may not suppress fat sufficiently in some areas. The image signals produced by fat and water can be reliably distinguished and separated using mDIXON techniques. Since almost no body fat is visible when using the "water images" for MRA scans, subtraction masks are not necessary for high-quality MR venograms.

Non-enhanced magnetic resonance angiography: Alternative methods have been developed that do not require the injection of contrast agents, as doing so may pose a risk to patients with compromised kidney function. These techniques are predicated on the variations in T_1, T_2, and chemical shifts of the various voxel tissues. Balanced steady-state free precession (bSSFP) imaging is a noteworthy non-enhanced technique for flow-independent angiography, as it naturally generates high signals from veins and arteries.

- **2D and 3D Acquisitions:** There are two distinct methods for obtaining the images. Both 2D and 3D images can generally be obtained. Cross sections at any view angle can be computed if 3D data is obtained. Although 2D data from various slices can also be combined to create 3D data, this method produces images with lower quality at view angles that differ from the original data acquisition. Moreover, projections can be computed using the 3D data in addition to being utilized to produce cross-sectional images. When dealing with complex vessel geometries where blood is flowing in all spatial directions, three-dimensional data acquisition might also be useful (sadly, this case also requires three different flow encodings, one in each spatial direction). TOF-MRA and PC-MRA both have benefits and drawbacks. Compared to TOF-MRA, PC-MRA allows for quantitative flow measurements and has fewer issues with slow flow. Low sensitivity is observed by PC-MRA when imaging non-uniform and pulsating flow.

Generally speaking, one of the main issues with flow-dependent MRA is slow blood flow. The blood signal and the static tissue signal diverge less as a result of it. This pertains to PC-MRA in which the blood-static tissue phase difference is smaller than with faster flow, or TOF-MRA in which the transverse blood magnetization and, consequently, the blood signal are smaller. Contrast agents can be used to increase blood signal. This is crucial because small vessels and those with very low flow velocities typically exhibit weak signals. Unfortunately, patients with impaired renal function may find using gadolinium-based contrast media dangerous. Recent research has looked into non-enhanced methods to prevent these complications and do away with the expense of contrast media.

- **Non-enhanced Techniques in Development:** Rather than relying on flow, flow-independent NEMRA techniques use variations in T_1, T_2, and chemical shifts to differentiate between blood and static tissue. A method of imaging known as "gated subtraction fast spin-echo" involves subtracting two fast spin echo sequences that were obtained at systole and diastole. In order to perform arteriography, the diastolic data set—which shows the arteries as bright—must be subtracted from the systolic data set, which shows the arteries as dark. calls for the application of ECG gating. This technology is also known by the trade names DeltaFlow (GE), native SPACE (Siemens), TRANCE (Philips), and Fresh Blood Imaging (Toshiba).
- **4D Dynamic MR Angiography (4D-MRA):** The vascular tree is extracted from the subsequent images using the first images as a subtraction mask before enhancement. gives the operator the ability to separate the venous and arterial phases of a blood groove while visualizing its dynamics. Compared to other MRA techniques, this one has received far less research attention to date.

Susceptibility weighted imaging (SWI), also known as BOLD venography, is a technique that uses the phase image to identify susceptibility differences between tissues. An image processing program combines the phase and magnitude data digitally to create an enhanced contrast magnitude image that is highly sensitive to venous blood, hemorrhage, and iron storage. This technique, known as blood-oxygen-level dependent (BOLD) venous blood imaging (SWI) was (and occasionally is) called BOLD venography. SWI is frequently used for high-resolution brain venographies and traumatic brain injuries (TBI) due to its sensitivity to venous blood.

Veins can be imaged using techniques similar to flow effect based MRA. In order to image the venous blood that has recently moved from the excited plane, magnetic resonance venography, or

MRV, for example, involves exciting a plane inferiorly while the signal is obtained in the plane immediately superior to the excitation plane. Variations in tissue signals may also be employed in MRA. This technique is based on the unique signal characteristics of blood, which are unaffected by MR flow effects and different from those of other bodily tissues. The balanced pulse sequences like bTFE or TrueFISP work best for this. BOLD imaging can also be utilized to evaluate the viability of tissue survival in stroke patients.

3.3.5.2. Artifacts

Generally speaking, turbulent flow causes a variety of different magnetized proton spins to lose phase coherence (intra-voxel dephasing phenomenon), which in turn causes a loss of signal in MRA techniques. Arterial stenosis may be overestimated as a result of this phenomenon. Additional artifacts seen in MRA consist of:

- **Phase-Contrast MRA:** Phase wrapping resulting from the image's maximum blood velocity being underestimated. The signal wraps from pi to -pi instead of the fast-moving blood about the maximum set velocity for phase-contrast MRA, aliasing the flow information. By using velocity encoding (VENC) values higher than the maximum measured velocity, this can be prevented. Another way to fix it is by using a technique known as phase-unwrapping.
- **Maxwell Terms:** results from the gradients field in the main field B_0 being switched. As a result, the over magnetic field becomes distorted and provides the flow with erroneous phase information.
- **Acceleration:** Phase-contrast imaging is not able to accurately encode accelerating blood flow, which can result in inaccurate blood flow measurements.
- **Saturation Artifact due to Laminar Flow:** Blood flow in many vessels is slower in the vicinity of the vessel walls than it is in the center. This can lower the vessel's apparent caliber by causing the blood close to the walls of the vessel to become saturated.
- **Venetian Blind Artifact:** The method can produce composed images with horizontal stripes if the flip angle across the slab is not uniform, as it acquires images in slabs (similar to multiple overlapping thin-slab acquisition, or MOTSA).

3.3.5.3. Visualization

On rare occasions, MRA directly creates (thick) slices that encompass the target vessel in its entirety. But more often than not, the acquisition produces a stack of slices that show a three-dimensional volume inside the body. This 3D dataset needs to be rendered using a method in order to be displayed on a 2D device, like a computer monitor. The most popular approach is maximum intensity projection (MIP), in which the highest value is chosen to be displayed on the screen while the computer mimics rays passing through the volume. The final pictures are similar to those obtained from traditional catheter angiography. An observer can better perceive depth and 3D structure if multiple projections of this type are integrated into a cine loop or QuickTime VR object. Direct volume rendering is a substitute for MIP in which the MR signal is converted to attributes such as color, opacity, and brightness before being employed in an optical model.

3.3.5.4. Clinical Use

Numerous arteries in the body have been successfully studied by MRA, including the renal arteries, the arteries in the lower limbs, the aorta and its major branches in the thorax and abdomen, and the cerebral and other vessels in the head and neck. However, MRA has not been as successful for the coronary arteries as either invasive catheter angiography or CT angiography. Atherosclerosis is most frequently the underlying cause, but other illnesses like aneurysms or aberrant vascular anatomy can also be identified.

One benefit of MRA over invasive catheter angiography is that it is a non-invasive test (no catheters need to be inserted into the body). An additional benefit over CT angiography and catheter angiography is the absence of ionizing radiation exposure for the patient. Furthermore, compared to contrast media used for CT and catheter angiography, those used for MRIs typically pose less of a risk of toxicity and allergic reactions. Furthermore, much less injections into the patient are required. The method's most significant shortcomings are its somewhat constrained spatial resolution and relatively high cost. Another concern with the scans is their duration; a CT scan is much faster. Additionally, it is not performed on patients for whom an MRI examination might be dangerous (such as those with pacemakers, metal in their eyes, or specific surgical clips).

The positioning for a typical MRI brain is the same as it is for MRA procedures to visualize cranial circulation. The patient will need to be immobilized inside the head coil. MRA typically takes an additional 10 minutes to the standard MRI protocol and is included in the entire MRI brain examination (Kuperman, 2000; Peter, Jezzard, Matthews Paul M, and Smith Stephen M, 2001; Edelman, 2006; Schröder, Leif, and Cornelius Faber, 2011).

3.4. How Does an MRI Scan Work?

An intense magnetic field is created around the patient by the large, cylindrical (tube-shaped) MRI machine, which also transmits radio wave pulses from a scanner. While some MRI machines are more open, others resemble tiny tunnels.

The atoms in your body align in the same direction due to the strong magnetic field produced by the MRI scanner. These atoms are then moved from their initial positions by radio waves that are sent by the MRI machine. The atoms return to their starting positions and emit radio signals when the radio waves are cut off. A computer receives these signals and transforms them into an image of the body part under examination. This image is displayed on a viewing screen. When studying organs or soft tissue, magnetic resonance imaging (MRI) may be utilized in place of computed tomography (CT). When it comes to differentiating between different kinds of soft tissues and between normal and abnormal soft tissues, MRI is superior. There is no chance of radiation exposure during an MRI procedure because ionizing radiation is not used.

Additional magnetic resonance technology has developed as a result of newer applications for magnetic resonance imaging. An examination called magnetic resonance angiography (MRA) is used to gauge how well blood flows through arteries. Additionally, vascular malformations, or anomalies of the blood vessels in the brain, spinal cord, or other parts of the body, can be found with MRA. These conditions include brain aneurysms.

The brain's functional magnetic resonance imaging, or fMRI, is used to pinpoint the precise area of the brain responsible for a given function, like speech or memory. Although the general regions of the brain where these functions take place are known, each individual may have a different precise location. You may be required to complete a task, like reciting the Pledge of Allegiance, during an fMRI of the brain. Doctors can arrange for surgery or other treatments for brain disorders by precisely locating the brain's functional center.

3.5. MRI Procedure

The duration of a magnetic resonance imaging (MRI) scan varies from 15 to 90 minutes, contingent upon the area under examination size and the quantity of images acquired. This is an innocuous process.

3.5.1. Before the Scan

Unless instructed otherwise, you should be able to eat, drink, and take any medications as usual on the day of your MRI scan. It is possible that you will be instructed to fast for up to four hours before the scan, and that you will also be asked to consume a substantial quantity of water. This is contingent upon the scanning area.

You will typically be asked to complete a questionnaire about your health and medical history when you first arrive at the hospital. This aids the medical team in making sure the scan is performed safely. Upon completion of the questionnaire, you will typically be required to sign a consent form before the scan can proceed. It's crucial to take out any metal objects from your body because the MRI scanner generates strong magnetic fields.

These include:

- watches
- jewelry, such as rings and necklaces
- piercings, such as ear, nipple and nose rings
- dentures (false teeth)
- hearing aids
- wigs (some wigs contain traces of metal)

While it's advisable to avoid bringing valuables to your scan, if you must, they can usually be kept in a locked locker. During the procedure, you might be required to wear a hospital gown, depending on the area of your body being scanned. Wearing clothing without metal zippers, fasteners, buttons, underwire (bras), belts, or buckles is advised if you are not required to wear a gown.

- **Contrast Agent:** A dye, or contrast agent, injection is required for certain MRI scans. This increases the clarity and detail of specific tissues and blood vessels. The contrast agent may occasionally have adverse effects like these.
- feeling or being sick
- a skin rash
- a headache
- dizziness

Most of the time, these side effects are minor and transient. In patients with severe renal disease, contrast agents may also result in damage to tissues and organs. To assess your kidney function and determine whether the scan is safe to proceed with, you might be offered a blood test if you have a history of kidney disease. Before receiving the injection, you should inform the staff of any past allergic reactions or issues with blood clotting.

- **Anesthesia and Sedatives:** Anesthesia, or painkilling medication, is typically not required for MRI scans because they are painless procedures. You can ask for a sedative to help you relax if you have claustrophobia. Asking your consultant well in advance of the scan is a good idea. You won't be able to drive for 24 hours after taking a sedative during the scan, so you'll need to make plans for a friend or family member to drive you home. A general anesthetic may be administered to infants and young children before an MRI scan. This is because, while they are awake, babies and young children frequently find it difficult to remain motionless during the scan.

3.5.2. During the Scan

A short cylinder with open ends is an MRI scanner. Inside the scanner, a motorized bed will be placed beneath you to lie on. Depending on which part of your body is being scanned, you will either put your feet or head through the scanner first. A frame might occasionally be positioned over the body portion being scanned, like the head or chest. To produce a higher-quality image, this frame has receivers that pick up the signals your body sends out during the scan. The magnetic resonance imaging scanner is run by a computer and is housed in a separate room to protect it from the scanner's magnetic field.

The person who runs the computer, the radiographer, will also be in a different room from you. However, you will be able to communicate with them, usually via an intercom, and they will always be able to see you through the viewing window and on a television monitor while the scan is in progress. You might be able to have a friend or relative stay with you while the scan is being done. Typically, parents can accompany their children.

You will ask anyone who stays with you if they have any metal objects in their body, such as a pacemaker. They will also have to adhere to the same rules about what to wear and what can be taken off that contains metal. It's crucial to remain motionless the entire scan until the radiographer tells you to relax to prevent blurry images. It could take a few seconds to three or four minutes for a single scan. During brief scans, you might be asked to hold your breath.

The entire process will take between 15 and 90 minutes, depending on the size of the area being scanned and the number of images taken. Throughout the process, there will be audible tapping sounds from the MRI scanner. This is the on-and-off electric current in the scanner coils. You will receive headphones or earplugs to wear. If you would like, you can typically bring your own CD and listen to music through headphones during the scan. When your scan is done, you will be taken out of the scanner.

3.5.3. After the Scan

Typically, an MRI scan is performed as an outpatient procedure. This implies that you won't have to spend the night in the hospital. You can get back to your regular activities right away after the scan. However, a friend or family member must drive you home and remain with you for the first 24 hours if you have taken a sedative. After taking a sedative, it is not safe to drive, operate heavy machinery, or consume alcohol for 24 hours. A radiologist, a medical professional skilled in interpreting scans and X-rays, needs to review your MRI scan and may need to consult with other specialists. This indicates that you probably won't receive the scan results right away. The physician who scheduled the scan will review the report from the radiologist with you. Unless they are required immediately, the results of an MRI scan typically take a week or two to arrive.

3.5.4. Risks

MRI uses a strong magnetic field, but it does not release the ionizing radiation that is present in CT and X-ray imaging. The magnetic field is strong enough to propel a wheelchair across the room and reaches beyond the machine to exert extremely strong forces on iron, some steel, and other magnetizable objects. Before having an MR scan, patients should inform their doctors of any medical conditions or implants.

The following things should be considered before undergoing an MRI scan:

- An MRI machine should not be used by people with pacemakers, vagus nerve stimulators, implanted cardioverter-defibrillators, insulin pumps, cochlear implants, deep brain stimulators, loop recorders, or capsules from capsule endoscopy.
- **Noise:** Certain MR scanners produce sound levels up to 120 decibels, which is a loud noise that is commonly referred to as clicking and beeping. This may necessitate the use of special ear protection.
- **Nerve Stimulation:** The MRI's quickly switching fields can occasionally cause a twitching sensation.
- **Contrast Agents:** Using certain gadolinium-containing agents, like gadodiamide and others, may increase the risk of nephrogenic systemic fibrosis, a rare but serious illness that is necessary for patients requiring dialysis due to severe renal failure. Current American guidelines advise dialysis patients to only receive gadolinium agents when absolutely necessary, and to begin dialysis as soon as possible after the scan to remove the agent from the body as soon as possible, even though a causal link has not been established.
- **Pregnancy:** Although there have been no effects shown on the fetus, it is advised to avoid MRI scans as a precaution, particularly during the first trimester when the fetus's organs are still developing and contrast agents, if used, may enter the fetal bloodstream.
- **Claustrophobia:** It may be difficult for some people to endure lengthy scan times inside the machine, even if their claustrophobia is mild. Patients are given tools to manage their discomfort through familiarization with the device and procedure, visualization methods, sedation, and anesthesia. Other coping techniques include covering or closing the eyes, holding a panic button, and watching a video or movie or listening to music. The patient is not completely encircled by the open MRI machine because it is open on the sides rather than a tube that is closed at one end. It was created to meet the needs of patients whose size or weight renders a traditional MRI impractical, as well as those who find the narrow tunnel and noises uncomfortable. High-quality images are available for many, but not all, types of examinations with the latest open MRI technology (Kuperman, 2000; Peter, Jezzard, Matthews Paul M, and Smith Stephen M, 2001; Edelman, 2006; Schröder, Leif, and Cornelius Faber, 2011).

3.6. Other Specialized Configurations

3.6.1. Magnetic Resonance Spectroscopy

Several single voxel or imaging-based methods can be used to measure the levels of various metabolites in bodily tissues using magnetic resonance spectroscopy (MRS). A spectrum of resonances is produced by the MR signal, and these resonances correlate to various isotope molecular configurations that are "excited." This signature is used to provide information on tumor metabolism and to diagnose specific metabolic disorders, particularly those that impact the brain.

Spectral and imaging techniques are combined in magnetic resonance spectroscopic imaging (MRSI) to generate spatially localized spectra from within the sample or patient. Although the available SNR limits the spatial resolution, each voxel's spectrum provides information on a large number of metabolites. Because MRSI uses the available signal to encode both spatial and spectral information, high SNR is only possible at higher field strengths (3 T and above). The popularity of MRIs with exceptionally high field strengths is hindered by their high acquisition and maintenance costs. Nonetheless, current software algorithms based on compressed sensing (e.g., SAMV) have been suggested as a way to attain super-resolution without needing such strong field intensities.

3.6.2. Real-time MRI

Continuous real-time imaging of moving objects, like the heart, is referred to as real-time magnetic resonance imaging. Since the early 2000s, numerous strategies have been developed, and one of them is based on iterative reconstruction and radial FLASH MRI. For images with an in-plane resolution of 1.5–2.0 mm, this results in a temporal resolution of 20–30 ms. While FLASH MRI produces a worse image contrast between the myocardium and blood pool, balanced steady-state free precession (bSSFP) imaging will cause severe banding artifacts when the B0 inhomogeneity is strong. Real-time MRI is likely to add valuable information on heart and joint diseases. It may also, in many cases, make MRI examinations easier and more comfortable for patients, particularly those with arrhythmias or patients who are unable to hold their breath.

3.6.3. Interventional MRI

MRI is a good option for interventional radiology, where the images generated by an MRI scanner are used to guide minimally invasive procedures because it has no negative effects on the patient or the operator. These processes don't require any ferromagnetic equipment. Intraoperative MRI is a growing subset of interventional MRI that involves the use of an MRI during surgery. Certain specialized MRI systems enable imaging to take place while the surgery is being performed. More often than not, the surgery is stopped briefly to allow for an MRI to evaluate the procedure's success or direct further surgical work.

3.6.4. Magnetic Resonance Guided Focused Ultrasound

High-intensity focused ultrasound (HIFU) beams are directed toward a tissue during guided therapy and are managed by magnetic resonance thermal imaging. The temperature rises to above 65°C (150°F) at the focus because of the high energy, totally destroying the tissue. With this technology, diseased tissue can be precisely destroyed. The target tissue can be seen in three dimensions with MR imaging, which makes it possible to precisely focus ultrasonic energy. Thermal, real-time, quantitative images of the treated area are provided by MR imaging. This enables the doctor to check whether the temperature produced by the ultrasound energy during each cycle is enough to cause thermal ablation in the targeted tissue, and if not, to adjust the parameters to guarantee a successful course of treatment.

3.6.5. Multinuclear Imaging

Because it is widely distributed in biological tissues and produces a strong signal due to its high gyromagnetic ratio, hydrogen has the most frequently imaged nucleus in magnetic resonance imaging (MRI). However, MRI may be able to image any nucleus that has a net nuclear spin. Helium-3, lithium-7, carbon-13, fluorine-19, oxygen-17, sodium-23, phosphorus-31, and xenon-129 are a few examples of these nuclei. Since ^{23}Na and ^{31}P are found in large amounts in the body naturally, they can be directly imaged. Because the nuclear density of gaseous isotopes, like ^{3}He or ^{129}Xe, is too low to produce a detectable signal under normal circumstances, they must first be hyperpolarized before being inhaled. It is possible to administer ^{17}O and ^{19}F in sufficient liquid dosages (e.g., ^{17}O-water), demonstrating that hyperpolarization is not required. Since helium and xenon are not typically found in biological tissues, using them has the advantage of reducing background noise and increasing contrast for the image itself.

Furthermore, heteronuclear magnetization transfer magnetic resonance imaging (MRI) may be used to image the high-gyromagnetic-ratio hydrogen nucleus rather than the low-gyromagnetic-ratio nucleus that is bonded to the hydrogen atom in any atom with a net nuclear spin that is bonded to an atom of hydrogen. Heteronuclear magnetization transfer magnetic resonance imaging (MRI) has the potential to identify the existence or absence of particular chemical bonds.

Currently, multinuclear imaging is mainly a research technique. Potential uses, however, include functional imaging and imaging of organs that are difficult to see on ^{1}H MRI (e.g., lungs and bones) or as substitutes for contrast materials. It is possible to image the distribution of air spaces within the lungs using inhaled hyperpolarized ^{3}He. For angiography and perfusion imaging, injectable solutions with ^{13}C or stabilized bubbles of hyperpolarized ^{129}Xe have been investigated as contrast agents. ^{31}P may be able to offer details on the composition and density of bones as well as brain function imaging. Lithium has the potential to be distributed throughout the human brain and is a crucial medication for treating conditions like bipolar disorder. Multinuclear imaging can help map this out.

3.6.6. Molecular Imaging by MRI

The benefits of magnetic resonance imaging (MRI) include its exceptional spatial resolution and proficiency in morphological and functional imaging. However, there are several drawbacks to MRI. Initially, the sensitivity of MRI can be very limited when compared to other imaging modalities, ranging from approximately 10^{-3} mol/L to 10^{-5} mol/L. The population difference between the nuclear spin states is extremely tiny at room temperature, which is the root of this issue. For instance, the difference between the high and low energy states at 1.5 Teslas, which is a typical field strength for clinical MRI, is about 9 molecules per 2 million. Increasing the magnetic field strength and producing hyperpolarization through optical pumping or dynamic nuclear polarization are two ways to improve MR sensitivity. Additionally, numerous chemical exchange-based signal amplification schemes boost sensitivity.

High specificity and high relaxivity (sensitivity) targeted MRI contrast agents are needed to achieve molecular imaging of disease biomarkers using MRI. Developing targeted MRI contrast agents has been the focus of numerous studies to date to accomplish molecular imaging by MRI. To accomplish targeting, peptides, antibodies, small ligands, and small protein domains—like HER-2 affibodies—have frequently been used. These targeting moieties are typically coupled to high payload MRI contrast agents or MRI contrast agents with high relaxivities in order to increase the sensitivity of the contrast agents. To demonstrate the gene action of distinct mRNA and gene transcription factor proteins, a new class of gene-targeting MR contrast agents has been developed. These new contrast agents can trace cells in living brains that have distinct mRNA, microRNA, and viral responses to inflammation in the tissue. The TaqMan analysis, optical, and electron microscopy all show a positive correlation with the changes in gene expression reported by the MR.

3.6.7. Parallel MRI

Gathering MRI data with successive applications of magnetic field gradients is a time-consuming process. There are physiologic and physical limits to the rate of gradient switching, even for the most efficient MRI sequences. By collecting some data concurrently rather than sequentially as is customary, parallel MRI gets around these restrictions. Arrays of radiofrequency (RF) detector coils, each with a unique "view" of the body, are used to achieve this. The residual spatial information is filled in by combining signals from different coils according to their established spatial sensitivity patterns after a smaller set of gradient steps is applied. The number of coils and the signal-to-noise ratio, which falls with increasing acceleration, are the two factors that limit the resulting acceleration. However, with appropriate coil array configurations, two to four-fold accelerations are frequently possible, and significantly higher accelerations have been shown with specialized coil arrays. Most MRI sequences can be used with parallel MRI. Following the introduction of the Simultaneous Acquisition of Spatial Harmonics (SMASH) technique in 1996–7, parallel imaging saw widespread development and application after several early suggestions for using arrays of detectors to accelerate imaging went largely unremarked in the MRI field. Currently, the most widely used parallel imaging techniques are Sensitivity Encoding (SENSE) and Generalized Autocalibrating Partially Parallel Acquisitions (GRAPPA). With the introduction of parallel MRI, the number of receiver channels on commercial MR systems increased quickly, and significant research and development were conducted in the areas of image reconstruction and RF coil design. Nowadays, parallel MRI is frequently utilized for clinical or research purposes as well as MRI exams in a variety of body parts.

3.6.8. Quantitative MRI

By creating spatial maps of relative variations in signal strength that are "weighted" by specific parameters, most magnetic resonance imaging (MRI) focuses on the qualitative interpretation of MR data. Alternatively, quantitative approaches try to measure specific spatial features or create spatial maps of precise tissue relaxometry parameter values or magnetic fields.

Here are some instances of quantitative MRI techniques:

- T1-mapping (notably used in cardiac magnetic resonance imaging)
- T2-mapping
- Quantitative susceptibility mapping (QSM)
- Quantitative fluid flow MRI (i.e., some cerebrospinal fluid flow MRI)
- Magnetic resonance elastography (MRE)

Although quantitative MRI has historically required longer scan times, its goal is to improve the reproducibility of MR images and interpretations. Sometimes, multi-parametric quantitative MRI—which maps several tissue relaxometry parameters in a single imaging session—is more precisely referred to as quantitative MRI (or qMRI). In an attempt to expedite the process of multi-parametric quantitative MRI, sequences that map multiple parameters simultaneously have been created. These sequences are the result of either fitting the evolution of the MR signal to a multi-parameter model or developing distinct encoding techniques for each parameter.

3.6.9. Hyperpolarized Gas MRI

Because there are fewer water molecules with protons that can be excited by the magnetic field, traditional MRI produces poor images of lung tissue. An MRI scan can detect lung ventilation defects using hyperpolarized gas. A patient is instructed to breathe in a mixture of hyperpolarized xenon and either nitrogen or helium as a buffer gas before the scan. Compared to a traditional MRI, the lung images that are obtained are of far higher quality (Kupeman, 2000; Norris, 2003; Zotev et al, 2008).

A Closer Look

Contrast Agents

Contrast agents are not necessary when using MRI to image anatomical structures or blood flow because the different characteristics of the tissues and blood naturally provide contrasts. Exogenous contrast agents, however, can be administered intravenously, orally, or intra-articularly for more specialized imaging modalities. The majority of contrast materials are either paramagnetic (e.g., negative contrast agents) or super-paramagnetic (SPIONs), which are used to shorten T_2 and T_2^* in healthy tissue by lowering its signal intensity. Examples of these materials include gadolinium, manganese, and europium. The most widely used intravenous contrast agents are based on highly paramagnetic gadolinium chelates. These substances have generally shown to be less dangerous than the iodinated contrast agents used in CT or X-ray radiography. Anaphylactoid reactions are rare, occurring in approx. Between 0 and 1%. Contrast-enhanced MRI scanning has become an option for patients with renal impairment who would not otherwise be able to undergo contrast-enhanced CT. Of particular interest is the lower incidence of nephrotoxicity, compared with iodinated agents, when given at usual doses.

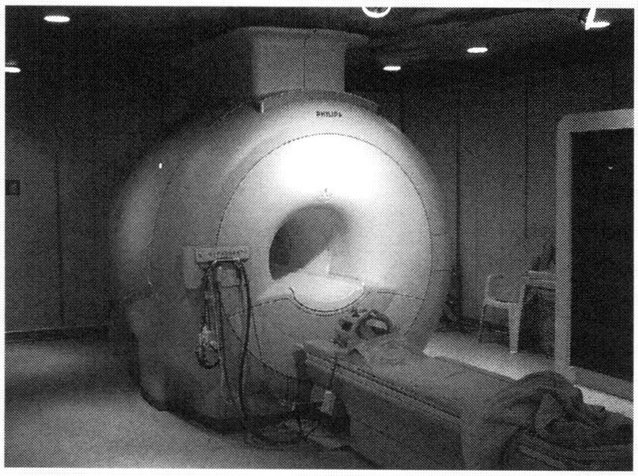

(By KasugaHuang, CC BY-SA 3.0, https://commons.wikimedia.org/w/index.php?curid=680466).

Octadentate complexes of gadolinium(III) are commonly used as contrast agents based on gadolinium. Since the complex is very stable (log K > 20), the concentration of uncomplexed Gd^{3+} ions in use should be less than the toxicity threshold. A water molecule that occupies the ninth position in the coordination sphere of the metal ion exchanges quickly with other water molecules in the reagent molecule's immediate vicinity, influencing the magnetic resonance relaxation time.

The United States Food and Drug Administration (FDA) declared in a drug safety communication in December 2017 that all gadolinium-based contrast agents (GBCAs) would now come with additional warnings. The FDA also demanded that gadolinium contrast suppliers perform more animal and clinical studies to evaluate the safety of these agents, in addition to increasing patient education. Gadolinium-containing agents have been shown to be beneficial for patients with renal impairment; however, in patients with severe kidney failure who need dialysis, there is a risk of nephrogenic systemic fibrosis, a rare but serious illness that may be related to the use of these agents. Although other agents have also been linked, gadodiamide has been linked the most frequently. Current American guidelines state that dialysis patients should only receive gadolinium agents when absolutely necessary, and that dialysis should be started as soon as possible after the scan to remove the agent from the body as soon as possible, even though a causal link has not been conclusively established.

In Europe, where there is a greater availability of gadolinium-containing agents, a risk classification of agents has been made public. 2008 saw the approval of gadoxetate, a novel contrast agent with the potential benefit of a dual excretion path under the brand names Eovist (US) and Primovist (EU).

Summary

- Subatomic particles have the quantum mechanical property of spin. Certain nuclei such as ^{1}H (protons), ^{2}H, ^{3}He, ^{23}Na or ^{31}P, have a non–zero spin and therefore a magnetic moment. In the case of the so-called spin-1/2 nuclei, such as ^{1}H, there are two spin states, sometimes referred to as *up* and *down*. Nuclei such as ^{12}C have no unpaired neutrons or protons, and no net spin; however, the isotope ^{13}C does.
- Quantum mechanics is required to accurately model the behavior of a single proton. However, classical mechanics can be used to describe the behavior of an ensemble of protons adequately.
- The decay of RF-induced NMR spin polarization is characterized in terms of two separate processes, each with their own time constants. One process, called T_1, is responsible for the loss of resonance intensity following pulse excitation. The other process, called T_2, characterizes the width or broadness of resonances.
- Bloch equations are used to calculate the nuclear magnetization $\mathbf{M} = (M_x, M_y, M_z)$ as a function of time when relaxation times T_1 and T_2 are present. Bloch equations are phenomenological equations that were introduced by Felix Bloch in 1946.
- MRI is the investigation of choice in the preoperative staging of rectal and prostate cancer and has a role in the diagnosis, staging, and follow-up of other tumors, as well as for determining areas of tissue for sampling in biobanking.
- Magnetic resonance imaging of the brain uses magnetic resonance imaging (MRI) to produce high quality two-dimensional or three-dimensional images of the brain and brainstem as well as the cerebellum without the use of ionizing radiation (X-rays) or radioactive tracers.
- Cardiac magnetic resonance imaging (cardiac MRI, CMR), also known as cardiovascular MRI, is a magnetic resonance imaging (MRI) technology used for non-invasive assessment of the function and structure of the cardiovascular system.
- Applications in the musculoskeletal system include spinal imaging, assessment of joint disease, and soft tissue tumors. Also, MRI techniques can be used for diagnostic imaging of systemic muscle diseases including genetic muscle diseases.
- Hepatobiliary MR is used to detect and characterize lesions of the liver, pancreas, and bile ducts. Focal or diffuse disorders of the liver may be evaluated using diffusion-weighted, opposed-phase imaging and dynamic contrast enhancement sequences.
- The MRI machine is a large, cylindrical (tube-shaped) machine that creates a strong magnetic field around the patient and sends pulses of radio waves from a scanner. Some MRI machines look like narrow tunnels, while others are more open.
- A magnetic resonance imaging (MRI) scan is a painless procedure that lasts 15 to 90 minutes, depending on the size of the area being scanned and the number of images being taken.

References

1. Blümich, B. (2000). *NMR Imaging of Materials*. Clarendon Press. DOI:10.1002/anie.198814061
2. Campeau, N. G., & Huston, J. (2012). Vascular disorders—magnetic resonance angiography: Brain vessels. *Neuroimaging Clinics of North America, 22*(2), 207–233, x. https://doi.org/10.1016/j.nic.2012.02.006. PMID 22548929.
3. Corfield, J. R., Wild, J. M., & Cowan, B. R. et al. (2008). MRI of postmortem specimens of endangered species for comparative neuroanatomy. *Nature Protocols, 3*(4), 597–605. https://doi.org/10.1038/nprot.2008.17.
4. Davis, S. M., Fisher, M., & Warach, S. (Eds.). (2003). *Magnetic Resonance Imaging in Stroke*. Cambridge University Press. ISBN: 9780521806831
5. Degen, C. L., Poggio, M., & Mamin, H. J. et al. (2009). Nanoscale magnetic resonance imaging. *Proceedings of the National Academy of Sciences*, in press. Proc Natl Acad Sci U S A. 2009 Feb 3;106(5):1313-7. doi: 10.1073/pnas.0812068106. Epub 2009 Jan 12. PMID: 19139397; PMCID: PMC2628306.
6. Dyverfeldt, P., Bissell, M., Barker, A. J., et al. (2015). 4D flow cardiovascular magnetic resonance consensus statement. *Journal of Cardiovascular Magnetic Resonance, 17*, 72. https://doi.org/10.1186/s12968-015-0174-5.
7. Edelman, R. R. (Ed.). (2006). *Clinical Magnetic Resonance Imaging* (3rd ed.). Saunder. PMCID: PMC7977829
8. Gaillard, F. (2017). Dynamic contrast enhanced (DCE) MR perfusion. *Radiopaedia*. Retrieved October 15, 2017, from: https://radiopaedia.org/articles/dynamic-contrast-enhanced-dce-mr-perfusion (accessed on 25 May 2024).
9. Hartung, M. P., Grist, T. M., & François, C. J. (2011). Magnetic resonance angiography: Current status and future directions. *Journal of Cardiovascular Magnetic Resonance, 13*(1), 19. https://doi.org/10.1186/1532-429X-13-19.
10. Huettel, S. A. (2009). *Functional Magnetic Resonance Imaging* (2nd ed.). Yale J Biol Med. 2009 Dec;82(4):233. Epub 2009 Dec. PMCID: PMC2794501.
11. Ishida, N., Koizumi, M., & Kano, H. (2000). The NMR Microscope: A unique and promising tool for plant science. *Annals of Botany, 86*(2), 259. https://doi.org/10.1006/anbo.2000.1181.
12. Jezzard, P., Matthews, P. M., & Smith, S. M. (Eds.). (2001). *Functional MRI: An Introduction to Methods*. Oxford University Press. DOI: 10.1093/acprof:oso/9780192630711.001.0001
13. Keshavamurthy, J., & Ballinger, R. et al. (2017). Phase contrast imaging. *Radiopaedia*. Retrieved October 15, 2017, from: https://radiopaedia.org/articles/phase-contrast-imaging (accessed on 25 May 2024).
14. Kramer, C. M., & Grist, T. M. (2012). Peripheral MR Angiography. *Magnetic Resonance Imaging Clinics of North America, 20*(4), 761–776. https://doi.org/10.1016/j.mric.2012.08.002. PMID 23088949.
15. Kuperman, V. (2000). *Magnetic Resonance Imaging: Physical Principles and Applications*. Academic Press. ISBN 978-0-08-053570, 182 pages.
16. Lee, S.-C. (2009). MR microscopy of micron scale structures. *Magn Reson Imaging* . 2009 Jul;27(6):828-33. doi: 10.1016/j.mri.2009.01.002. Epub 2009 Mar 17.

17. Logothetis, N. K. (2008). What we can do and what we cannot do with fMRI. *Nature, 453*, 869–878. https://doi.org/10.1038/nature06976.

18. Logothetis, N. K., Pauls, J., Augath, M., Trinath, T., & Oeltermann, A. (2001). Neurophysiological investigation of the basis of the fMRI signal. *Nature, 412*, 150–157. https://doi.org/10.1038/35084005.

19. Lotz, J., Meier, C., Leppert, A., & Galanski, M. (2002). Cardiovascular flow measurement with phase-contrast MR imaging: Basic facts and implementation. *Radiographics, 22*, 651–671.

20. Manning, W. J. (2010). *Cardiovascular Magnetic Resonance* (2nd ed.). Clin Cardiol. 2006 Sep;29(9 Suppl 1):I34-48. doi: 10.1002/clc.4960291306. PMID: 17009576; PMCID: PMC6654515.

21. Markl, M., Frydrychowicz, A., Kozerke, S., et al. (2012). 4D Flow MRI. *Journal of Magnetic Resonance Imaging, 36*, 1015–1036.

22. Mathew, R. C., Löffler, A. I., & Salerno, M. (2018). Role of cardiac magnetic resonance imaging in valvular heart disease: Diagnosis, assessment, and management. *Current Cardiology Reports, 20*(11), 119. https://doi.org/10.1007/s11886-018-1057-9.

23. Modo, M. M. J. J., & Bulte, J. W. M. (2011). *Magnetic Resonance Neuroimaging: Methods and Protocols*. Humana Press. DOI:10.1007/978-1-61737-992-5, ISBN: 978-1-61737-991-8.

24. Muja, N. (2008). Magnetic resonance imaging of cells in experimental disease models. Prog Nucl Magn Reson Spectrosc. 2009 July ; 55(1): 61–77. doi:10.1016/j.pnmrs.2008.11.002.

25. Myerson, S. G. (2009). *Cardiovascular Magnetic Resonance*. Oxford University Press. ISBN: 9780199682928.

26. Nakada, T., Matsuzawa, H., & Kwee, I. L. (2008). High-resolution imaging with high and ultra-high-field magnetic resonance imaging systems. *NeuroReport, 19*(1), 7–13. https://doi.org/10.1097/WNR.0b013e3282f2e00b.

27. Nayak, K. S., Nielsen, J. -F., Bernstein, M. A., et al. (2015). Cardiovascular magnetic resonance phase contrast imaging. *Journal of Cardiovascular Magnetic Resonance, 17*, 71.

28. Norris, D. G. (2003). High field human imaging. *Journal of Magnetic Resonance Imaging, 18*(5), 519–529. https://doi.org/10.1002/jmri.10390.

29. Schröder, L., & Faber, C. (2011). *In Vivo NMR Imaging: Methods and Protocols*. Humana Press. DOI:10.1007/978-1-61779-219-9, ISBN: 978-1-61779-218-2

30. Stankovic, Z., Allen, B. D., Garcia, J., et al. (2014). 4D flow imaging with MRI. *Cardiovascular Diagnosis and Therapy, 4*, 173–192.

31. Turnbull, L. W. (2009). Dynamic contrast-enhanced MRI in the diagnosis and management of breast cancer. *NMR in Biomedicine, 22*(1), 28–39. https://doi.org/10.1002/nbm.1273. PMID 18654999. S2CID 5305422.

32. Zotev, V. S., Volegov, P. L., Matlashov, A. N., et al. (2008). Parallel MRI at microtesla fields. *Journal of Magnetic Resonance, 192*, 197–208. https://doi.org/10.1016/j.jmr.2008.02.015.

Chapter

POSITRON EMISSION TOMOGRAPHY

4

Contents

Introduction

Nuclear medicine imaging includes PET imaging, sometimes referred to as a PET scan or PET imaging. Radiotracers, which are trace amounts of radioactive material, are used in nuclear medicine. Physicians diagnose, assess, and treat a wide range of illnesses using nuclear medicine. These consist of ailments like cancer, heart disease, neurological, gastrointestinal, or endocrine problems, among others. Exams in nuclear medicine identify molecular activity. They may be able to detect illness in its early stages as a result. They can also demonstrate how well you are healing from your condition. It is noninvasive to practice nuclear medicine. It is usually painless, except intravenous injections. Radiopharmaceuticals, also known as radiotracers, are radioactive substances that are used in these tests to help diagnose and evaluate medical conditions. Molecules designated with a small quantity of radioactive material are known as radiotracers. They gather in inflammatory areas or tumors. They can attach to particular body proteins. One of the most widely used radiotracers is F-18 fluorodeoxyglucose (FDG), which is a glucose-like molecule. Due to their increased metabolic activity, cancer cells may take up glucose more quickly. PET scans reveal this increased rate. This enables your physician to identify illness before other imaging tests reveal it. FDG is merely one of several radiotracers that are being developed or used.

Typically, the radiotracer will be administered via injection. Alternatively, depending on the exam, you might inhale it as a gas or swallow it. It builds up in the area that is being studied. Gamma-ray emissions from the radiotracer are picked up by a specialized camera. In addition to producing images, a computer and camera provide molecular data. To create unique views, several imaging centers combine nuclear medicine images with computed tomography (CT) or magnetic resonance imaging (MRI). It is referred to by physicians as co-registration or image fusion. Through image fusion, a physician can integrate and analyze data from two distinct exams on a single image. As a result, more accurate data and a diagnosis are produced. Both exams can be conducted simultaneously by single photon emission CT/CT (SPECT/CT) and positron emission tomography/CT (PET/CT) units. One new imaging technology is PET/MRI. It's not accessible everywhere right now. A PET scan measures vital bodily processes like metabolism. It aids in the assessment of organ and tissue function by medical professionals. CT imaging creates several images of the inside of the body by using specialized X-ray equipment and, occasionally, a contrast agent. These images are viewed and interpreted by a radiologist via a computer monitor. CT imaging offers superior anatomical data. Nowadays, nearly all PET scans are done using combined PET/CT scanners. When the two scans are done together, they may help identify abnormal metabolic activity and yield a more accurate diagnosis than when they are done separately.

Orientation and Directional Terms

Term	Definition	Illustration
Nuclear medicine	Nuclear medicine uses radioactive material inside the body to see how organs or tissue are functioning (for diagnosis) or to target and destroy damaged or diseased organs or tissue (for treatment).	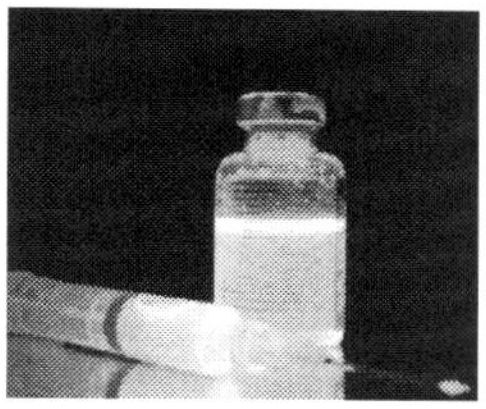
Medical Scintillography	A special type of nuclear medicine procedure that uses small amounts of radioactive material to diagnose and assess the severity of a variety of bone diseases and conditions, including fractures, infection and cancer.	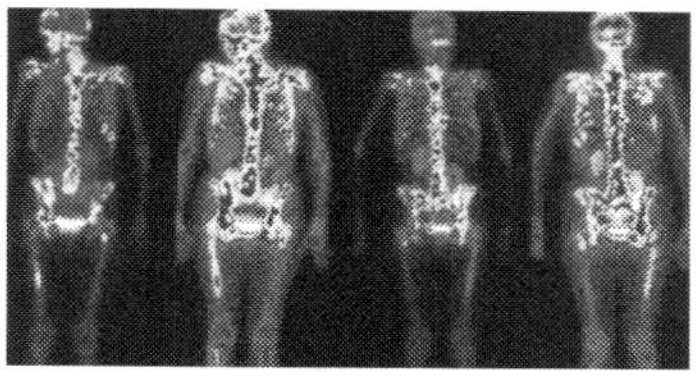
Magnetic Resonance Imaging (MRI)	Magnetic resonance imaging (MRI) is a type of scan that uses strong magnetic fields and radio waves to produce detailed images of the inside of the body.	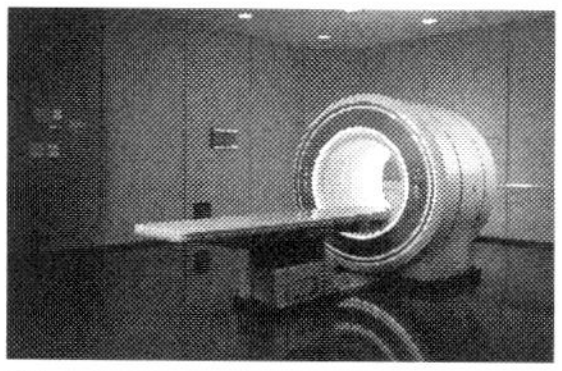
Intravenous	A medical technique that administers fluids, medications and nutrients directly into a person's vein.	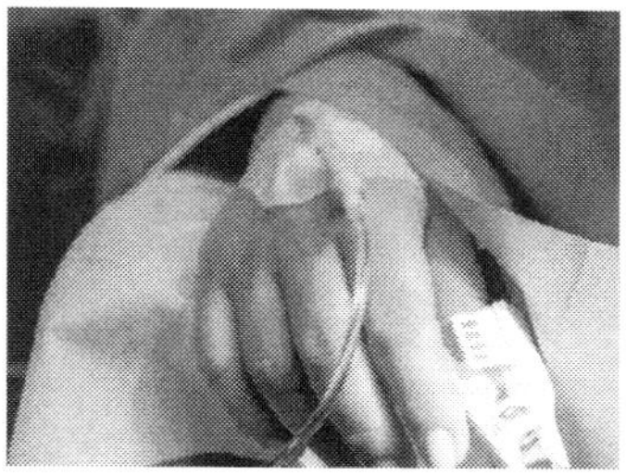
Avalanche photodiodes	A highly sensitive semiconductor photodiode detector that exploits the photoelectric effect to convert light into electricity.	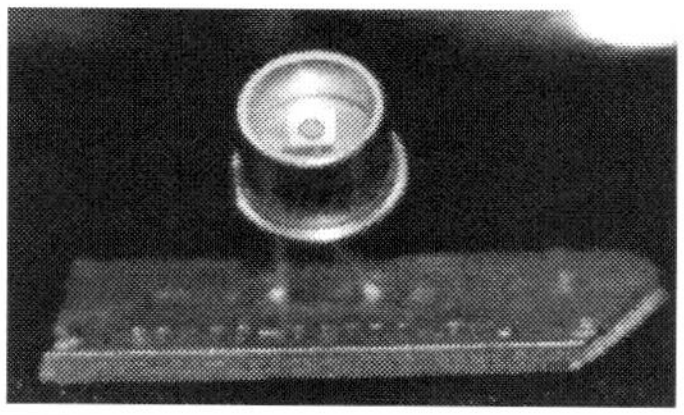

4.1. Fundamental Of Positron Emission Tomography

Using radioactive materials known as radiotracers, positron emission tomography (PET) is a functional imaging modality that visualizes and quantifies alterations in physiological activities such as blood flow, absorption, and regional chemical composition as well as metabolic processes. Various tracers are employed for different imaging applications, based on the target physiological process.

For example:

- Fluorodeoxyglucose ([^{18}F]FDG or FDG) is commonly used to detect cancer;
- [^{18}F]Sodium fluoride (Na^{18}F) is widely used for detecting bone formation;
- Oxygen-15 (^{15}O) is sometimes used to measure blood flow.

PET is a widely used medical scintillography method in nuclear medicine imaging. As a tracer, a radiopharmaceutical—a radioisotope linked to a medication—is injected into the body. A positron is released when the radiopharmaceutical experiences beta plus decay. Two gamma rays are released in opposite directions when the positron and a regular electron interact. Two gamma cameras detect these gamma rays and combine them to create a three-dimensional image. PET-CT scanners are those that combine a PET scanner with a computed tomography (CT) scanner. It is possible to reconstruct PET scan images from a CT scan that was taken in the same session using a single scanner. A PET scanner's high initial and continuing operating costs are among its drawbacks. A type of nuclear medicine procedure called PET scans body tissues to determine how metabolically active individual cells are. In actuality, PET combines nuclear medicine with biochemical analysis. PET is primarily used to visualize biochemical changes occurring in the body, such as the metabolism of the heart muscle (the process by which cells convert food into energy after it is digested and absorbed into the blood). PET is most commonly used in patients with cancer, heart disease, and brain disorders. In contrast to other nuclear medicine exams, which measure the quantity of a radioactive material obtained in a particular location within body tissue to assess the function of the tissue, PET measures metabolism within bodily tissues.

As a nuclear medicine procedure, PET uses a small quantity of radioactive material known as radiopharmaceutical, also known as a radionuclide or radioactive tracer, to help examine the tissue being studied. PET studies assess an organ or tissue's metabolism in particular, providing insights into the structure, physiology, and biochemical characteristics of the tissue or organ under study. As a result, PET can identify biochemical changes in a tissue or organ that may indicate the beginning of a disease process before other imaging modalities, like computed tomography (CT) or magnetic resonance imaging (MRI), can reveal anatomical changes associated with the disease. Physicians who specialize in treating cancer, neurologists and neurosurgeons, and cardiologists, who treat the brain and nervous system, are the medical professionals who use PET the most frequently. However, this process is starting to be applied more frequently in other fields as long as PET technologies continue to advance.

To obtain more precise information about malignant (cancerous) tumors and other lesions, PET may also be used in conjunction with other diagnostic procedures like computed tomography (CT) or magnetic resonance imaging (MRI). More recent technology creates PET/CT scanners, which combine PET and CT into one unit. In addition to evaluating epilepsy, Alzheimer's disease, and coronary artery disease, PET/CT holds great promise for the diagnosis and treatment of lung cancer. Originally, PET procedures were carried out in special PET centers because, in addition to the PET scanner, the equipment needed to make the radiopharmaceuticals had to be available. This included a cyclotron and a radiochemistry lab. Currently, all that is needed to conduct a PET scan is a scanner because radiopharmaceuticals are produced across a wide region and sent to PET centers. Gamma camera systems, which scan patients after receiving small doses of radionuclide injections and are currently utilized in other nuclear medicine procedures, are a technological advancement that further expands the availability of PET imaging. For use in PET scan procedures, these systems have been modified. Compared to a traditional PET scan, the gamma camera system can finish a scan faster and for less money (Laruelle, 2000; Malmgren and Thom, 2012; Cendes and Fernando, 2013).

4.1.1. Uses

In pre-clinical and clinical settings, PET is employed as a medical and research instrument. It is widely used in the clinical diagnosis of some diffuse brain diseases, such as those that cause different types of dementia, as well as in the imaging of tumors and the search for metastases by clinical oncologists. PET is an invaluable research tool that helps advance our understanding of how the heart and brain normally function as well as aid in the development of new drugs. PET is also employed in animal-based pre-clinical research. The number of animals needed for a given study is significantly decreased, and it permits repeated investigations into the same subjects over time where subjects can function as their control. With this strategy, research projects can increase the statistical quality of their findings while requiring a smaller sample size. Anatomical changes in the body are a result of physiological processes. PET can provide molecular-level information well in advance of any obvious anatomic changes because it can detect both the expression of certain proteins and biochemical processes. To achieve this, PET scanning uses radiolabeled molecular probes, the uptake rates of which vary based on the type and function of the involved tissue. Using an injected positron emitter in a PET scan, regional tracer uptake in different anatomic structures can be seen and somewhat measured.

PET imaging is typically done with a dedicated PET scanner, but it can also be done with a conventional dual-head gamma camera with a coincidence detector. However, the quality of the images and the time it takes to acquire them are not as good with a gamma camera compared to a PET scanner. Despite these drawbacks, using a gamma camera is a lower-cost option for institutions with low PET scanning demand. Another option for these institutions is to refer patients to another facility or have a mobile scanner come to them. Other medical imaging options include SPECT, CT, MRI, fMRI, and ultrasound. SPECT is similar to PET in that it uses radioligands to detect molecules in the body, but it is less expensive and provides lower-quality images than PET.

4.1.2. PET Work Procedure

PET detects photons—subatomic particles—emitted by a radionuclide in the organ or tissue under study using a scanning device, which is a machine with a large hole in the middle. The radioactive atom is joined to chemical compounds that are naturally utilized by the specific organ or tissue during its metabolic process to create the radionuclides used in PET scans. For instance, because glucose is used by the brain for metabolism, a radioactive atom is added to glucose (blood sugar) to create the radionuclide fluorodeoxyglucose (FDG) in PET scans of the brain. The use of FDG in PET scanning is common. Depending on the goal of the scan, other materials may be used for PET scanning. A radioactive form of oxygen, carbon, nitrogen, or gallium may be used as the radionuclide if the blood flow and perfusion of a particular organ or tissue are of interest.

An intravenous (IV) line is used to inject the radionuclide into a vein. The body portion under examination is then gradually passed over by the PET scanner. The radionuclide breaks down to release positive ions. When positrons collide with electrons close to the decay event, gamma rays known as annihilation photons are produced. The annihilation photons are then detected by the scanner when they coincidentally arrive at the detectors 180 degrees apart. These gamma rays are analyzed by a computer, which then uses the data to produce an image map of the tissue or organ under study. The quantity of radionuclides accumulated in the tissue determines the degree of organ or tissue function and impacts the brightness of the tissue on the image.

4.1.3. Oncology

Clinical oncology frequently uses PET scanning with the radiotracer [^{18}F]fluorodeoxyglucose (FDG). FDG is a glucose analog that is absorbed by cells that use glucose and phosphorylated by hexokinase, the mitochondrial form of which is markedly increased in malignant tumors that grow quickly. The PET scan is made possible by the radioactive glucose molecule's metabolic trapping. Because the local glucose uptake correlates with tissue metabolic activity, the concentrations of the imaged FDG tracer show this. FDG is used to investigate the potential for cancer metastasis—the spread of cancer to other parts of the body. 90% of all FDG PET scans performed today are used in standard medical care to detect cancer metastases. Different types of dementia can also be diagnosed with the same tracer. Less frequently, the tissue concentrations of various types of interesting molecules inside the body are imaged using other radioactive tracers, which are typically but not always labeled with fluorine-18 (18F) (Figure 4.1).

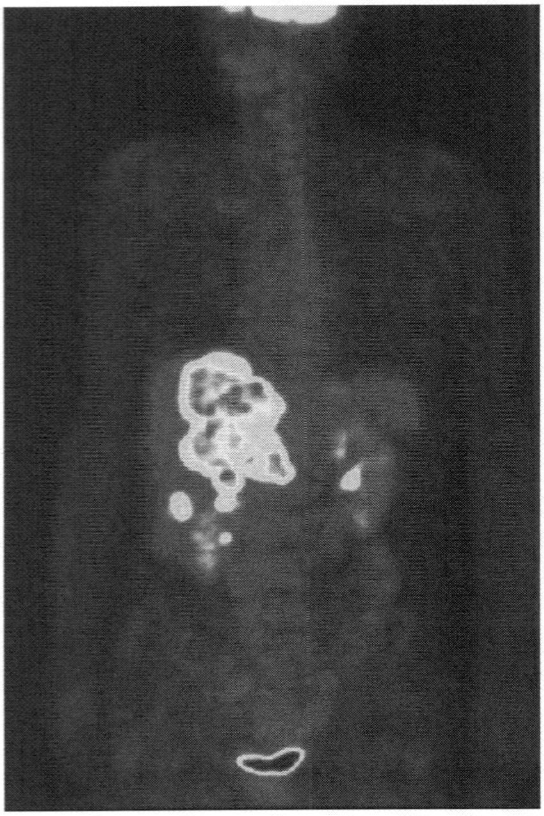

Figure 4.1. *Whole-body PET scan using 18F-FDG (fluorodeoxyglucose). The normal brain and kidneys are labeled, and radioactive urine from the breakdown of the FDG is seen in the bladder. In addition, a large metastatic tumor mass from colon cancer is seen in the liver.*

Source: https://upload.wikimedia.org/wikipedia/commons/3/3d/PET-MIPS-anim.gif.

A standard dose of FDG used in an oncological scan exposes the patient to 7.6 mSv of radiation. FDG, which replaces a hydroxy group with fluorine-18, halts further reactions in glucose metabolism within cells. This is because the phosphate added by hexokinase cannot be removed by most tissues, leading to FDG being trapped in cells until it decays. This results in intense radiolabeling of tissues with high glucose uptake, such as the normal brain, liver, kidneys, and most cancers. FDG-PET is commonly used for diagnosing, staging, and monitoring treatment in cancers like Hodgkin lymphoma, non-Hodgkin lymphoma, and lung cancer due to their elevated glucose uptake compared to normal tissue.

Negative results in interim PET scans are associated with better overall survival and progression-free survival, according to a 2020 review of studies on the use of PET for Hodgkin lymphoma. The certainty of the evidence was, however, very low for progression-free survival and moderate for survival. Oncology is gradually incorporating a few more isotopes and radiotracers for particular uses. For example, tumors of adrenocortical origin have been identified using 11C-labeled metomidate, or 11C-metomidate. Furthermore, it has been shown that Fluorodopa (FDOPA) PET/CT, also known as F-18-DOPA PET/CT, is a more sensitive method than Iobenguane (MIBG) scan for identifying and localizing pheochromocytomas.

4.1.4. Why is PET Performed?

PET scans are generally useful for assessing the presence of disease or other conditions in organs and/or tissues. PET can also be used to assess how well organs like the heart or brain are functioning. PET is most frequently used in the diagnosis of cancer and the assessment of cancer treatment.

More specific reasons for PET scans include, but are not limited to, the following:

- To diagnose dementias (conditions that involve deterioration of mental function), such as Alzheimer's disease, as well as other neurological conditions such as:
    - Parkinson's disease. A progressive disease of the nervous system in which a fine tremor, muscle weakness, and a peculiar type of gait are seen.
    - Huntington's disease. A hereditary disease of the nervous system, which causes increasing dementia, bizarre involuntary movements, and abnormal posture.
    - Epilepsy. A brain disorder involving recurrent seizures.
    - Cerebrovascular accident (stroke)
- To locate the specific surgical site before surgical procedures of the brain
- To evaluate the brain after trauma to detect hematoma (blood clot), bleeding, and/or perfusion (blood and oxygen flow) of the brain tissue
- To detect the spread of cancer to other parts of the body from the original cancer site
- To evaluate the effectiveness of cancer treatment
- To evaluate the perfusion (blood flow) to the myocardium (heart muscle) as an aid in determining the usefulness of a therapeutic procedure to improve blood flow to the myocardium
- To further identify lung lesions or masses detected on chest X-ray and/or chest CT
- To assist in the management and treatment of lung cancer by staging lesions and following the progress of lesions after treatment
- To detect recurrence of tumors earlier than with other diagnostic modalities

4.1.5. Neuroimaging

4.1.5.1. Neurology

Blood flow to the brain is indirectly measured by oxygen-15 PET imaging. According to this method, a higher radioactivity signal means that blood flow is higher, and higher blood flow is thought to be correlated with higher brain activity. For such applications, oxygen-15 has a 2-minute half-life, so it has to be piped straight from a medical cyclotron, which is challenging. Using FDG in PET imaging capitalizes on the brain's natural ability to use glucose quickly. Standard FDG PET scans of the brain can be used to diagnose neuropathologies and measure the amount of glucose used regionally (Laruelle, 2000; Malmgren and Thom, 2012; Cendes and Fernando, 2013) (Figure 4.2).

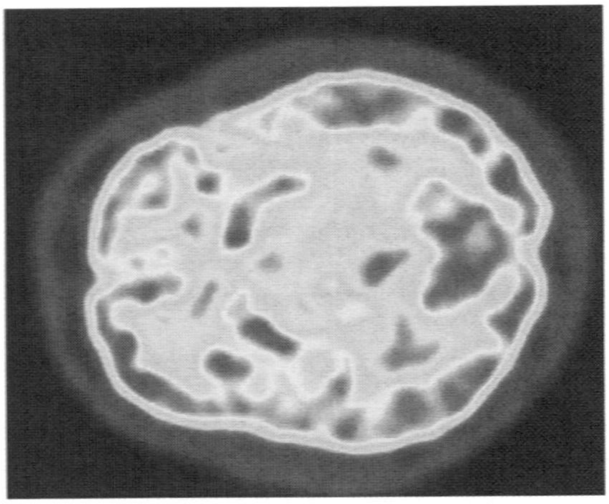

Figure 4.2. *PET scan of the human brain.*

Source: https://upload.wikimedia.org/wikipedia/commons/thumb/c/c6/PET-image.jpg/800px-PET-image.jpg.

Brain diseases like Alzheimer's disease (AD) significantly reduce the ability of the brain to metabolize oxygen and glucose simultaneously. As a result, early Alzheimer's disease diagnosis and effective distinction of Alzheimer's disease from other dementing processes may both be achieved with FDG PET of the brain. FDG PET has the benefit of being much more widely available for these applications. Pittsburgh compound B (PiB), florbetapir, flutemetamol, and florbetaben are a few fluorine-18-based radioactive tracers used to detect amyloid-beta plaques, a possible biomarker for Alzheimer's in the brain.

PET imaging with FDG can also be used for localization of "seizure focus." A seizure focus will appear as hypometabolic during an interictal scan. Several radiotracers (i.e., radioligands) have been developed for PET that are ligands for specific neuroreceptor subtypes such as [^{11}C] raclopride, [^{18}F]fallypride and [^{18}F]desmethoxyfallypride for dopamine D2/D3 receptors; [^{11}C]McN5652 and [11C]DASB for serotonin transporters; [^{18}F]mefway for serotonin 5HT1A receptors; and [^{18}F]Nifene for nicotinic acetylcholine receptors or enzyme substrates (e.g., 6-FDOPA for the AADC enzyme). These agents permit the visualization of neuroreceptor pools in the context of a plurality of neuropsychiatric and neurologic illnesses.

The hippocampal sclerosis that causes epilepsy can also be diagnosed with PET. For this purpose, FDG and the less popular tracers flumazenil and MPPF have been investigated. If the sclerosis is unilateral (affecting either the right or left hippocampal region), FDG uptake can be compared to the healthy side. PET may be used to diagnose a condition even if MRI is difficult to interpret. Amyloid imaging is getting close to clinical use thanks to the development of several new probes for non-invasive, in-vivo PET imaging of neuroaggregate in the human brain. The University of California, Los Angeles's [^{18}F] FDDNP and the University of Pittsburgh's Pittsburgh compound B (PiB) were the first amyloid imaging probes. These probes enable the identification of amyloid plaques in Alzheimer's patients' brains, which may help medical professionals confirm a positive pre-mortem diagnosis of AD and advance the creation of innovative anti-amyloid treatments. As a substrate for acetylcholinesterase, [^{11}C] polymethylpentene (PMP) is a novel radiopharmaceutical used in PET imaging to measure the activity of the acetylcholinergic neurotransmitter system. Acetylcholinesterase levels in post-mortem examinations of AD patients have been found to be lower. [^{11}C] Acetylcholinesterase activity in the brain is mapped using PMP, which may help with premortem AD diagnosis and treatment monitoring. Using PET scans, Avid Radiopharmaceuticals has created and commercialized florbetapir, a compound that detects amyloid plaques using the longer-lasting radionuclide fluorine-18.

- **Neuropsychology or Cognitive Neuroscience:** To examine links between specific psychological processes or disorders and brain activity.
- **Psychiatry:** Many substances have been radiolabeled with C-11 or F-18 to indicate that they bind selectively to neuroreceptors of interest in biological psychiatry. Successful use of radioligands in studies involving human subjects has been demonstrated for those that bind to dopamine receptors (D1, D2, reuptake transporter), serotonin receptors (5HT1A, 5HT2A, reuptake transporter), opioid receptors (mu and kappa), cholinergic receptors (nicotinic and muscarinic), and other sites. Research studies on patients with schizophrenia, drug addiction, mood disorders, and other psychiatric conditions have compared the condition of these receptors in patients to that of healthy controls.
- **Stereotactic Surgery and Radiosurgery:** PET can also be used in image-guided surgery for the treatment of intracranial tumors, arteriovenous malformations and other surgically treatable conditions.

4.1.5.2. Cardiology

Research on cardiovascular disease, atherosclerosis, and vascular disorders: FDG PET can be used to detect myocardium that is hibernating. It's unclear, though, whether PET is more cost-effective than SPECT for this purpose. It is also possible to identify patients at risk of stroke through FDG PET imaging of atherosclerosis. It can also be used to evaluate the effectiveness of new treatments for atherosclerosis.

4.1.5.3. Infectious Diseases

Molecular imaging technologies can enhance treatment follow-up and diagnosis by providing better images of infections. In clinical settings, FDG imaging of bacterial infections has been extensively employed by PET to detect the inflammatory response linked to the infection. To image bacterial infections in vivo, three distinct PET contrast agents have been developed: [^{18}F] maltose, [^{18}F]maltohexaose, and [^{18}F]2-fluorodeoxysorbitol (FDS). The additional advantage of FDS is its ability to specifically target Enterobacteriaceae.

4.1.5.4. Bio-distribution Studies

A novel medication may be injected into animals and radiolabeled during pre-clinical trials. Biodistribution studies are the term used to describe these scans. Compared to the more traditional method of killing and dissecting the animals, the information regarding drug uptake, retention, and elimination over time can be obtained quickly and affordably. Usually, studies comparing the ability of radiolabeled compounds to bind selectively to a site and unlabeled drugs to do so can be used to indirectly infer drug occupancy at a putative site of action. This allows testing several possible drug candidates for the same target with a single radioligand. An associated method is using radioligands to compete with an endogenous (naturally occurring) substance at a specific receptor to show that the drug releases the endogenous substance (Laruelle, 2000; Malmgren and Thom, 2012; Cendes and Fernando, 2013).

4.1.5.5. Small Animal Imaging

A tiny animal PET has been created that is suitable for scanning a completely conscious rat. Animals can be scanned with this RatCAP (Rat Conscious Animal PET) without the confusing effects of anesthesia. PET scanners marketed for use in academic and pharmaceutical research are those made especially for imaging rodents, or microPETs as they are also known as scanners for small primates. The microminiature scintillators and amplified avalanche photodiodes (APDs) utilized in the scanners are based on a single-chip silicon photomultiplier system. The first veterinary facility to use a small clinical PET scanner for clinical (as opposed to research) animal diagnosis was the UC Davis School of Veterinary Medicine in 2018. Veterinary PET scanning is anticipated to be scarce in the near future due to cost and the limited benefit of identifying cancer metastases in companion animals, which is this modality's primary use.

4.1.5.6. Musculo-Skeletal Imaging

PET imaging has been used for imaging muscles and bones. FDG is the most commonly used tracer for imaging muscles, and NaF-F18 is the most widely used tracer for imaging bones.

- **Muscles:** PET is a practical method for researching the skeletal muscles during physical activity. In addition, PET can offer information on muscle activation concerning deep-lying muscles (like the gluteus minimus and vastus intermedialis) in contrast to methods like electromyography, which are limited to superficial muscles that are directly beneath the skin. However, because PET must be measured after the exercise is over, it has the drawback of not providing any timing information regarding muscle activation. This is because FDG takes time to build up in the muscles that are activated.
- **Bones:** Together with [^{18}F] sodium floride, PET for bone imaging has been in use for 60 years for measuring regional bone metabolism and blood flow using static and dynamic scans. Researchers have recently started using [^{18}F] sodium floride to study bone metastasis as well (Laruelle, 2000; Malmgren and Thom, 2012; Cendes and Fernando, 2013).

4.2. Approaches Of Positron Emission Tomography (PET) Scan

One imaging test that can help reveal the metabolic or biochemical function of your tissues and organs is a positron emission tomography (PET) scan. Tracers, which are radioactive drugs, are used in PET scans to display both normal and abnormal metabolic activity. Before the disease manifests on other imaging tests, such as computerized tomography (CT) and magnetic resonance imaging (MRI), a PET scan can frequently identify the abnormal metabolism of the tracer in diseases. Most frequently, a vein in your hand or arm is used to inject the tracer. The tracer will subsequently accumulate in bodily regions with elevated metabolic or biochemical activity levels. This helps to identify the exact location of the illness. The images obtained from PET are commonly paired with CT or MRI to form PET-CT or PET-MRI scans. An imaging test that creates pictures of your organs and tissues in action is called a positron emission tomography (PET) scan. A PET scanner and a safe, injectable radioactive chemical known as a radiotracer are used in this test. Large-scale radiotracer absorption by diseased cells, a sign of a possible health issue, is picked up by the scanner. PET scans are widely used by medical professionals to aid in the diagnosis and evaluation of cancer treatments. The scan can also be used to evaluate specific heart and brain problems (Figure 4.3).

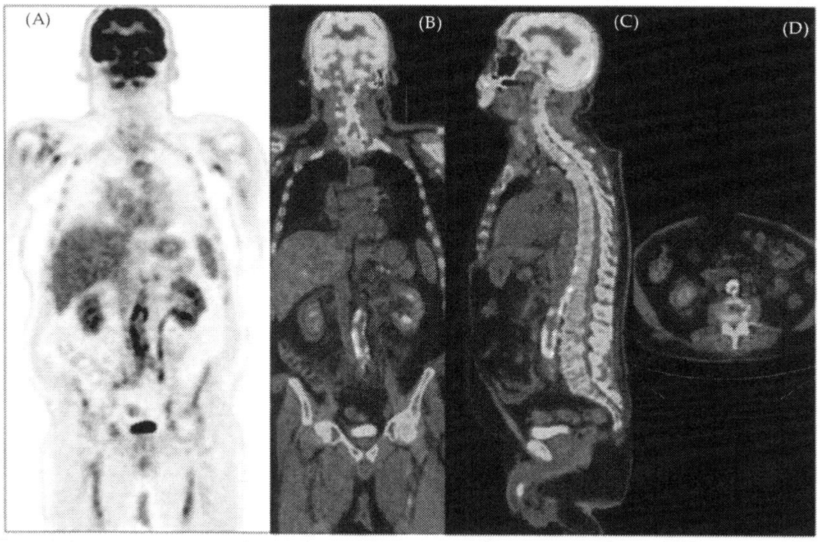

Figure 4.3. *A positron emission tomography (PET) scan uses a safe injectable radioactive chemical called a radiotracer and a device called a PET scanner to show images of your organs and tissues at work.*

Source: *Antunovic L, Artesani A, Coniglio M, Oyen WJG, Ciccarelli M, Selmi C, Chiti A, Sollini M. [^{18}F] FDG PET/CT in Large Vessel Vasculitis: The Impact of Expertise and Confounders on Image Analysis. Diagnostics. 2022; 12(11):2717. https://doi.org/10.3390/diagnostics12112717.*

4.2.1. When Would I Need a PET Scan?

Generally speaking, a PET scan can assess vital signs like blood flow, oxygen consumption, and glucose metabolism. Additionally, it can detect malfunctioning tissues and organs. A PET scan, which can identify cancer and/or make a diagnosis, will probably be recommended if your doctor believes you may have the disease.

If you've already been diagnosed with cancer, your provider may recommend more than one PET scan throughout your treatment to:

- Determine whether the cancer has spread in your body (metastasized).
- Assess the effectiveness of treatment.
- Determine if the cancer has returned after treatment (recurred).
- Evaluate the prognosis (outlook) of the cancer.

If you're having heart issues, your provider may recommend a PET scan to:

- Determine the effects of a heart attack on areas of your heart.
- Identify areas of the heart muscle that would benefit from angioplasty or coronary artery bypass surgery.

If you're experiencing neurological symptoms, your provider may recommend a PET scan to evaluate possible brain abnormalities, such as tumors, seizures and other central nervous system conditions.

4.2.2. PET scan Performance

You will receive tracers prior to the scan via an inhalation of gas, a drinkable solution, or a vein in your arm. You will have to wait for about an hour before the scan starts because your body needs time to absorb the tracers. Depending on the part of your body being scanned, it will take a certain amount of time for your body to completely absorb the tracer. You should avoid moving too much, unwind, and make an effort to stay warm while you wait. You should refrain from watching TV, listening to music, and reading while having a brain scan.

The scan will then take place, and it could take 30 to 45 minutes. This entails lying on a slender table that is connected to a PET machine that resembles the capital letter "O." To perform the scan, the table is gently lowered into the device. It could take longer—up to three hours—if you are having several tests. During the scan, you will have to lie still. You will be informed by the technician when you must remain motionless. It might be necessary for you to hold your breath for a few seconds. Throughout the test, you'll hear clicking and buzzing sounds. You'll slide out of the machine after it has recorded all the required images. At that point, the test is over. Generally, you can resume your day after the test, unless your doctor instructs you otherwise. However, you should limit your contact with pregnant people and infants during this time, as radioactive material can stay in your body for a few hours to days. After the test, sip on lots of liquids to aid in the removal of the tracers from your body. Your doctor will receive the information from a qualified specialist who has interpreted the PET scan images in the interim. Your doctor can typically receive the results in a few days. The results will be discussed with you by your doctor during your follow-up visit.

4.2.3. What Happens During the Scan?

A healthcare professional and a nuclear medicine technologist usually perform the scan in a hospital or at a PET center using special equipment.

- Over your arms, legs, and chest, the technologist will apply tiny metal disks, or electrodes. Electrocardiogram (ECG or EKG) machines are connected to wires on the disks. Throughout the test, the ECG monitors your heart rate and notifies the computer when a scan is needed.
- You will have an intravenous line (IV) placed in your arm. The tracer will be injected through the IV line.
- You'll lie on a flat table that's connected to the PET scanner and a computer. The table will slide into the scanner, which is shaped like a giant doughnut.
- Detectors in the PET scanner capture the radioactive patterns of the cardiac tracer. The data is converted into visual representations on a computer display. To provide images of thin slices of your entire

heart from every angle, multiple scans are performed over time. It's crucial that you remain motionless and raise your arms above your head during every scan.

- Your healthcare team will take a baseline picture of your heart before the tracer is injected. This takes about 15 to 30 minutes.
- Next, the tracer will be injected and your heart will be scanned again.
- In the event of a nuclear chemical stress test (also known as a pharmacologic stress test), you will be prescribed medication that stimulates your heart's blood flow in a manner akin to that of physical activity. Adenosine, dobutamine, and dipyridamole (Persantine) are a few examples of these medications. The medical staff will check how well your heart absorbs the tracer both before and after the medication. The tracer won't show up in certain parts of your heart that don't receive enough blood during stress if you have severe coronary artery disease.
- The test takes between 1 and 3 hours.

4.2.4. PET Scan vs. Other Tests

PET scans reveal cellular metabolic alterations taking place within an organ or tissue. This is crucial since illnesses frequently start at the cellular level. Cellular issues cannot be detected by MRIs or CT scans. PET scans are able to identify very early cell changes.

When a disease modifies the structure of your organs or tissues, CT scans and MRIs are only able to identify changes later on. Detection of illness at the cellular level gives your doctor the best view of complex systemic diseases, such as:

- coronary artery disease (CAD)
- brain tumors
- memory disorders
- seizure disorders

Sometimes these tests are used along with PET scans to give doctors a clearer picture of the inside of your body. This is often called PET/CT or a PET/MRI scan. In this case, the tests are performed at the same time.

- On its own, a CT scan uses special X-ray equipment to produce pictures of the inside of the body.
- MRI scans use magnetic fields and radio frequency pulses to create images of internal structures such as organs, soft tissues, and bone.

These two scans produce a phenomenon known as image fusion when they are combined with a PET scan. The two scan images are combined by a computer to produce a three-dimensional image, which offers more details and enables a more accurate diagnosis. PET scans and gallium scans are comparable. They entail injecting a radioactive tracer called gallium citrate. Gallium scans are a multi-day procedure that are usually carried out one to three days following the administration of the tracer. Although certain gallium scan types are combined with more modern testing, like PET scans, these scans aren't as frequently used for cancer detection.

4.2.5. Risks Involved with a PET Scan

Despite the low level of radiation exposure, radioactive tracers are used in PET scans. Your body faces minimal risks because of the tracer's tiny radiation dosage. The Food and Drug Administration (FDA) has standards for tracer performance and safety that must be met. Tracers are classified as radiopharmaceuticals. However, talking to your doctor about potential risks is a good idea. Since the test's results can be very helpful in diagnosing serious medical conditions, the test's risks are also negligible. With the radioactive component attached, the tracer is basically glucose. Even if you have a history of diabetes or kidney disease, this makes it very simple for your body to naturally remove the tracers following the test.

- **People with Allergies and Other Health Conditions:** It's possible to have an allergic reaction to the tracer. People who are allergic to iodine, aspartame, or saccharin should let their doctor know.

Those who can't have an iodine tracer typically receive a tracer made of diluted barium sweetened with saccharin.

Those most likely to have an allergic reaction to the iodine tracer include people with:

- a history of allergic reactions to PET scans
- allergies
- asthma
- heart disease
- dehydration
- the blood cell disorders sickle cell anemia, polycythemia vera, and multiple myeloma
- kidney disease
- a drug regimen that includes beta-blockers, nonsteroidal anti-inflammatory drugs (NSAIDs), or interleukin-2 (IL-2)
- **People Who Are Pregnant:** Radiation is not considered safe for developing fetuses. If you're pregnant or think you may be pregnant, you should not get a PET scan.
- **People Getting a PET/CT Scan:** If you're receiving a PET/CT scan, additional tracer will be needed. This can be harmful to people who have kidney disease or who have elevated creatinine levels from medications they're already taking.
- **Other risks:** Other risks of the test include discomfort if you're claustrophobic or uncomfortable with needles.

The injection may also lead to symptoms such as bleeding, bruising, or swelling.

4.3. Detectors in Positron Emission Tomography

The highly sensitive molecular imaging technique known as positron emission tomography relies on the simultaneous detection of annihilation photons following positron decay. The most popular detector uses light sensors to read out dense, quick, and bright scintillators.

4.3.1. Requirements for PET Detectors

Positrons lose energy in the surrounding tissue after emission during positron decay, and they ultimately annihilate with an electron. The technique of Positron imaging depends on the simultaneous back-to-back emission of two photons, each with an energy of 511 keV, during the annihilation process. It is possible to determine a line-of-response (LOR) without the need for geometrical collimation, which is necessary for gamma camera-based single photon emission tomography imaging, by detecting these photons within a very short time window. Positron emission tomography (PET) has excellent sensitivity because of this coincidence mode of acquisition.

Several requirements for the detection system follow from this basic principle:

- Detection efficiency for photons with 511 keV needs to be high since the coincidence efficiency is the product of efficiencies of two channels.
- For effective reduction of scattered radiation in the measured signal, the detectors need to provide accurate information on the energy deposited in a detector element.
- The detectors need to be fast to operate with short coincidence windows, reducing the number of random coincidences and potentially providing time-of-flight information.
- The detection elements need to be small since their size determine the achievable spatial resolution.

The kind of detectors that still best meet these criteria are scintillation detectors. They rely on a scintillator component that is detected by a light sensor. Research on light sensors and scintillation crystals has greatly enhanced PET detectors and system performance since the initial PET designs.

4.3.1.1. Scintillation Crystals

The above-mentioned prerequisites correspond to the characteristics of scintillation crystals: high atomic number, dense materials provide high photofraction and interaction probability. Photon statistics has a significant impact on energy resolution; therefore, bright scintillators are favored. Furthermore, readout schemes other than a one-to-one coupling between the scintillation crystal and the light sensor are made possible by high light yield. Exact time stamping of events is achieved through the rapid emission of scintillation light. With minimal self-absorption within the crystal element, the scintillation wavelength must fall within the light sensor's optimal detection range. Additionally, minimal light loss between the crystal and the light sensor is guaranteed by matching indices of refraction. The benefit of rugged materials is that they don't break when cut into tiny, individual pieces. Because some scintillation materials are hygroscopic, extra caution needs to be used when encasing them.

The first positron imaging machines relied on sodium-iodine (NaI(Tl)) crystals doped with thorium, a material widely recognized from Anger gamma cameras. A photomultiplier tube was used to read out each crystal, thereby reducing the size of individual detection elements. A 2D projection of the positron emitter density in the brain was produced by operating pairs of NaI(Tl) detectors ($3 \times 3 \times 4$ cm^3) simultaneously and translating them laterally in the first device used for in vivo scanning. Although NaI(Tl) is a bright scintillator, its detection efficiency for 511 keV photons is low due to its density of 3.67 g/cm^3 and effective atomic number of only 51. As a result, when the high-Z scintillator bismuth germanate (BGO) became accessible in the early 1970s, it gained attention as a PET scintillator substitute and was the preferred scintillator for a long time in PET equipment.

A new generation of PET scanners was created about 20 years later as a result of the development of quick, bright crystals. The growth of cerium-doped lutetium oxyorthosilicate (LSO:Ce) was established in the early 1990s. Subsequently, LYSO:Ce was unveiled, necessitating a lower melting temperature during the crystal growth process. Both LSO and LYSO are much brighter and faster than BGO, but they have slightly lower atomic numbers and comparable densities to BGO. Consequently, without significantly lowering the detection efficiency, much better timing and energy resolution could be accomplished. These two scintillation materials, barium fluoride (BaF_2) and cesium fluoride (CsF), decay even more quickly. The first time-of-flight PET scanners with coincidence timing resolution of 500–750 ps were already using them in the 1980s. Compared to BGO-based scanners, both materials perform less well in terms of detection efficiency and light yield, which lowers system performance. In addition to having a short decay time, $LaBr_3$:Ce scintillation material offers good light yield and energy resolution. Unfortunately, its atomic number and density are comparable to those of CsF and BaF_2, which limits the detection efficiency. Nevertheless, a tomograph based on $LaBr_3$:Ce was constructed to demonstrate how timing and energy resolution affect the quality of the image. Some characteristics of scintillators used for PET are summarized in Table 4.1.

Table 4.1. Basic Properties of Common Scintillation Crystals Used in PET Scanners

Property	NaI (Tl)	**BGO**	**GSO**	**LSO**	**LYSO**	**$LaBr_3$**	**GAGG**
Chemical Formula	NaI	$Bi_4Ge_3O_{12}$	Gd_2SiO_5	Lu_2SiO_5	$Lu_{2(1-x)}Y_{2x}SiO_5$	$LaBr_3$	$Gd_3(Ga, Al)_5O_{12}$
Z_{eff}	51	74	59	66	60	47	48
Density (g/cm^3)	3.67	7.13	4.89	7.4	7.2	5.3	6.63
Light output (ph/keV)	41	9	10	31	30	67	54
Wavelength (nm)	410	480	440	420	420	370	540
Decay time (ns)	230	300	60	40	41	25	94
Hygroscopic?	Yes	No	No	No	No	Yes	No

Source: *Yu X, Zhang X, Zhang H, Peng H, Ren Q, Xu J, Peng Q, Xie S. Requirements of Scintillation Crystals with the Development of PET Scanners. Crystals. 2022; 12(9):1302. https://doi.org/10.3390/cryst12091302.*

4.3.1.2. Light Sensors

It is necessary to transform the weak scintillation light into an electrical signal so that its arrival time and total amount of light can be measured. As a result, the characteristics of the scintillation light must be taken into consideration when choosing the light sensors for a detection system. Most crucially, the scintillation light's detection efficiency, e.g., the signal rise time should be as short as possible, and charge amplification and wavelength (420 nm in LSO:Ce) need to be high. Furthermore, a linear response in relation to the scintillation light output is presumed. The photomultiplier tube has been the conventional light sensor used in PET detectors. While silicon-based light sensors have also been around for a long time, it is only recently that these light sensors have been integrated into large-scale PET systems that exhibit superior performance.

4.3.1.3. Photomultiplier tubes

The majority of PET detectors manufactured thus far have been built around photomultiplier tubes (PMTs). A PMT is a vacuum glass tube that has an anode, a set of electrodes called dynos that have progressively higher voltages, and a photocathode. The photocathode and incident photons that enter through the glass window collide to produce photoelectrons (efficiency at 420 nm is approximately 30%). The voltage differential between the photocathode and the first dynode accelerates these primary photoelectron travel in the direction of the first dynode. Secondary electrons are produced when the electrons reach the dynode. Afterwards, depending on the PMT design, this process is repeated at each progressive dynode, producing a signal amplification of up to 106. The advantage of PMTs over solid-state sensors comes from their vacuum environment, which allows for a relatively low dark count rate (tens of counts per second)—the number of output pulses produced by randomly emitted electrons from the photocathode and dynosdes per unit of time. Furthermore, signal rise times are usually very brief. The creation of position-sensitive, square multi-anode PMTs (PSPMT, flat panel PMT) with e.g., 64 readout channels covering an area of approx. A new era of high-resolution detectors was made possible by 5 × 5 cm^2. These light sensors were essential for the development of organ-specific PET systems and small animal PET instrumentation because of their small size and low housing requirements (Laruelle, 2000; Malmgren and Thom, 2012; Cendes and Fernando, 2013).

4.3.1.4. Avalanche Photodiode

Analyzed as light sensors for PET detectors, avalanche photodiodes (APD) were once solid-state photon sensors with suitable properties. When an incident photon enters a regular p-i-n photodiode, it only produces one electron-hole pair; however, an APD offers internal signal amplification, which is necessary for PET applications. An APD occurs when an electron from the incident photon is accelerated by a high reverse voltage, colliding with the lattice to create a new pair of electrons and holes. The newly created electron and the original electron can then repeat this process, causing a significant avalanche effect and signal amplification. On the other hand, compared to PMTs, the average internal gain of APDs used in PET is substantially lower, typically around 100.

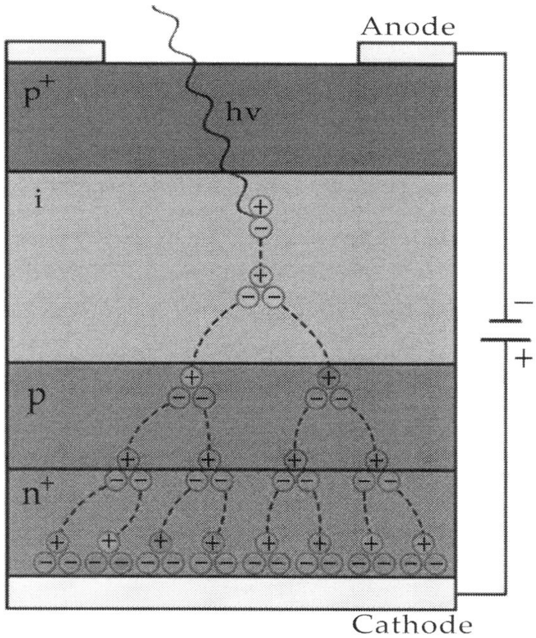

Figure 4.4. *An avalanche photodiode.*

Source: *Lozovoy, K. A., Douhan, R. M. H., Dirko, V. V., Deeb, H., Khomyakova, K. I., Kukenov, O. I., Sokolov, A. S., Akimenko, N. Y., Kokhanenko, A. P. Silicon-Based Avalanche Photodiodes: Advancements and Applications in Medical Imaging. Nanomaterials. 2023; 13(23), 3078. https://doi.org/10.3390/nano13233078.*

Furthermore, APDs' timing resolution is less precise than PMTs,' ranging from several ns to several s. APDs in PET operate in proportionate mode, i.e., the reverse voltage is adjusted so that the signal produced is proportionate to the scintillation light that is incident. APDs can be used in high magnetic fields and have a substantially higher quantum efficiency (80% versus 30%) than PMTs, which makes them suitable for combined PET/MR imaging. APDs are the foundation of the first commercial simultaneous PET/MR system intended for clinical use. Furthermore, they can be produced as compact arrays of individual small APDs (Figure 4.4).

4.3.2. Silicon Photomultiplier

The goal of silicon photomultipliers (SiPMs) is to combine the advantages of APDs and PMTs. SiPMs require only moderate reverse voltage (below 100 V), and they yield gains that are on par with or higher than those of PMTs. Like APDs, SiPMs can be used in PET/MR imaging because they are resistant to magnetic fields. SiPMs have better timing resolution than APDs below 1 ns, which qualifies them for time-of-flight PET. An array of parallelly connected APDs operating in Geiger mode makes up a SiPM, i.e., utilizing a voltage higher than the breakdown. This voltage produces a strong enough electric field across the depletion region to support the impact ionization process on its own. Even when only one incident photon is present, these Geiger-mode APDs produce a sizable output signal.

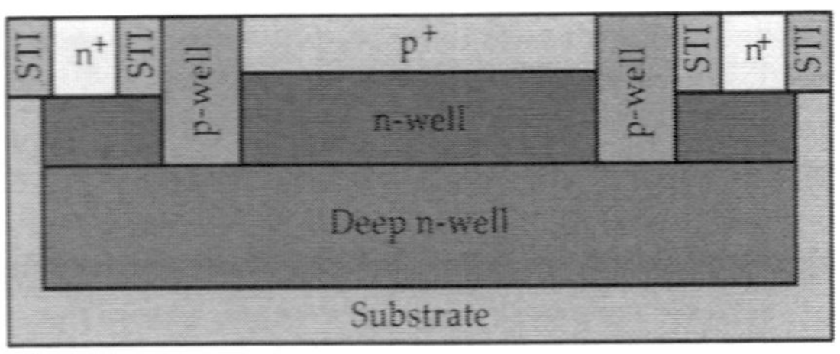

Figure 4.5. *Cross-section of the APD with a guard ring*

Source: *Lozovoy, K. A., Douhan, R. M. H., Dirko, V. V., Deeb, H., Khomyakova, K. I., Kukenov, O. I., Sokolov, A. S., Akimenko, N. Y., Kokhanenko, A. P. Silicon-Based Avalanche Photodiodes: Advancements and Applications in Medical Imaging. Nanomaterials. 2023; 13(23), 3078. https://doi.org/10.3390/nano13233078.*

As a result, another name for them is single-photon APDs (SPADs). Therefore, a single SPAD cannot estimate the quantity of incident photons. This problem is solved by a SiPM by employing a range of minuscule SPADs (Figure 4.5). If there are more available SPADs than photons entering the array, the SiPM signal is proportional to the number of photons reaching the SiPM surface after adding the signals from each SPAD in the array. This might not hold true for bright scintillators, in which case non-linear response must be taken into account.

Similar to PMTs, SiPMs have an analog output signal that is proportional to the quantity of scintillation light that is detected. To obtain energy and timing information, this signal must be read out and converted to digital form using the proper electronics. In contrast, digital SiPMs incorporate counting electronics directly onto the SiPM wafer, thereby decreasing the sensitive area. As a result, the output is the number of fired SPADs, negating the requirement for analog readout electronics. These digital SiPMs have recently been applied to the development of a large axial field-of-view tomograph. They are the light sensors found in a clinical PET/CT device.

4.3.3. Types of Detectors

Several schemes of combining scintillation crystals with light sensors have been developed since the first prototype PET scanners (Figure 4.6).

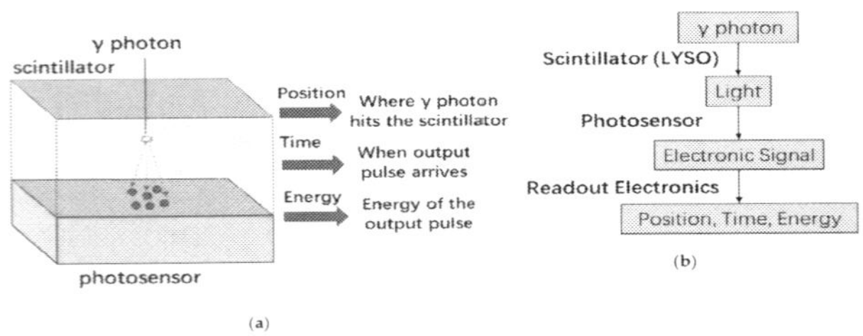

Figure 4.6. *Development of PET detector design.*

Source: Lozo Jiang, W., Chalich, Y., & Deen, M. J. Sensors for Positron Emission Tomography Applications. Sensors. 2019; 19(22), 5019. https://doi.org/10.3390/s19225019.

4.3.3.1. One-to-One Coupled Detectors

The earliest PET detectors were made up of a single PMT and scintillation crystal. The size of the crystal cross-section determines the system's intrinsic spatial resolution. As a result, to increase resolution, one would need to decrease crystal size while keeping sensitivity constant by increasing the total number of detectors. The size reduction is limited by the bulkiness of PMTs, and the cost of the system rises with the number of detectors used. This issue was resolved by the block detector. However, one-to-one coupling is used in certain contemporary preclinical systems. SiPMs are used in these scanners in place of PMTs to reduce size.

4.3.3.2. Block Detectors

The next development in PET detector technology was the block detector, which produced modules with tiny crystal elements that were closely packed. A photodetector array (originally PMTs) and a cubic scintillation crystal connected optically make up a typical block detector. Starting from the frontal surface, the scintillator features perpendicular cuts. There is a reflective substance inside the incisions. To produce a linear light distribution among the PMTs, the depth of the cuts increases in the direction of the corners, beginning at about half of the crystal depth and continuing to nearly full depth. Anger logic is used to estimate the position of a scintillation event, with events clustered at particular points that correspond to the individual scintillator elements. A lookup table derived from the scintillator's uniform irradiation can be used to associate each event with a specific scintillator element.

A typical configuration consists of 8 × 8 individual crystal elements read out by only four PMTs. Such a design significantly reduces the number of readout channels and system cost compared to the one-to-one coupling (Laruelle, 2000; Malmgren and Thom, 2012; Cendes and Fernando, 2013),

4.3.3.3. Continuous Detectors

Continuous detectors work similarly to block detectors in that they use a large scintillation crystal without any cuts that is optically coupled to a photodetector array (PSPMT or APD/SiPM array). Because there are no individual components with gaps in between, this method seeks to maximize sensitivity while also further lowering system costs due to lower manufacturing costs. By examining the shape of the light distribution, the event position can be estimated. Three categories of positioning techniques exist: machine learning-based, statistical, and analytical. Both two- and three-dimensional light distribution models are used in the analytical techniques. The statistical techniques include maximum likelihood, nearest neighbors, chi-square, and least squares. Support vector machines, neural networks, and gradient tree boosting are a few machine learning-based techniques.

Since the cross-section size of monolithic crystals does not limit the resolution, it is possible to achieve a sub-millimeter spatial resolution in modern continuous detectors. When employing statistical positioning algorithms, one drawback of using continuous detectors is the requirement for a protracted detector calibration, which typically necessitates complex algorithms and significant processing power, followed by a hardware setup. Furthermore, the position of Compton interaction in monolithic crystals is difficult to estimate. A further difficulty is the scintillation light truncation near the crystal edges. To counteract this effect, several strategies were put forth, such as using trapezoid crystals, double-sided readout, optical absorbers on the crystal edges, and letting light pass into nearby monolithic crystals.

4.3.3.4. Depth-of-Interaction Detectors

Since the size of the subject to be scanned and the amount of injected activity is much smaller in preclinical PET scanners than in clinical systems, depth-of-interaction (DOI) estimation becomes necessary when one aims to achieve high sensitivity while maintaining high spatial resolution. Using long, narrow scintillation crystals is one method of achieving high sensitivity. However, this has the drawback that, if a source is positioned at a specific radial offset from the field-of-view center, the generated annihilation photons may pass the first crystal without interacting and subsequently produce a scintillation deep within the adjacent crystal. If a specific place is designated for the interactions, e.g., the crystal entrance or center, as is the case in systems without DOI encoding, these lines-of-response will be erroneously positioned. The radial component of spatial resolution degrades as a result of what is known as the parallax effect.

Using 3D localization algorithms based on the light distribution across the light sensor array and monolithic scintillators is one method of estimating the DOI. For 20 mm thick monolithic scintillators, DOI resolution of less than 3 mm was attained. An alternative is to use two or more scintillation crystals coupled to one another along their axis with an optical grease and varying decay times and pulse shapes. A phoswich detector is another name for this type of design. The height of each individual crystal that makes up the detector is approximately equal to the DOI resolution of such a device. It does, however, require the right electronics and materials with sufficiently varied light emission times. Alternative methods involve the utilization of multi-layer offset crystal designs or multi-layer crystals with edge readout.

Utilizing double-sided readout without altering the scintillators themselves is an additional method of calculating the DOI. Since the lateral sides of the crystals are left rough in this design, the ratio of scintillation light observed at the two ends of the crystals is proportionate to the DOI. This approach produces highly accurate DOI estimations. This configuration makes it possible to use a single SiPM array to detect light emitted in both directions. When employing a machine learning-based positioning algorithm, the average DOI resolution obtained by this method was demonstrated to be 3 mm for an 8 × 8 array of 1.53 × 1.53 × 15 mm^3 of Ce:LYSO crystals. To make the pulse shape DOI-dependent, the crystals in another single-sided readout method have phosphor coatings applied to their sides (Table 4.2).

Table 4.2. Some Commercial/Tested APDs for PET Applications

Sensors	Crystal	Crystal Size (mm^3)	CRT FWHM (ns)	Energy Resolution @511 keV FWHM (%)	**Spatial Resolution FWHM (mm)**
Hamamatsu S8664-55 (2 × 2 Array)	LSO	2 × 2 × 20 (9 × 9 Array)	2.47	20.9	2
Hamamatsu S8550	LSO	2 × 2 × 15 (Four Crystals)	2.15 ± 0.11	12.8 ± 0.6	-

LabPET detector	LYSO/LGSO phoswich pair	2 × 2 × 10/12 (Single of Each)	6.6 [b] 10.7 [c]	24 ± 6 (LYSO) 25 ± 6 (LGSO)	1.3–1.4
LabPET II detector (two 4 × 8 arrays)	LYSO	1.2 × 1.2 × 12 (8 × 8 Array)	3.6 ± 0.3	20 ± 1	0.81 ± 0.04
RMD PSAPD detector	LYSO	0.9 × 0.9 × 1 (8 × 8 Array)	15.7 ± 0.2	10.62 ± 0.04	0.84 ± 0.02
Hamamatsu S8550-02	LYSO:Ce	21.4–23.5 × 18.5 × 10 (Monolithic) [a]	27	13.2	2.12–2.64

[a] Double-layer trapezoidal crystals varying in the transverse direction (21.4/22.4 for one, 22.5/23.5 for the other). [b] LYSO/LYSO coincidence. [c] LGSO/LGSO coincidence.

Source: *Jiang, W., Chalich, Y., & Deen, M. J. Sensors for Positron Emission Tomography Applications. Sensors. 2019; 19(22), 5019. https://doi.org/10.3390/s19225019.*

4.3.3.5. Time-of-Flight Detectors

Time-of-flight (TOF)-PET is a technology aiming at limiting the region along the line of response within which the positron annihilation occurred. TOF-PET estimates the position of the annihilation event by measuring the difference in the arrival times between the two annihilation photons in the opposing detectors (Figure 4.7).

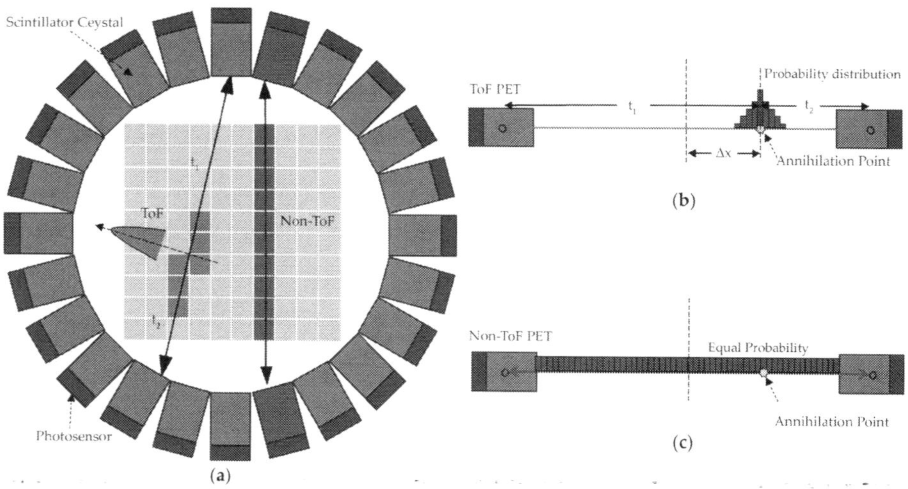

Figure 4.7. *TOF-PET concept: By measuring the difference in arrival times the position of the annihilation event along the line-of-response can be determined.*

Source: *Jiang, W., Chalich, Y., & Deen, M. J. Sensors for Positron Emission Tomography Applications. Sensors. 2019; 19(22), 5019. https://doi.org/10.3390/s19225019.*

The PET detector must meet certain requirements in order to allow TOF measurements. The light pulse profile should rise and decay instantaneously during the scintillation process. Although there isn't a perfect material as of yet, TOF-PET detectors have employed L(Y)SO:Ce, BaF_2, CsF, and $LaBr_3$:Ce. The photodetector should exhibit low noise, rapid rise and decay of the charge pulse profile, low charge transit time spread, and high scintillation light detection efficiency. Tof-PET detectors are currently made using both PMTs and SiPMs. Clinical PET scanners can achieve a few hundred ps timing resolution when they are equipped with the right electronic readout.

4.3.4. Systems

Clinical PET systems have developed over time, starting with two detector elements that measured one coincidence line at a time and ending with systems that acquired nearly 10^{11} lines-of-response, covering the entire human body at once with 564,480 crystals. In the Explorer project, the concept of creating a PET device with maximum solid angle coverage that could reach sensitivity ranges that would enable very low-activity examinations was brought to the clinical setting. Driven by this achievement, numerous research endeavors and products are being developed that offer PET with a large axial field of view, ranging from 1 to 2 meters, or total body PET.

Apart from the exceptional scalability of SiPM-based detectors, the new systems' exceptional time resolution value of 210 ps is also advantageous for total-body PET. This translates into a 3 point 2 cm spatial uncertainty of the emission point along the line-of-response. The time-of-flight information in the image reconstruction reduces image noise, which is frequently equated with an effective increase in system sensitivity, even though this does not directly improve the tomograph's spatial resolution. Furthermore, TOF-PET is not a novel concept; it was first applied in the 1980s. The development of customized, integrated electronics with numerous synchronized, parallel readout channels, rapid, low-cost light sensors with high sensitivity, and appropriate scintillators are the only things that could enable TOF-PET to be used in clinical applications. Excellent time resolution and TOF in image reconstructions may also lead to better opportunities for systems with partial ring geometry, which are necessary for proton therapy's in-beam PET. The development of PSPMTs has greatly benefited high-resolution PET system designs for small animal imaging, providing excellent interaction position identification within arrays of very small crystals (1 to 1.5 mm side length). SiPM readout has been the basis for several preclinical systems, not just for simultaneous PET/MR.

4.4. Physical Basis of Positron Emission Tomography

The physical characteristics of isotopes, or radioactive forms of simple atoms like hydrogen, oxygen, fluorine, etc., serve as the foundation for Positron Emission Tomography, or PET.)—decaying and releasing positrons. Isotopes are obtained in PET centers using cyclotrons. More complex molecules such as those of oxygen, water, glucose, etc., are composed of simpler atoms. PET centers use specialized radiochemical laboratories, or "hot cells," to conduct these chemical reactions. The radioactive material is injected into the patient's blood during PET scan measurements, and circulation carries it to the brain. Cells in the brain either absorb the radioactive material (such as oxygen or glucose) or cellular receptors bind the appropriate ligand. In the first scenario, more radioactive material accumulates and more glucose (or oxygen) is consumed in proportion to the activity of a particular brain region. In the second scenario, the amount of ligand bound to these receptors increases with receptor density. Isotopes are radioactive forms of simple atoms, such as hydrogen, oxygen, fluorine, etc., and PET is based on their physical characteristics. As they decompose, they release positrons. To obtain isotopes, cyclotrons are used in PET centers. Components of more complex molecules, such as glucose, oxygen, and water molecules, are assembled from simpler atoms. In particular radiochemical labs of PET centers, known as "hot cells," these chemical reactions are conducted. Radioactive material is injected into the patient's blood during PET scan measurements, and the material travels through the bloodstream to the brain. The radioactive material (such as oxygen or glucose) is either consumed by brain cells or bound by corresponding ligand by cellular receptors. In the first scenario, greater amounts of glucose (or oxygen) are consumed and more radioactive material is accumulated in proportion to the activity of a particular brain area. The second scenario involves a greater amount of ligand bound to receptors that have a higher receptor density.

Positron emissions are released by the radioactive material when it accumulates in a particular region of the brain. Positron-electron annihilation releases two gamma quantums per interaction. The number of gamma quantum encounters recorded by specialized detectors positioned all over the subject's head is directly correlated with the metabolic activity of the brain region under study.

The number of events that result in the emission of two gamma quantums is the source parameter for PET. Several detectors in a PET scanner register gamma quantum waves, and these detectors are arranged in layers, rings, or cylinders that encircle the subject's head. Special mathematical reconstruction techniques are used, akin to MRI techniques, to restore a 3D pattern of radioactive substance distribution density. It should be noted that the PET method's spatial resolution is noticeably less than the MRI's. PET is a costly and invasive procedure. A cyclotron and a specialized radiochemical laboratory are required for its application. Relatively little isotope is given to the subject to lower the radiation dose they are exposed to; this results in a PET image that is of lower quality. However, PET appears to be the only technique currently available for some scientific tasks (such as studying the density receptors of dopamine reuptake).

4.4.1. Characteristics of Positron Emission

The phenomenon of spontaneous positron emission by the nuclei of some unstable ultra-short-lived radionuclides (USLRs), in which there are more protons than neutrons, is the basis for the positron emission tomography (PET) technique. When the positron and electron annihilate, two gamma-photons with the same energy (511 keV) are released and travel in opposite directions, nearly 180° apart (almost collinearly).

Since the positron needs to lose its kinetic energy first, annihilation cannot occur in the orbit of its own atom. The positron's flight length from the emission point to the annihilation point is determined by both its energy and the environment's density. It is subject to variation over a broad range. For instance, it varies between 1 and 8 mm in the muscle. This is one of the causes of PET's lower resolving power in comparison to certain other radiodiagnostic techniques (MRI, CT). The physical limit of the method's resolving capacity has likely been reached in contemporary positron emission scanners, where space resolution is 1–6 mm (FWNM) (Rudd et al, 2002; Brix et al, 2005).

4.4.2. Principles of Detection of Positron Decay

A PET scanner's primary parts include a gantry, a bed that can be moved to position a patient in the ring, computer stations for gathering and storing raw data (also known as sinograms), and the ability to reconstruct, process, and store images in addition to producing hard copies. The detector block, which is made up of multiple crystals connected to a group of photomultipliers in one instance, is a crucial part of the detector ring. The size, shape, and composition of the materials that make up the crystals in the detector block, as well as the diameter of the detector ring, have a significant impact on the physical attributes of the scanner. The crystal scintillates as a result of the interaction between the gamma-photon and the latter. A computer complex can detect and process the electric pulse that the photomultiplier produces in response to scintillation.

Two sets of extremely sensitive detectors are housed in rings and are used to look for coincidences in the PET scanner's detector ring. The annihilation point is on the line that connects two detectors that are opposite one another (the coincidence line) if the detectors detect two gamma photons within the coincidence range. Annihilation does not always have to happen precisely in the center of the detectors. For this reason, the so-called "coincidence window," which allows for a brief diversion of radiation detection by pairs of detectors from 4.2 to 12 ns, is employed in PET. In a sinogram, the event is identified and captured as polar coordinates (the angle and the radius). A sinogram is a curve that shows how many occurrences are on file for each coincidence line. Every crystal has a space representation in the computer's electronic matrix, which establishes the radiation point's space coordinates. An annihilation point's coordinates can be found precisely by identifying multiple lines that pass through it. The quantity of pulses obtained in a particular crystal is determined by the radioactive source's physical characteristics, which also reflect the source's qualitative features. The computer processes (reconstructs) the sinogram to show the object under examination and to ascertain the radioactivity distribution in the slice.

In addition to true coincidences, dispersed and random coincidences that arise from various annihilations are found. Dispersed coincidences are associated with the Compton effect, which causes them to shift in direction of motion. A 511 keV energy window is used to distinguish between random and scattered photons with lower energy and actual radiation. The aforementioned features of PET allow for the identification and separation of a true signal, meeting time and energy requirements. "Electronic collimation" was the term used to describe the suggested method of detecting the signal realized in positron tomographs. Physical collimators are no longer used; instead, electronic collimation is used. As a result, PET's sensitivity increased by a factor of ten or more when compared to single photon emission computer tomography, making it feasible to accurately measure quick biochemical reactions on tomographic slices of any organ or tissue.

The "dead time" is the amount of time, albeit not much, that must pass before the detector can no longer process the signal and detect new events. The amount of radioactivity in the tomograph's field of view and the scanner's speed both affect how much signal is lost as a result of dead time. Modern PET scanners can continue to operate at a variety of computing rates without experiencing appreciable reductions in resolution. Limiting screens made of lead or tungsten (septa) are used in PET scanners to lower the quantity of dispersed and random coincidences. A two-dimensional (2D) regime is used for radiation detection when a septum is present; in the absence of a septum, the process is referred to as a three-dimensional (3D) regime. It is possible to obtain images with the highest resolving capacity and minimal noise by using the 2D mode. But in this instance, the tomograph's sensitivity (i.e.the relationship between the number of annihilation acts found in the tomograph's field of view and their actual number in the field of vision) decreases multiple times; the characteristics of the detector blocks, the detector ring's diameter, the mode of data acquisition (2D or 3D), and the scanning duration all determine the scanner's sensitivity. In the 3D mode, scanning without a septum yields the highest positron scanner sensitivity (Figure 4.13b). But in this instance, dead time losses rise and the noise level doubles. When compared to the 3D mode, the 2D mode allows for higher quantitative analysis accuracy and treatment efficiency control. So, a specific clinical task influences the scanning mode selection. Currently, hybrid PET-CT scanners that only operate in 3D mode and lack a septum are manufactured.

Photon absorption correction, also known as attenuation correction, is a feature of PET scanners that corrects for the irregularities in the tissues' absorption of ionizing radiation from radioactive transmission sources of 68Ge and 137Cs. In order to achieve a higher accuracy in reproducing the distribution of the radionuclide label in tissues and to offset radiation distortion, attenuation correction is required. Modern tomographs have integrated transmission sources within the detector ring. Because the control is remote, personnel are less exposed to radiation and security is maintained. For example, we present pictures of a homogeneous 68Ge photon both with and without attenuation. The image demonstrates that without absorption irregularity correction, it is impossible to reproduce the radioactive label distribution accurately in a tomographic slice. The quantitative analysis of PET images also requires the correction of the irregularity of radiation absorption by tissues. Digital data acquired through CT are used in PET-CT combined scanners for this purpose. In CT, the effective beam energy of X-rays is between 70 and 80 keV. As a result, images produced using radioactive sources with an energy of 511 keV are different from images corrected for PET using CT attenuation correction. For the same reason, non-linear attenuation coefficients produced by PET-CT data processing distort the true distribution and cause radiation buildup in dense tissues—especially the bones—to be overstated. Consequently, there may be a 1–2x difference in quantitative measurements of the same formations and tissues obtained using PET and PET-CT scanners. The use of contrast agents in CT causes additional distortions and causes artifacts to appear on PET images, greatly inflating the true radioactivity value in the contrast agent accumulation focus.

Because the tomograph was so big and needed its own room, with first-generation PET scanners, part of the apparatus was located outside the tomograph. Concerning conditioning, screening, and speed, there were issues. PET scanners' primary parts can now be made substantially smaller and more efficiently constructed thanks to advancements in video technology, hardware, and the development of personal computers. Modern scanners are therefore designed with their most crucial components right in the detector ring. Tomographs as a result of this situation grew in size; as a result, they became faster and more stable, reliable, and protected (Figure 4.8).

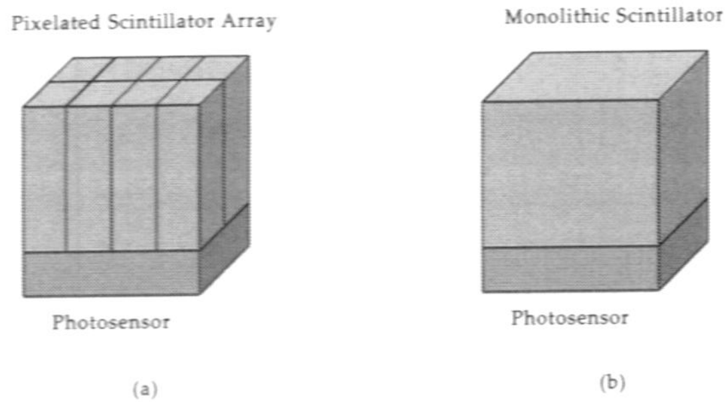

Figure 4.8. *Illustration of a positron emission tomography (PET) detector: (a) pixelated scintillator (2 × 4 array) mounted on a photosensor; (b) monolithic scintillator mounted on a photosensor.*

Source: *Jiang, W., Chalich, Y., & Deen, M. J. Sensors for Positron Emission Tomography Applications. Sensors. 2019; 19(22), 5019. https://doi.org/10.3390/s19225019.*

4.4.3. Reconstruction of Images, Data Processing, and Analysis

The computer gathers the first raw PET data in the form of sinograms for the object under examination. An image based on sinograms can be obtained through the reconstruction process. There are various approaches to reconstruction. The specific reconstruction method chosen will depend on the organ under examination as well as the task at hand. The technique known as filtered back-projection, or iterative method, is typically employed for image reconstructions of organs like the heart and brain. MLE, OSE, and RAMLA are a few of the modifications to the iterative method. The OSEM iterative reconstruction algorithm is most commonly used for whole-body exams because its smoothing feature ensures the best possible image quality. It is favored to use less complex filters when examining the brain and heart because they lessen the distortion of the true distribution of radiopharmaceuticals (RPs) in the slices. It should be remembered, though, that inadequate smoothing—especially when paired with low statistics—can exacerbate image heterogeneity, making it more challenging to interpret the findings. An image's informativity may be lost if there is excessive smoothing, which lowers resolution. Because most scanner manufacturers' instructions are complex, they usually advise using factory protocols and reconstruction installations. The principles of image reconstruction and other physical aspects of the PET method are described in detail in many reports.

The specific clinical task will determine how further image processing (postprocessing) is carried out and how hard copies of the images are obtained. Three projections are used for visual analysis in the first stage of PET image processing: axial, sagittal, and coronal projections. During a whole-body examination, 3D image analysis is utilized to obtain a more precise understanding of the location and anatomical connections of the inspected region. Each organ's image standardization process is covered in detail in the corresponding chapters of this book. Accurate understanding of the pharmacokinetics and normal distribution of the employed RPs is a prerequisite for a successful analysis. Each RP has a unique definition of the physiologic (normal) distribution, which varies depending on its characteristics. As a result, the results are presented with the state of the unaffected organs under examination or the entire body as well as the lesion area's characteristics, such as its location, scintigraphic size, RP distribution regularity, contour accuracy, and relationship to unaffected tissues. Typically, threshold level, color scales, and image contrast range are used to solve these problems. Certain issues with the interpretation of scintigraphic images arise from the functional images' lack of anatomic reference points. For this reason, precise matching or fusion of images with various modalities is required in several scenarios. In order to accurately localize the changes that have been revealed anatomically, matching functional PET images with data from structural imaging (CT, MRI) is first necessary. It is also necessary when there are notable physiological (individual) fluctuations in the levels of RP uptake in tissues. Furthermore, superimposition is required when the size of the formation is small and near the tomograph's resolving capacity as well as when the structure of the formation is highly heterogeneous.

Quantitative or semiquantitative PET-image analysis in absolute and relative values is used in the second stage. Standardized uptake value (SUV) is a dimensionless value used for semiquantitative analysis of the objects examined in whole-body examination and, more recently, in brain examination. SUV is defined as the relationship between the amount of added radioactivity per kilogram of body mass (MBq/kg) and the specific radioactivity in the measured zone (kBq/cm3). The scanner's software automatically calculates SUV while accounting for the radionuclide's physical half-life. It should be noted that when using SUV for image analysis, inaccurate data regarding the patient's height and weight, the amount of radioactivity introduced and when it was introduced, and detector drift can all lead to significant errors. For this reason, an SUV change that is more than 25% of the initial value during treatment is acknowledged to be significant. The relationship between radioactivity accumulated in the affected area and radioactivity in unaffected tissues (referent zones) is expressed using the tumor/nontumor (T/NT) ratio. In certain situations, it is appropriate to use mathematical models that suggest dynamic scanning of the organ under examination in order to determine the arterial blood "input function," or activity-time curve. It is most convenient to scan the left ventricle in order to measure blood radioactivity. Mathematical models are frequently used in heart exams because, while the left ventricular cavity's presence in the tomograph's field of view makes it easier to obtain the inline function, the high variability of metabolic processes in this organ limits the applicability of simple quantitative analysis methods.

4.4.4. PET Data Quality Control

The three categories of PET data quality control techniques are parameter changes of the tomograph during operation, regular control, and acceptance trials. Acceptance testing is carried out while the equipment is being installed. Early information about the scanner's operating parameters is obtained during the trial process, and this information is subsequently used as a model for daily or recurring technical state control. Modern scanners come equipped with dependable and user-friendly controls, image quality correction, and quantitative data reproducibility methods like cross-calibration and normalization. The automatic calculation of the deviation of the detector readings from the mean during daily control allows for the assessment of the devices' condition, highlighting deviations from the allowable parameters and pinpointing and locating errors. If there is a deviation of more than 2.5% from the admissible deviation of the sensitivity of the opposite pairs of detectors, normalization is performed. A standard calibration phantom with specified radioactivity is brought into the scanner's field of view for this purpose. The so-called "blank scan," which is produced during normalization, is required to align the scanner's field of view as closely as possible during image reconstruction. The calibration factor (ECF), an integrated factor representing detector drift, physical decay of calibration sources, and a few other parameters affecting measurement precision, is also computed during normalization. The ECF value is unique to a particular tomograph model and is determined by the way it is built. This factor is also employed as a quantitative data reproducibility criterion. For instance, each detector block's field of vision needs to be aligned when the ECF value deviates more than 5% from its initial value (set up). Utilizing positron-emitting radionuclides (^{68}Ge, ^{137}Cs) with a half-life of 1–10 years, homogenous calibration phantoms are created. The phantom should have a uniform distribution of radionuclides. Using a curiemeter, measurements of radionuclides can only be made prior to their introduction into the phantom. A specific PET center measures the radioactivity of the RPs that are injected into the patient as aqueous solutions. When changing calibration sources, recalibration is done for the factory ^{68}Ge phantom and a water phantom of known specific activity prepared in the PET center. The calibration factor (ECF) and the results of the quantitative analysis in a particular scanner are influenced by the precision of recalibrating the sources.

For the method to be used clinically, dependable PET data image and reproducibility quality control are therefore ensured by the hardware arsenal that is currently available. Biological, control, hardware, software, and mixed artifacts are all possible. Hardware issues are typically discovered during the daily checkup, which makes it possible to assess the extent of the damage. For this, sinogram analysis is also employed. Breakdowns in analog processors or bucket controllers are the most common causes of hardware malfunctions. A stripe that precisely matches the damaged processor appears on the sinogram when an analog processor malfunctions. The stripe is broader and encompasses all of the controller's processors when a controller is damaged. The daily calibration process reveals damage to the detector block. Through scanning following a unique program or through a "set-up" procedure, the damaged block is identified. Finding mixed or program errors is a trickier issue. Applying a specific program, for instance, is used to remove radioactive calibration sources from containers. The radioactive sources shut off due to a malfunction in its operation. This may appear to be a malfunction in the system forcing them to vacate.

Through the introduction of the necessary changes into the sinogram header and its subsequent repeated reconstruction, errors made by the operator (incorrect patient or radioactive introduction information) can be rectified. Errors in patient positioning or the data collection procedure, however, cannot be fixed after the fact. Injection mistakes, in which part or all of the RP is left in the injection site, can also produce artifacts. For example, radioactive material can leak out of a vein along with blood and land on a dirty dressing. Another possibility is contamination from radioactive urine. Radiation can spread to the patient's arms, clothing, and, in some cases, the tomograph bed when it reaches the patient's bedside. When one or more uptake foci with superficial locations show up on the image, it can lead to false-positive diagnoses of certain diseases, like melanoma. There is usually some challenge in detecting contamination. Consequently, following the methodology and having a precise notion of the likelihood and location of an artifact's appearance are crucial when handling them. If there's a chance that the tomograph may have been contaminated, try cleaning the radioactive material off your skin, taking off any contaminated clothing, changing the linen, and wiping down the surface. Moving or scanning organs while the patient is displaced can also result in artifacts e.g., cardiac or pulmonary excursion, resulting in an imprecise representation (Rudd et al, 2002; Brix et al, 2005) (Table 4.3).

Table 4.3. Comparative Table of Fast Scintillators Which Can Be Considered for ToF-PET

Comparative Table of Fast Scintillators Which Can Be considered for ToF-PET						
	LSO(Ce)	LSO (Ce, Ca)	LYSO(Ce)	$LaBr_3$	BaF_2	Plastic
Density ($gcm^3 gcm^3$)	7.40	similar to LSO	similar to LSO	5.29	4.89	1.03
Effective atomic number (Z)	66	similar to LSO	similar to LSO	46	54	12
Rise time (ns)	≤ 0:5	similar to LSO	similar to LSO	0.2–0.5	~0.03	0.7–1
Decay time (ns)	40	31@0.4% Ca	similar to LSO	15–26	0.8/620	2–5
Photon yield/keV	20–30	~35	similar to LSO	63	1.8/10	10
Refractive index (n)	1.82	1.82	1.82	1.90	1.56	1.58
Hygroscopic	No	No	No	Yes	Slightly	No
Peak emission wavelength (nm)	420	420	similar to LSO	380	220/310	Various

Source: Spanoudaki, V. C., & Levin, C. S. Photo-Detectors for Time-of-Flight Positron Emission Tomography (ToF-PET). Sensors. 2010; 10(11),10484–10505. https://doi.org/10.3390/s101110484.

A Closer Look

Hybrid Imaging

The integration of Positron Emission Tomography (PET) with other imaging modalities such as Computed Tomography (CT) and Magnetic Resonance Imaging (MRI) has revolutionized diagnostic imaging, offering synergistic benefits that surpass the capabilities of each modality alone. PET/CT and PET/MRI combine the functional and molecular information provided by PET with the anatomical details offered by CT and MRI, respectively. PET/CT combines PET's sensitivity to biochemical processes with CT's high spatial resolution, enabling precise localization and characterization of abnormalities. This hybrid approach is particularly valuable in oncology, where it enhances cancer detection, staging, treatment planning, and monitoring. The integration of PET with CT allows for the accurate anatomical localization of PET-avid lesions, facilitating more informed clinical decisions. Moreover, PET/CT reduces imaging time and improves patient comfort by acquiring both functional and structural images in a single session, enhancing workflow efficiency and patient throughput in clinical practice.

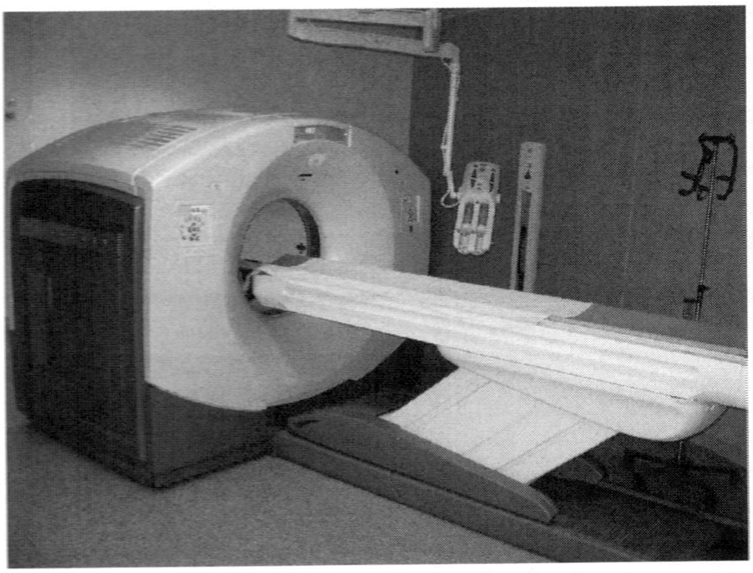

Source: *By Hg6996 – Own work, Public Domain, https://commons.wikimedia.org/w/index.php?curid=8322582.*

On the other hand, PET/MRI combines PET's molecular imaging capabilities with MRI's excellent soft tissue contrast and multi-parametric imaging capabilities without ionizing radiation exposure. This hybrid modality is particularly advantageous in neuroimaging and musculoskeletal imaging, where MRI excels in visualizing soft tissues and anatomical structures with high contrast resolution. PET/MRI enables the simultaneous acquisition of metabolic, functional, and anatomical information, providing comprehensive insights into various pathologies with superior soft tissue characterization and spatial resolution compared to PET/CT. Additionally, PET/MRI allows for advanced imaging protocols, such as dynamic contrast-enhanced MRI, diffusion-weighted imaging, and spectroscopy, which can further enhance diagnostic accuracy and provide additional functional information.

Both PET/CT and PET/MRI offer complementary strengths, allowing for more comprehensive assessments in various clinical scenarios. In cardiology, PET/CT can provide information on myocardial perfusion and metabolism, while PET/MRI can offer insights into cardiac function, tissue characterization, and myocardial viability. In neurology, PET/CT can assess cerebral metabolism and neuroreceptor binding, while PET/MRI can evaluate brain structure, connectivity, and functional activity with high spatial and temporal resolution.

Moreover, the combination of PET with CT or MRI facilitates the development of novel imaging biomarkers and quantitative imaging techniques, allowing for more accurate disease characterization, treatment response assessment, and patient stratification in clinical trials. Additionally, the integration of PET with advanced image analysis algorithms and artificial intelligence techniques further enhances the diagnostic and prognostic utility of multimodal imaging approaches.

Summary

- Positron emission tomography, also called PET imaging or a PET scan, is a type of nuclear medicine imaging. Nuclear medicine uses small amounts of radioactive material called radiotracers. Doctors use nuclear medicine to diagnose, evaluate, and treat various diseases.
- Positron emission tomography (PET) is a functional imaging technique that uses radioactive substances known as radiotracers to visualize and measure changes in metabolic processes and in other physiological activities including blood flow, regional chemical composition, and absorption.
- PET is both a medical and research tool used in pre-clinical and clinical settings. It is used heavily in the imaging of tumors and the search for metastases within the field of clinical oncology, and for the clinical diagnosis of certain diffuse brain diseases such as those causing various types of dementias.
- PET scanning with the radiotracer [^{18}F] fluorodeoxyglucose (FDG) is widely used in clinical oncology. FDG is a glucose analog that is taken up by glucose-using cells and phosphorylated by hexokinase (whose mitochondrial form is significantly elevated in rapidly growing malignant tumors).
- PET imaging with oxygen-15 indirectly measures blood flow to the brain. In this method, increased radioactivity signal indicates increased blood flow which is assumed to correlate with increased brain activity.
- PET imaging has been used for imaging muscles and bones. FDG is the most commonly used tracer for imaging muscles, and NaF-F18 is the most widely used tracer for imaging bones.
- A positron emission tomography (PET) scan is an imaging test that can help reveal the metabolic or biochemical function of your tissues and organs. The PET scan uses a radioactive drug called a tracer to show both typical and atypical metabolic activity
- PET scans show metabolic changes occurring at the cellular level in an organ or tissue. This is important because diseases often begin at the cellular level. CT scans and MRIs cannot reveal problems at the cellular level.
- Positron emission tomography is a highly sensitive molecular imaging modality, based on the coincident detection of annihilation photons after positron decay. The most used detector is based on dense, fast, and luminous scintillators read out by light sensors.
- Silicon photomultipliers (SiPMs) aim to combine the benefits of PMTs and APDs. SiPMs produce gains equal or greater to those of PMTs, while requiring only moderate reverse voltage (below 100 V).

References

1. Agdeppa, E. D., Kepe, V., Liu, J., Flores-Torres, S., Satyamurthy, N., Petric, A., et al. (2001). Binding characteristics of radiofluorinated 6-dialkylamino-2-naphthylethylidene derivatives as positron emission tomography imaging probes for beta-amyloid plaques in Alzheimer's

disease. *The Journal of Neuroscience, 21*(24), RC189. https://doi.org/10.1523/JNEUROSCI.21-24-j0001.2001.

2. Azad, G. K., Siddique, M., Taylor, B., Green, A., O'Doherty, J., & Gariani, J., et al. (2019). 18F-Fluoride PET/CT SUV? *Journal of Nuclear Medicine, 60*(3), 322–327. https://doi.org/10.2967/jnumed.118.215384.
3. Brix, G., Lechel, U., Glatting, G., Ziegler, S. I., Münzing, W., Müller, S. P., & Beyer, T. (2005). Radiation exposure of patients undergoing whole-body dual-modality 18F-FDG PET/CT examinations. *Journal of Nuclear Medicine, 46*(4), 608–613.
4. Buchsbaum, M. S., Christian, B. T., Lehrer, D. S., Narayanan, T. K., Shi, B., Mantil, J., et al. (2006). D2/D3 dopamine receptor binding with [F-18] fally pride in thalamus and cortex of patients with schizophrenia. *Schizophrenia Research, 85*(1–3), 232–244. https://doi.org/10.1016/j.schres.2006.04.026.
5. Catafau, A. M., Searle, G. E., Bullich, S., Gunn, R. N., Rabiner, E. A., Herance, R., et al. (2010). Imaging cortical dopamine D1 receptors using [11C]NNC112 and ketanserin blockade of the 5-HT2A receptors. *Journal of Cerebral Blood Flow & Metabolism, 30*(5), 985–993. https://doi.org/10.1038/jcbfm.2009.256.
6. Cendes, F. (2013). Neuroimaging in investigation of patients with epilepsy. *Continuum, 19*(3 Epilepsy), 623–642. https://doi.org/10.1212/01.CON.0000431379.23240.56.
7. de Jong, P. A., Tiddens, H. A., Lequin, M. H., Robinson, T. E., & Brody, A. S. (2008). Estimation of the radiation dose from CT in cystic fibrosis. *Chest, 133*(5), 1289–1291. https://doi.org/10.1378/chest.07-2850.
8. Gowrishankar, G., Namavari, M., Jouannot, E. B., Hoehne, A., Reeves, R., Hardy, J., & Gambhir, S. S. (2014). Investigation of 6-[18F]-fluoromaltose as a novel PET tracer for imaging bacterial infection. *PLOS ONE, 9*(9), e107951. https://doi.org/10.1371/journal.pone.0107951.
9. Hodolic, M., Topakian, R., & Pichler, R. (2016). 18 F-fluorodeoxyglucose and 18 F-flumazenil positron emission tomography in patients with refractory epilepsy. *Radiology and Oncology, 50*(3), 247–253. https://doi.org/10.1515/raon-2016-0018.
10. Kelloff, G. J., Hoffman, J. M., Johnson, B., Scher, H. I., Siegel, B. A., Cheng, E. Y., et al. (2005). Progress and promise of FDG-PET imaging for cancer patient management and oncologic drug development. *Clinical Cancer Research, 11*(8), 2785–2808. https://doi.org/10.1158/1078-0432.CCR-04-2626.
11. Kuhl, D. E., Koeppe, R. A., Minoshima, S., Snyder, S. E., Ficaro, E. P., Foster, N. L., et al. (1999). In vivo mapping of cerebral acetylcholinesterase activity in aging and Alzheimer's disease. *Neurology, 52*(4), 691–699. https://doi.org/10.1212/WNL.52.4.691.
12. Laruelle, M. (2000). Imaging synaptic neurotransmission with in vivo binding competition techniques: a critical review. *Journal of Cerebral Blood Flow & Metabolism, 20*(3), 423–451. https://doi.org/10.1097/00004647-200003000-00001.
13. Levivier, M., Massager, N., Wikler, D., Lorenzoni, J., Ruiz, S., Devriendt, D., et al. (2004). Use of stereotactic PET images in dosimetry planning of radiosurgery for brain tumors: clinical experience and proposed classification. *Journal of Nuclear Medicine, 45*(7), 1146–1154.
14. Luster, M., Karges, W., Zeich, K., Pauls, S., Verburg, F. A., Dralle, H., et al. (2010). Clinical value of 18F-fluorodihydroxyphenylalanine positron emission tomography/computed tomography

(18F-DOPA PET/CT) for detecting pheochromocytoma. *European Journal of Nuclear Medicine and Molecular Imaging, 37*(3), 484–493. https://doi.org/10.1007/s00259-009-1314-7.

15. Malmgren, K., & Thom, M. (2012). Hippocampal sclerosis – origins and imaging. *Epilepsia, 53*(Suppl 4), 19–33. https://doi.org/10.1111/j.1528-1167.2012.03611.x.

16. Mathis, C. A., Bacskai, B. J., Kajdasz, S. T., McLellan, M. E., Frosch, M. P., Hyman, B. T., et al. (2002). A lipophilic thioflavin-T derivative for positron emission tomography (PET) imaging of amyloid in brain. *Bioorganic & Medicinal Chemistry Letters, 12*(3), 295–298. https://doi.org/10.1016/S0960-894X(01)00785-2.

17. Mukherjee, J., Christian, B. T., Dunigan, K. A., Shi, B., Narayanan, T. K., Satter, M., & Mantil, J. (2002). Brain imaging of 18F-fallypride in normal volunteers: blood analysis, distribution, test-retest studies, and preliminary assessment of sensitivity to aging effects on dopamine D-2/D-3 receptors. *Synapse, 46*(3), 170–188. https://doi.org/10.1002/syn.10134.

18. Oi, N., Iwaya, T., Itoh, M., Yamaguchi, K., Tobimatsu, Y., & Fujimoto, T. (2003). FDG-PET imaging of lower extremity muscular activity during level walking. *Journal of Orthopedic Science, 8*(1), 55–61. https://doi.org/10.1007/s007760300009.

19. Rudd, J. H., Warburton, E. A., Fryer, T. D., Jones, H. A., Clark, J. C., Antoun, N., et al. (2002). Imaging atherosclerotic plaque inflammation with [18F]-fluorodeoxyglucose positron emission tomography. *Circulation, 105*(23), 2708–2711. https://doi.org/10.1161/01.CIR.0000020548.60110.76.

20. Weinstein, E. A., Ordonez, A. A., DeMarco, V. P., Murawski, A. M., Pokkali, S., MacDonald, E. M., et al. (2014). Imaging Enterobacteriaceae infection in vivo with 18F-fluorodeoxysorbitol positron emission tomography. *Science Translational Medicine, 6*(259), 259ra146. https://doi.org/10.1126/scitranslmed.3009815.

Chapter 5

X-RAY DETECTORS

Contents

Introduction

X-ray detectors are essential instruments in many domains, such as industry, research, security, and medicine. They are essential to the taking and processing of X-ray pictures, which helps doctors identify illnesses, make sure safety precautions are followed, examine objects, and carry out research. X-ray detectors are vital parts of radiography, fluoroscopy, and computed tomography (CT) scans in medical imaging. When X-ray photons enter the patient's body, these detectors are made to catch them and turn them into electrical signals. Usually, semiconductor technology or scintillation materials are used to accomplish this conversion process. Materials like cesium iodide or gadolinium oxysulfide, which release light when hit by X-ray photons, are used in scintillation detectors. Once this light is detected, photodetectors such as photodiodes or photomultiplier tubes transform it into electrical signals. Conversely, semiconductor detectors make use of substances like silicon or amorphous selenium, which use the photoelectric effect to directly convert X-ray photons into electrical charges. Medical imaging has undergone a revolution thanks to the development of digital X-ray detectors, which provide better workflow efficiency, reduced radiation doses, and higher image quality. Digital detectors enable instantaneous image acquisition and electronic storage by doing away with the need for conventional film-based X-ray systems. They also provide post-processing features like image enhancement and manipulation, which improve patient care and diagnostic accuracy.

X-ray detectors are essential for security screening tasks like cargo scanning at ports and baggage inspection at airports, even outside the healthcare industry. By spotting forbidden objects like guns, explosives, and contraband, these detectors are essential in spotting possible threats. Security X-ray detectors use semiconductor or scintillation technology to transform X-ray signals into useful information, much like medical imaging does. Sophisticated algorithms and machine learning techniques are frequently incorporated into these systems to improve threat detection capabilities and reduce false alarms. X-ray detectors are used in industrial settings for non-destructive testing (NDT), which examines the integrity of components and materials without causing harm. Engineers can measure dimensions, find flaws, and evaluate structural integrity in a variety of materials, including metals, composites, and ceramics, by using nondestructive testing (NDT) techniques like computed tomography and radiography. In industrial applications, X-ray detectors need to have high sensitivity and resolution to accommodate different sample sizes and shapes and detect minute defects.

Moreover, X-ray detectors are essential to scientific study, especially in disciplines like chemistry, physics, and materials science. Scientists examine the atomic and molecular composition, structure, and characteristics of materials using X-ray diffraction (XRD) and X-ray fluorescence (XRF) techniques. XRD detectors quantify the X-rays that crystalline materials scatter, offering important information about the phase composition and crystal structure. On the other hand, XRF detectors measure the fluorescence released when X-rays interact with the atoms of the material to determine the elemental composition of the sample. X-ray detectors are adaptable tools with many uses in a wide range of fields and businesses. In the fields of industrial inspection, scientific research, and medical diagnosis, among others, these detectors are essential for driving technological advancements, enhancing safety, and deepening our comprehension of the environment. The capabilities of detectors are expected to be further enhanced by ongoing innovation, opening up new applications and promoting advancement across a variety of fields (Kotter and Langer, 2002; Lança, Luís; Silva, Augusto, 2013).

Orientation and Directional Terms

Term	Definition	Illustration
Tomography	Tomography is an X-ray technique in which shadows of superimposed structures are blurred out by a moving X-ray tube.	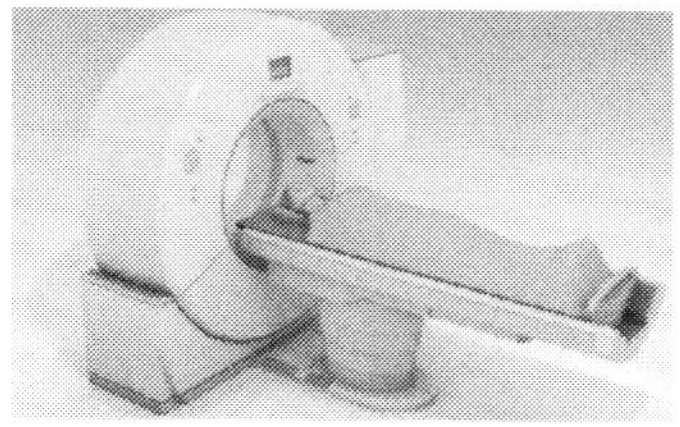
X-ray diffraction	It is a versatile non-destructive analytical technique used to analyze physical properties such as phase composition, crystal structure and orientation of powder, solid and liquid samples.	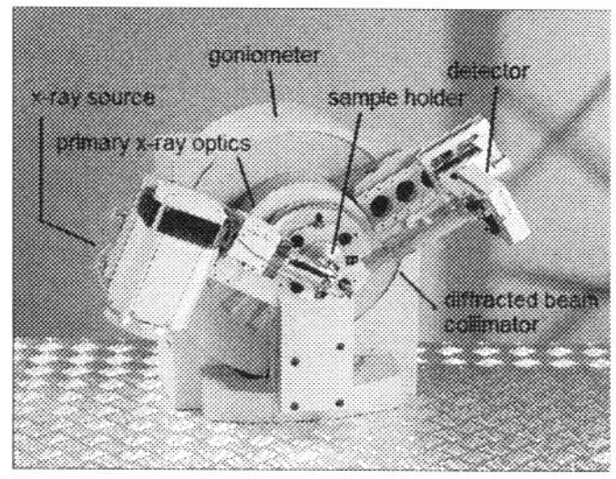
Photostimulable phosphor plate	Photostimulable phosphor plates (PSPs). Under a protection layer is a photo sensitive phosphor plate.	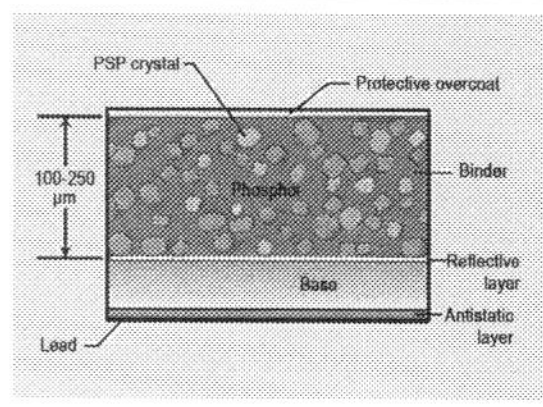 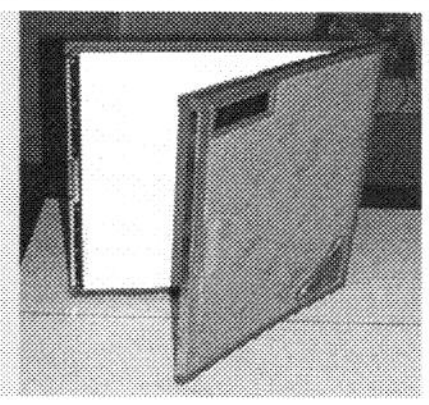
Fluoroscopy	Fluoroscopy is a type of medical imaging that shows a continuous X-ray image on a monitor, much like an X-ray movie.	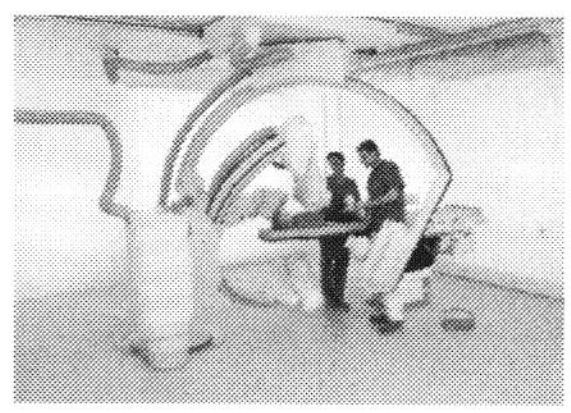
Silicon drift detectors	Silicon drift detectors (SDDs) are X-ray radiation detectors used in X-ray spectrometry (XRF and EDS) and electron microscopy.	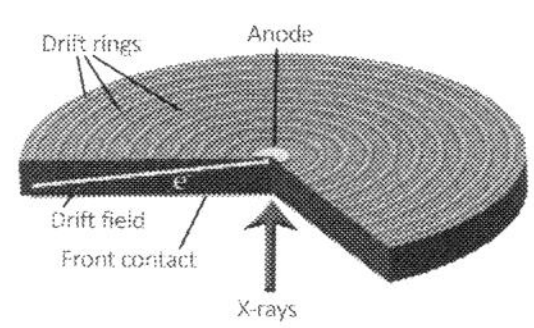

5.1. Overview of X-ray Detectors

Devices called X-ray detectors are used to measure an X-ray's flux, spectrum, spatial distribution, and/or other characteristics. Detectors fall into two main categories: dose measurement devices i.e., ionization chambers, Geiger counters, and dosimeters used to measure the local radiation exposure, dose, and/or dose rate, for example, to confirm that radiation protection equipment and procedures are effective continuously and imaging detectors (photographic film and X-ray plates, which are now mostly replaced by various digitizing devices like image plates or flat panel detectors).

5.1.1. X-ray Imaging

To capture an image using an image detector, the area of the patient that needs to be X-rayed is positioned between the X-ray source and the image receptor. This creates a representation of the internal structure of the specific body part in the form of a shadow. Denser tissues, like bone, partially obstruct (attenuate) the X-rays, while softer tissues allow them to pass through more easily. When the X-rays hit a certain area, it darkens upon development, making bones appear lighter in comparison to the surrounding soft tissues (Figure 5.1).

To highlight specific vessels, radiopaque contrast compounds containing barium or iodine can be injected into veins or arteries (for example, barium). High atomic number elements found in contrast compounds, such as bone, effectively block X-rays, making the formerly hollow organ or vessel easier to see. Numerous kinds of high atomic number elements were assessed in the search for nontoxic contrast materials. Certain elements that were selected turned out to be hazardous. For instance, thorium, which was once used as a contrast agent (Thorotrast), was found to be toxic and resulted in a very high cancer incidence decades after use. Although it is impossible to predict who might be sensitive to contrast, modern contrast materials have improved and there is a low risk of severe allergic reactions.

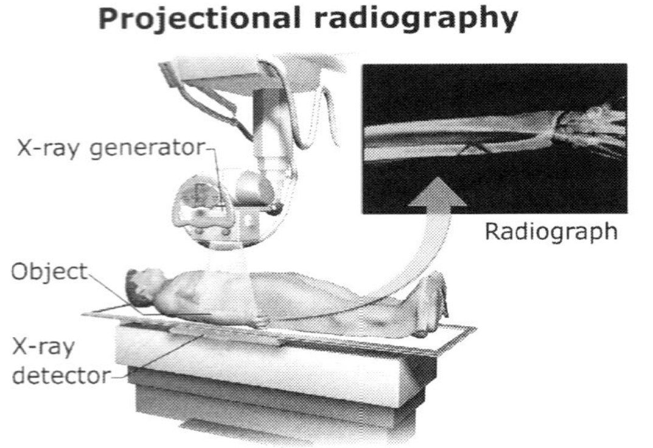

Figure 5.1. *Acquisition of projectional radiography, with an X-ray generator and an imaging detector.*

Source: https://upload.wikimedia.org/wikipedia/commons/thumb/d/db/Projectional_radiography_components.jpg/800px-Projectional_radiography_components.jpg.

5.1.2. X-ray Imaging Systems

Early X-ray sky images were created using collimated X-ray detectors, which involved placing a metal tube (known as a collimator) in front of the detector to limit the viewing direction to a small area. To achieve higher spatial resolution at X-ray energies, an imaging system is needed to focus the X-rays. Unlike visible light, X-ray photons cannot be focused using refraction or single scattering from a mirror at a normal angle, as X-rays will penetrate most materials. However, scattering at a grazing angle can help focus X-rays. The simplest X-ray telescope mirror design is a paraboloid shape, allowing X-rays along the axis to be focused by scattering at a grazing angle. While this type of mirror was used on the SAS-2 (Copernicus) satellite, it can only bring on-axis rays to focus, limiting the field of view due to aberrations for off-axis sources. Multiple scattering can focus X-rays both on-axis and off-axis at near grazing incidence. The "Wolter type I" configuration, which is comprised of concentric pairs of paraboloid–hyperboloid cylindrical mirror shells, is the most widely utilized mirror geometry in X-ray astronomy (Figure 5.2). Usually made of finely polished glass with a thin layer of dense material—like gold or iridium—that has a high enough X-ray reflectivity, the mirrors are constructed. The paraboloid–hyperboloid shell pairs are nested to provide a maximum scattering surface for the incident X-rays in order to maximize the scattering area.

When X-rays enter the mirror parallel to its axis, they first scatter off the paraboloid shells, which are followed by the hyperboloid shells, which focus the beam. The mirror collecting area, also known as the "effective area," is sensitive to photon energy and off-axis angle and is usually much less than one square meter in all situations. For instance, the largest X-ray telescope ever flown, the XMM-Newton Observatory, has an effective area that varies from approximately 0.6 square meters near 0.1 keV to 0.1 square meters near 10 keV. Because of the energy dependence of the scattering angle, the mirror focal length is dependent on photon energy (Kotter and Langer, 2002; Lança, Luís; Silva, Augusto, 2013).

Since the focal plane is typically curved, images captured with a plane parallel detector, for instance, will exhibit progressively more distortion as the off-axis angle increases. Even though a telescope's spatial resolving power is inversely related to photon wavelength, X-ray telescopes typically have far lower spatial resolution than optical telescopes with comparable collecting areas due to the practical challenges of focusing X-rays. The best X-ray imaging telescope ever flown is housed in the *Chandra* X-ray observatory; its absolute limiting resolution is roughly 0.5 seconds of arc. For comparison, the theoretical diffraction limit at 1 keV for *Chandra* is about 2.5×10^{-4} seconds of arc (Körner et al, 2007; Grupen, Claus; Buvat, Irène, 2012; Dance et al, 2014).

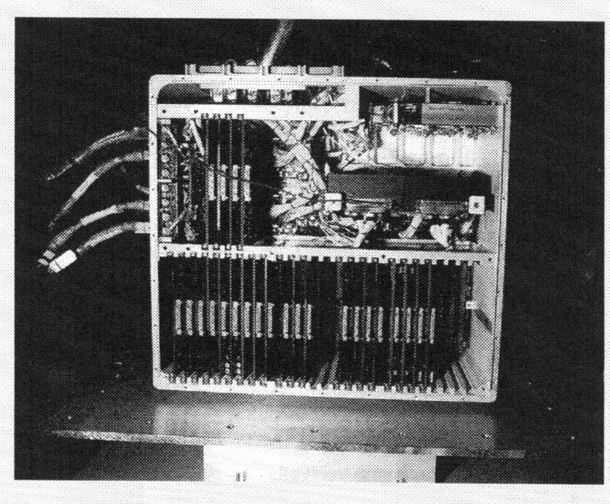

Figure 5.2. *HRC flight unit of Chandra*

Source: By NASA – http://chandra.harvard.edu/resources/chandraMission.html, Public Domain, https://commons.wikimedia.org/w/index.php?curid=23137241.

Wolter type I X-ray mirrors are often expensive to produce and launch due to the need for high tolerances in polishing and their heavy weight. To reduce costs, some mirrors use nested sets of thin, lightweight, conical aluminum foil shells to approximate the reflecting surface. While these thin-foil mirrors may sacrifice some angular resolution, they can provide greater throughput across a wide energy range by nesting hundreds of foils in a single mirror. This technology was first used by the Broad-band X-ray Telescope during the ASTRO-1 mission and later by the ASCA X-ray observatories.

5.1.2.1. X-ray Film

- **Mechanism:** Silver halide crystal grains, usually silver bromide, are present in typical X-ray film. It is possible to modify the grain size and composition to change the characteristics of the film, such as increasing the developed image's resolution. A latent image is formed when the film is exposed to radiation, which ionizes the halide and traps free electrons in crystal defects. These defects draw silver ions, which are then reduced to form clusters of transparent silver atoms. These are changed into opaque silver atoms during the developing process, which creates the visible image. The darkest area is where the greatest radiation was found. To stop further exposure, additional developing steps should be taken to remove unsensitized grains and stabilize the sensitized grains (e.g., from the visible light).

- **Replacement:** The action of X-rays on sensitized glass photographic plates produced the first radiographs, or X-ray images. Glass plates were quickly replaced by X-ray film, also known as photographic film, which has been used for decades to capture and present industrial and medical images. Digital computers eventually developed the capacity to display and store large enough amounts of data to enable digital imaging. While film technology is still widely used in industrial radiography processes, computerized and digital radiography have been the norm in medical and dental applications since the 1990s to examine the welded joints). Although it is easily recovered from used X-ray film, silver, which was once essential to the radiography and photography industries, is a non-renewable resource. Modern digital technologies do not require wet processing facilities, in contrast to X-ray films. Digital image preservation also reduces the need for physical storage.

5.1.2.2. Photostimulable Phosphors

Phosphor plate radiography uses photostimulated luminescence (PSL) to record X-rays, instead of traditional photographic plates. A photostimulable phosphor plate (PSP) is utilized in this method, with excited electrons in the phosphor material remaining 'trapped' in 'color centers until stimulated by a laser beam. The light emitted during laser stimulation is captured by a photomultiplier tube, and the resulting signal is converted into a digital image using computer technology. The PSP plate is reusable and can be used with existing X-ray equipment without any modifications. This technique is also referred to as computed radiography (CR).

5.1.2.3. Image Intensifiers

Additionally, X-rays are utilized in real-time procedures like contrast studies of the hollow organs (e.g., angiography). Fluoroscopy for a barium enema of the small or large intestine. X-ray-sensitive contrast is a key component of angioplasty, a medical procedure that treats arterial systemic diseases, to identify lesions that may be treated (Figure 5.3).

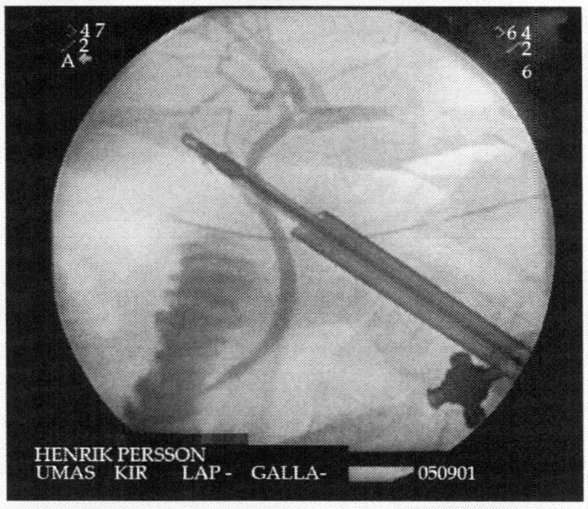

Figure 5.3. *Radiograph taken during cholecystectomy.*

Source: https://upload.wikimedia.org/wikipedia/commons/thumb/c/c7/Laprascopy-Roentgen.jpg/689px-Laprascopy-Roentgen.jpg.

5.1.2.4. Semiconductor Detectors

Solid state detectors detect X-rays by means of semiconductors. Because they directly convert X-ray photons to electrical charge and a digital image, direct digital detectors get their name. Intervening steps, such as first converting X-ray photons to visible light and then an electronic signal, may be present in indirect systems. In both systems, the electronic signal is read out and converted to a digital image using thin film transistors. Both systems are direct in the sense that they don't require manual scanning or a development step to produce a digital image, unlike film or CR. Comparing both kinds of systems to CR, the quantum efficiency is significantly higher.

- **Direct Detectors:** Si(Li) or Ge(Li) doped silicon or germanium semiconductor detectors have been developed since the 1970s. In the semiconductor, X-ray photons are transformed into electron-hole pairs, which are then obtained to detect X-rays. This technique, known as energy-dispersive X-ray spectroscopy (EDX or EDS), is frequently employed in tiny X-ray fluorescence spectrometers and allows for the direct determination of the X-ray energy spectrum when the temperature is low enough (the detector is cooled by Peltier effect or even cooler liquid nitrogen). Conventionally fabricated semiconductors are used to create silicon drift detectors (SDDs), which offer a high resolving power radiation measurement at a reasonable cost. In contrast to traditional X-ray detectors like Si(Li), they don't require liquid nitrogen cooling. These detectors are only effective at low energies and are seldom used for imaging.

Early in the new millennium, medical imaging began to see practical application. Because of its high spatial resolution and X-ray-absorbing qualities, amorphous selenium is utilized in commercial large area flat panel X-ray detectors for mammography and general radiography. However, because of the low atomic number of selenium, a thick layer is needed to obtain adequate sensitivity.

The semiconductor materials cadmium telluride (CdTe) and its zinc alloy, cadmium zinc telluride, are thought to be among the most promising for X-ray detection because of their high quantum number and wide band-gap, which enable high efficiency at room temperature operation. SPECT and bone densitometry are two current uses, but radiographic imaging-ready flat panel detectors are not yet on the market. Energy-resolving pixel detectors, like the HEXITEC detector from the Science and Technology Facilities Council and the Medipix detector from CERN, are the subject of current research and development. When exposed to an X-ray beam, common semiconductor diodes like 1N4007 or PIN photodiodes will generate a tiny amount of current in photovoltaic mode.

- **Indirect Detectors:** A scintillator is used in indirect detectors to convert X-rays into visible light, which a TFT array reads. Although there may be a resolution trade-off, this can offer sensitivity advantages over the current (amorphous selenium) direct detectors. Today, indirect flat panel detectors, or FPDs, are widely used in industrial, dental, veterinary, and medical settings.

  An amorphous or disordered layer of silicon is applied thinly to a glass sheet to form the TFT array. Millions of transistors are imprinted on the silicon at a microscopic level in an extremely ordered array that resembles the grid on a piece of graph paper. Every single pixel (picture element) is comprised of a light-absorbing photodiode, to which a thin-film transistor (TFT) is connected. When photons enter the photodiode, they split into electron-hole pairs, which are two types of electrical charge carriers. As the intensity of incoming light photons will determine how many charge carriers are produced, an electrical pattern is formed that can be quickly transformed into a voltage and then a digital signal, which is then processed by a computer to create a digital image. Despite its exceptional electronic qualities, silicon is not a very effective X-ray photon absorber. Because of this, scintillators composed of materials like gadolinium oxysulfide or caesium iodide are first affected by X-rays. The X-rays are absorbed by the scintillator, which then transforms them into photons of visible light that are transferred to the photodiode array (Körner et al, 2007; Grupen, Claus; Buvat, Irène, 2012; Dance et al, 2014).

5.1.3. Dose Measurement

5.1.3.1. Gas Detectors

A gas will become ionized when X-rays pass through it, creating free electrons and positive ions. According to its energy, an arriving photon will produce a certain number of these ion pairs. Ions and electrons in the gas chamber will move in different directions if there is an electric field present, which will result in a detectable current. The applied voltage and the chamber's geometry will determine how the gas behaves. Ionization chambers extract all ions and electrons before their recombination using a comparatively low electric field of approximately 100 V/cm. As a result, the current is constant and proportionate to the dose rate that the gas is exposed to. To measure radiation dose levels, ion chambers are frequently used as portable radiation survey meters.

A thin, positively charged anode wire is positioned in the center of a cylindrical chamber in proportional counter geometry. The majority of the gas volume will function as an ionization chamber, but the electric field is strong enough to cause gas molecules to become ionized in the area nearest to the wire. An avalanche effect will result, significantly boosting the output signal. The amount of charge accumulated is proportional to the number of ion pairs produced by the absorbed X-ray because each electron causes an avalanche that is roughly the same size. This enables the energy of each incoming photon to be measured.

UV photons are produced by Geiger-Müller counters by using an even higher electric field. These initiate fresh avalanches, which ultimately cause the gas surrounding the anode wire to become completely ionized. As a result, the signal is amplified but there is a dead time following each event, which prevents the X-ray energies from being measured. Gas detectors are typically single-pixel detectors that only measure the number of interacting photons or the average dose rate over the gas volume, as previously mentioned. However, by placing numerous crossed wires in a wire chamber, it is possible to make the detectors spatially resolving.

5.1.3.2. Silicon PN Solar Cells

The ability of silicon PN solar cells to detect all types of ionizing radiation, including hard X-rays, soft X-rays, and extreme UV, was proven in the 1960s. Photoionization, the process by which ionizing radiation strikes an atom and releases a free electron, is how this type of detection works. A solar cell, an ammeter, and a visible light filter that lets in unwanted wavelengths but blocks ionizing radiation from reaching the solar cell are needed for this kind of broadband ionizing radiation sensor.

5.1.3.3. Radiochromic Film

Self-developing radiochromic film can provide very high resolution measurements, for dosimetry and profiling purposes, particularly in radiotherapy physics.

5.1.4. Production and Detection of X-rays

5.1.4.1. Production of X-rays

The acceleration of a charged particle, atomic transitions between discrete energy levels, and the radioactive decay of some atomic nuclei are the three common processes that produce X-rays. Every mechanism produces an X-ray radiation spectrum that is unique to it. Accelerating electric charges produce electromagnetic waves, according to the theory of classical electromagnetism. An intense electron beam strikes a solid target in the most prevalent terrestrial X-ray source, the X-ray tube. The beam's fast-moving electrons are repeatedly deflected and slowed as they interact with the target atoms' electrons and nuclei. Bremsstrahlung, or "braking radiation" in German, is a continuous spectrum of electromagnetic radiation with a peak intensity in the X-ray region that is emitted by the beam electrons during this sudden deceleration. This continuous spectrum contains the majority of the energy emitted by an X-ray tube. Synchrotron particle accelerators and storage rings are sources of a continuum of X-rays that are far more potent (and larger). Strong magnets confine charged particles (usually electrons or positrons) to a closed orbit after they are accelerated to extremely high energies (billions of electron volts) in a synchrotron. The charged particles emit what is known as synchrotron radiation when they are deflected by the magnetic fields, which accelerates them due to the change in motion direction. The intensity and frequency distribution of this continuum are dictated by the strength of the magnetic fields and the energy of the circulating particles. X-ray investigations of materials are conducted worldwide using specially engineered synchrotron light sources.

The target material in an X-ray tube emits a spectrum of discrete X-ray emission lines in addition to the continuous spectrum of radiation produced by the decelerating electrons. This "characteristic radiation" is produced when the target atoms are excited by collisions with the swiftly moving electrons. Usually, an atom's tightly bound inner-shell electron is expelled first by a collision, and a loosely bound outer-shell electron enters the inner shell to fill the vacancy. A single photon with an energy equal to the difference between the inner-shell and outer-shell vacancy states is released by the atom during this process. In the X-ray region of the spectrum, photon wavelengths typically correspond to this energy difference. When a target material is exposed to a primary X-ray beam, it can also produce characteristic X-ray radiation. The series of electron transitions that lead to the emission of secondary X-ray photons is started by the primary X-ray photons.

Atomic changes can occasionally result in the production of X-rays as a byproduct. The atomic nucleus absorbs an inner-shell atomic electron during the electron capture process, which reduces the atomic number by one and starts the conversion of a nuclear proton into a neutron. An outer-shell electron swiftly fills the empty inner-shell orbit, resulting in the production of a distinctive X-ray photon. An X-ray photon can also occasionally be released when an excited nucleus relaxes to a lower energy state. But the photons released in the majority of these kinds of nuclear transitions are even more energetic than X-rays; they belong to the gamma-ray region of the electromagnetic spectrum.

Over the past 50 years, a large number of astronomical sources of X-rays have been found; taken as a whole, they represent a wealth of data regarding the universe (X-ray sources). The hot corona of the Sun and the coronas of other common stars in the Milky Way Galaxy both emit X-rays. There are a lot of binary star systems that release a lot of X-rays; the most powerful ones generate over 1,000 times the solar energy in the X-ray region alone. Another powerful source of X-rays is supernova remnants, which are occasionally linked to atomic emissions from extremely hot gases (in the range of 10 million kelvins) or synchrotron radiation from high-energy charged particles circling in strong magnetic fields. Strong extragalactic X-ray sources, such as quasars, galactic clusters, and active galaxies, are presently the subject of intensive scientific investigation; however, in certain instances, the precise mechanisms underlying X-ray production remain unclear or unclear. Since the Earth's atmosphere absorbs X-rays heavily, satellites in orbit are required to make astronomical observations in the X-ray region.

5.1.4.2. Detection of X-rays

Röntgen was one of the first people to use photographic film as an X-ray detector, and this straightforward method is still widely used in medical applications. Radiation-sensitive silver halide crystals in an emulsion on the film surface are exposed by X-ray photons, which causes a photochemical change in the affected crystals that darkens the exposed area.

Even though photographic methods have advanced significantly since Röntgen's day and are still very helpful for qualitative applications, they are not ideal for more precise measurements of X-ray intensities and spectral content. Many more potent detection techniques have been created. Atoms in a gas-filled volume are ionized by incoming X-ray photons in a Geiger-Müller tube, also known as a Geiger counter. A high voltage is applied to cause additional ionizations from collisions between freed electrons and neutral atoms, which results in an easily detectable electrical pulse and an avalanche of charged particles. More advanced detection techniques that distinguish between X-rays of various energies rely on the ionization of gas atoms. Other widely used detection techniques rely on capacity of the X-rays to separate charges in semiconductors and cause visible fluorescence in crystals.

5.1.5. Digital X-ray Detector

5.1.5.1. 2D Digital Radiography X-ray Detectors

A digital radiography device that instantly generates a digital image on a computer screen is called a digital X-ray detector. It is used for X-ray inspection of objects. Digital radiography (DR) gathers information about an object while it is being imaged using X-ray-sensitive plates or a digital detector array. Without the need for an intermediary system, the data can be sent in real time to a computer, producing high-quality images with an enhanced signal-to-noise ratio. Many industrial applications use digital X-ray detectors because the non-destructive method produces high-quality images fast, effectively, and affordably.

The photodiode, readout electronics, and scintillator are the main parts of a digital X-ray detector. X-rays are converted into visible light by the scintillator after they have passed through the object being scanned. The light is subsequently transformed by the photodiode into an electrical signal that the electronic readout can use to create a digital image that shows the scanned object's results.

5.1.5.2. Advantages of Digital X-ray Detectors

There are several benefits that digital X-ray detectors have over traditional film imaging methods. One major advantage is that digital X-ray detectors scan objects much faster than analog ones, providing high-quality images in a matter of seconds. Another benefit is that digital X-ray detectors are more efficient at capturing X-rays, which means less radiation is used by the machine to create the final image. To summarize, the main benefits of digital X-ray detectors are:

- High-quality images
- Faster capture and results
- In-line and at-line capabilities for production environments
- Lower radiation emissions
- Can be enhanced with computed tomography (CT)

5.1.5.3. Applications of Digital X-ray Detectors

Digital X-ray detectors are advantageous in both industrial and medical contexts for a broad range of industries and applications. But unlike medical equipment, the industrial X-ray solutions covered in this blog are different. Industrial radiography is used for metrology measurements both internally and externally, defect detection, quality control, and process optimization on manufactured components. In industries like aerospace, automotive, medical devices, and electronics where quality is critical and manufactured parts safety is paramount, this inspection method is invaluable (Körner et al, 2007; Grupen, Claus; Buvat, Irène, 2012; Dance et al, 2014).

5.2. X-ray Generation and Detection

The production and detection of X-rays depend on a number of critical factors that are essential to the reliability and security of medical imaging. The X-ray tube, which produces X-rays through electron acceleration towards an anode, is the central component of X-ray technology. The anode material, tube voltage (kVp), and tube current (mA) are the parameters that control this process. The energy of the X-rays generated is determined by tube voltage (kVp). Elevated voltages produce more X-rays that penetrate deeper, which is essential for imaging denser tissues like bone. The amount of electrons passing through the tube in a given amount of time is determined by the tube current (mA), which has a direct impact on the X-ray beam's intensity. Radiographers can balance patient dose and image quality while customizing imaging to meet unique clinical requirements by modifying these parameters.

An additional crucial component is filtration. Low-energy photons are preferentially absorbed by the body as X-rays pass through it, decreasing image contrast and raising patient dose. These low-energy photons are selectively removed by filters, which are usually composed of aluminum or other materials. This improves image quality while lowering needless radiation exposure. Selecting the right anode material is essential. Because of its high melting point and effective X-ray production, tungsten is widely used. The anode target's rotation speed and angle, among other things, have an impact on heat dissipation and the effectiveness of X-ray production.

X-ray detectors are essential in the detection process. Digital detectors, which can be flat-panel detectors or computed radiography (CR) systems, have largely replaced traditional film-based detectors. For interpretation, these detectors transform X-rays into electrical signals or digital pictures. Radiation dose and image quality are directly impacted by detector size, material, and efficiency.

The term "spatial resolution" describes an imaging system's capacity to discern minute structures. Improved visualization of minute details, which is essential for identifying subtle abnormalities, is made possible by higher spatial resolution. Conversely, contrast resolution describes the system's capacity to distinguish between tissues with various X-ray attenuation characteristics. Optimizing both forms of resolution improves the precision of the diagnosis. In X-ray imaging, noise and scatter radiation present major challenges. Image quality can be lowered by noise, which can come from statistical fluctuations or electronic interference. Algorithms for image processing and signal averaging are two strategies that reduce noise. The interaction of X-rays with bodily tissues produces scatter radiation, which lessens the contrast and clarity of images. Using a grid and properly collimating reduces scatter, which enhances image quality. A precise parameter balance is required for both X-ray generation and detection optimization to produce high-quality images with the least amount of radiation exposure. For diagnostic imaging in healthcare to be safe and effective, it is imperative to comprehend and manage these parameters.

5.2.1. Key Parameters

Key parameters involved in X-ray generation and detection include:

1. **X-ray Tube Voltage (kVp)**: The voltage applied across the X-ray tube determines the energy of the X-rays produced. Higher voltages generate higher energy X-rays, capable of penetrating denser materials.
2. **X-ray Tube Current (mA)**: The tube current represents the flow of electrons within the X-ray tube. Higher tube currents result in more X-rays being produced, leading to increased image brightness.
3. **Filtration**: X-ray beams often pass through filters to remove lower-energy photons, reducing patient dose and improving image quality by reducing scatter.
4. **Anode Material**: The material of the anode affects the X-ray spectrum. Common materials include tungsten

due to its high melting point and efficient X-ray production.

5. **Exposure Time**: The duration for which X-rays are emitted from the tube. Longer exposure times generally result in higher radiation doses but can improve image quality in certain cases.
6. **X-ray Detector Efficiency**: Efficiency of the detector in converting incident X-rays into electrical signals. Higher efficiency detectors produce clearer images with lower radiation exposure.
7. **Detector Material**: Different materials are used for X-ray detectors, including scintillator materials (such as cesium iodide or gadolinium oxysulfide) and semiconductor materials (such as amorphous selenium or silicon). Each material has its own characteristics affecting sensitivity, resolution, and cost.
8. **Contrast Resolution**: The ability of the imaging system to differentiate between tissues with different X-ray attenuation properties. Higher contrast resolution allows for better differentiation between structures with similar densities.
9. **Noise**: Undesirable variations in the image caused by factors such as electronic interference or statistical fluctuations in the number of X-rays detected. Minimizing noise is crucial for achieving high image quality.
10. **Scatter Radiation**: X-rays that deviate from the primary beam path and interact with surrounding materials. Scatter radiation reduces image contrast and can obscure details, so techniques such as collimation and grid use are employed to minimize its effects.

Understanding and controlling these parameters are essential for optimizing X-ray imaging for diagnostic purposes while minimizing patient dose and maximizing image quality.

5.2.2. Image Receptor Format

The size and form of the medium used to capture X-ray images are determined by the image receptor format, which is an essential component of medical imaging systems. In radiology departments, the choice of image receptor format has a major impact on image quality, diagnostic precision, and workflow efficiency. In contemporary radiology, one of the most widely used image receptor formats is the digital flat-panel detector (FPD), which has essentially supplanted older film-based and computed radiography (CR) systems. An array of photodiodes or thin-film transistors (TFTs) is used in FPDs to capture the emitted light or charge and convert it into a digital signal. The scintillator layer transforms X-rays into visible light or directly into electric charge.

Comparing digital FPDs to conventional film-based systems reveals a number of benefits. First of all, they offer instantaneous image capture and display, which cuts down on the time needed for film processing and overall examination. In busy radiology departments, this quick turnaround time improves workflow efficiency and patient throughput. In addition, compared to film, digital FPDs have a larger dynamic range and are more sensitive to X-rays, producing images with better contrast and detail resolution. Additionally, digital images are simple to electronically store, retrieve, and transmit, making them useful for archiving, integration with picture archiving and communication systems, and remote consultations (PACS). The physical size, or active area, of an image receptor format is another crucial factor. Larger detectors have a larger surface area, which makes it possible to image larger anatomical regions in a single exposure and minimizes the need for the patient to be repositioned during image acquisition. This reduces radiation exposure and motion artifacts while simultaneously increasing patient comfort and the effectiveness of the examination.

Furthermore, optimizing image composition and visualization is greatly influenced by the aspect ratio of the image receptor format. For imaging structures like the chest or abdomen, for instance, where a panoramic view is frequently needed to capture the entire area of interest, a wide aspect ratio is beneficial. On the other hand, an almost square or square shape might be better for imaging the extremities since it makes better use of the detector's space and exposes the surrounding tissues to less radiation than is necessary.

Moreover, the image receptor assembly's thickness is a crucial factor to take into account, especially for portable or mobile imaging systems. More flexibility and maneuverability are provided by thinner detectors, which facilitate patient positioning and access in a variety of clinical settings, such as operating rooms, emergency rooms, and intensive care units. Furthermore, thinner detectors reduce geometric distortion and maximize image sharpness by minimizing the distance between the X-ray source and the image receptor.

Advanced image receptor technologies, including photon-counting detectors and amorphous selenium (a-Se) direct-conversion detectors, have become increasingly popular in recent years. Photon-counting detectors provide improved energy resolution and noise performance, allowing for spectral imaging and material decomposition techniques that enhance tissue characterization and contrast. Additionally, a-Se detectors convert X-rays directly into electrical charge without a scintillator layer, leading to higher detective quantum efficiency (DQE) and better image quality while minimizing radiation exposure.

A vital part of medical imaging systems, the image receptor format has a big impact on workflow effectiveness, diagnostic precision, and image quality. The choice of an appropriate format for an image receptor should take into account elements like thickness, aspect ratio, physical size, and detector technology in order to maximize image interpretation and acquisition while reducing radiation exposure to the patient and lengthening the examination period. Image receptor technology developments keep radiology innovative by opening up new imaging modalities and applications for better patient care.

5.2.3. Spatial Resolution

In medical imaging, the term "spatial resolution" describes an imaging system's capacity to distinguish minute details or structures inside an object that is being imaged. It is an important parameter since it directly affects the final image's sharpness and clarity, which influences the capacity of clinicians to make precise diagnoses.

In the context of spatial resolution, there are two main components to consider: intrinsic resolution and system resolution.

1. **Intrinsic Resolution**: This is the imaging system's intrinsic spatial resolution limit, which is established by variables like the detector pixel size, the X-ray focal spot size, and the separation between the X-ray source and the object being imaged. A smaller focal spot size in X-ray imaging results in a narrower X-ray

beam, which sharpens image details and improves spatial resolution. Higher spatial resolution can also be achieved by using smaller detector pixels to capture finer details.

2. **System Resolution**: System resolution includes all elements—X-ray source, detectors, electronics, and image processing algorithms—that have an impact on the overall imaging system's spatial resolution. A few examples of the variables that affect system resolution are geometric magnification, noise, scatter radiation, and image reconstruction methods. Maximizing spatial resolution and image quality requires optimizing these factors.

Several techniques can be employed to improve spatial resolution in X-ray imaging:

- **Focal Spot Size Optimization**: Using X-ray tubes with smaller focal spots can enhance spatial resolution by reducing the blurring effect caused by the finite size of the focal spot.
- **Detector Pixel Size Reduction**: Decreasing the size of detector pixels allows for finer details to be captured, improving spatial resolution. However, this must be balanced with the need to maintain sufficient signal-to-noise ratio and detector efficiency.
- **Geometric Magnification**: Increasing the distance between the X-ray source and the detector, or by placing the object closer to the X-ray source, can magnify the image and enhance spatial resolution. This technique is commonly used in mammography to visualize small breast lesions.
- **Image Processing Algorithms**: Advanced image processing techniques such as edge enhancement, deconvolution, and iterative reconstruction can help improve spatial resolution by enhancing image sharpness and contrast.
- **Scatter Radiation Control**: Minimizing scatter radiation through the use of anti-scatter grids, collimators, and beam filters can improve spatial resolution by reducing background noise and improving image contrast.

The capacity to see minute anatomical details and identify minute abnormalities is directly impacted by the crucial X-ray imaging parameter known as spatial resolution. Through the optimization of various factors like focal spot size, detector pixel size, geometric magnification, and image processing techniques, medical imaging professionals can enhance their diagnostic accuracy and attain higher spatial resolution.

5.2.4. Frame Rate

Frame rate, usually measured in frames per second (fps), is the quantity of individual frames or images shown or recorded per unit of time.

In medical imaging, frame rate plays a crucial role in various modalities, such as fluoroscopy, ultrasound, and certain types of dynamic imaging.

1. **Fluoroscopy**: Fluoroscopy is a real-time visualization technique that uses a continuous X-ray beam to see moving anatomical structures, like the digestive

system during a barium swallow or the cardiovascular system during a cardiac catheterization. In fluoroscopy, the frame rate controls the smoothness of the motion display. Increased frame rates lead to improved temporal resolution and smoother motion, which facilitate quicker procedural guidance and more precise dynamic process assessment.

2. **Ultrasound**: The speed at which individual ultrasound frames are recorded and shown, each representing a distinct moment in time, is referred to as the frame rate in ultrasound imaging. Better visualization of quick physiological processes, like blood flow dynamics or cardiac motion, is made possible by a higher frame rate. This is especially significant for echocardiography and vascular imaging, where accurate timing is essential for determining abnormalities in blood flow and diagnosing diseases like arrhythmias.
3. **Dynamic Imaging**: In dynamic imaging methods like computed tomography (CT) perfusion studies and magnetic resonance imaging (MRI), where successive images are collected over time to evaluate tissue perfusion or contrast enhancement patterns, frame rate is also crucial. A higher frame rate enables more precise temporal resolution, which is useful for diagnosing diseases like tumors or strokes because it captures fast changes in tissue perfusion dynamics.

In medical imaging, achieving the ideal frame rate necessitates striking a balance between many variables, including data storage capacity, temporal and spatial resolution, and imaging modality. A higher frame rate usually calls for faster image processing and acquisition capabilities, which could mean more advanced imaging methods or more powerful hardware.

The right frame rate in clinical practice is determined by the particular imaging application and the clinical question being answered. For instance, higher frame rates are usually needed in cardiac imaging—where rapid motion is involved—to clearly see cardiac function and identify abnormalities. In contrast, frame rate might not be as important in some static imaging applications, like radiography or non-contrast CT, and more focus might be on enhancing other aspects of image quality, like spatial resolution or contrast resolution.

The quality and clinical utility of dynamic imaging studies are directly impacted by the frame rate, a fundamental parameter in medical imaging. Healthcare providers can obtain high-quality imaging data that improves patient care and diagnostic accuracy by optimizing frame rates to suit particular clinical applications.

5.2.5. The Direct and Indirect Mode of Operation

In digital radiography (DR) systems, there are two different ways to transform X-ray photons into digital signals for processing and image capture: the direct mode and the indirect mode. Each of these modes has pros and cons of its own and varies in how it detects and transforms X-ray energy into electrical signals.

5.2.5.1. Direct Mode of Operation

In the direct mode, a high atomic number and density detector material, such as cadmium telluride (CdTe) or amorphous selenium (a-

Se), directly converts X-ray photons into electrical signals. When incident X-ray photons create electron-hole pairs in these materials, a phenomenon known as photoconductivity occurs, resulting in a detectable electrical current.

Advantages of the direct mode include:

- High efficiency in converting X-ray energy into electrical signals, resulting in excellent detective quantum efficiency (DQE) and image quality.
- Minimal light scattering, which helps preserve spatial resolution and contrast.
- Simplified detector structure, potentially leading to lower manufacturing costs and improved reliability.

However, the direct mode also has limitations:

- **Limited Material Availability:** Materials suitable for direct conversion are often expensive and challenging to manufacture.
- **Thickness Constraints:** Direct conversion detectors need to be relatively thick to capture sufficient X-ray energy, which can limit spatial resolution and increase manufacturing complexity.

5.2.5.2. Indirect Mode of Operation

In the indirect mode, a scintillator material, such as cesium iodide (CsI) or gadolinium oxysulfide (Gd2O2S), absorbs X-ray photons first and then reacts to the exposure to X-rays by emitting visible light photons. An array of photo-detectors, usually thin-film transistors (TFTs) or amorphous silicon (a-Si) photodiodes, is then used to convert these light photons into electrical signals. The advantages of the indirect mode include:

- Greater flexibility in scintillator material selection, allowing for optimization of properties such as X-ray absorption efficiency, light output, and cost.
- Improved spatial resolution compared to direct conversion detectors, as scintillator thickness can be optimized independently of X-ray absorption requirements.
- Compatibility with existing detector technologies, facilitating the integration of indirect conversion systems into conventional radiographic equipment.

However, the indirect mode also has some drawbacks:

- Light scattering within the scintillator material can degrade spatial resolution and contrast, particularly in thicker detectors.
- Additional noise sources associated with the conversion of light photons to electrical signals may reduce overall image quality.
- Lower DQE compared to direct conversion detectors, resulting in reduced signal-to-noise ratio and potentially inferior image quality, especially at lower radiation doses.

In digital radiography, the direct and indirect modes of operation present particular benefits and drawbacks. The selection of one of these modes is contingent upon various factors, including the intended image quality, financial constraints, and particular clinical uses. Improvements in both modes are being driven by advances in detector technology, which aims to improve patient safety, efficiency, and image quality in digital radiography systems.

5.2.6. Principles of the Direct-Conversion Digital X-ray Image Detector

A crucial part of contemporary digital radiography systems is the direct-conversion digital X-ray image detector, which is made to convert incident X-ray photons straight into electrical signals without the need for any intermediate steps that involve light emission. Compared to indirect-conversion detectors, this method has many benefits, such as increased efficiency, better spatial resolution, and lower noise. The basic idea behind how direct-conversion detectors work is that X-ray photons interact with a semiconductor material, usually amorphous selenium (a-Se), to produce electron-hole pairs that are subsequently obtained to produce an electrical signal.

The key principles of the direct-conversion digital X-ray image detector:

1. **Photoelectric Effect**: The direct-conversion detector relies on the photoelectric effect, where X-ray photons are absorbed by the semiconductor material, leading to the ejection of inner-shell electrons from atoms within the material. This process occurs preferentially at lower X-ray energies and is highly efficient in materials with high atomic number and density, such as a-Se.
2. **Electron-Hole Pair Generation**: The ejected electrons create electron-hole pairs within the semiconductor material as they move through the crystal lattice. These electron-hole pairs represent the conversion of X-ray energy into electrical charge, which serves as the primary signal for image formation.
3. **Charge Collection**: Once generated, the electron-hole pairs are separated by an applied electric field within the detector, with the electrons drifting towards the positively biased electrode and the holes towards the negatively biased electrode. This charge separation process ensures that the electrical signal produced is proportional to the incident X-ray energy, enabling accurate detection and quantification of X-ray photons.
4. **Charge Integration**: As X-ray photons are continuously absorbed by the detector during the exposure, the generated electron-hole pairs accumulate, resulting in a net electrical charge proportional to the total X-ray exposure. This accumulated charge represents the raw image signal and is subsequently read out and digitized for image reconstruction and display.
5. **Amorphous Selenium Structure**: Direct-conversion detectors typically utilize amorphous selenium as the semiconductor material due to its high atomic number, high X-ray absorption efficiency, and low dark current. The a-Se layer is typically deposited on a conductive substrate and biased to create the necessary electric field for charge collection and transport.
6. **Thin-Film Transistor (TFT) Array**: Direct-conversion detectors often incorporate a thin-film transistor (TFT) array for pixel-level readout and signal processing. Each pixel in the detector array is

connected to a TFT switch, allowing for independent readout and manipulation of the electrical signal from each detector element.

Direct-conversion digital X-ray detectors provide better image quality, efficiency, and dose performance than indirect-conversion detectors because they make use of the photoelectric effect and charge transport within semiconductor materials. Modern digital radiography systems rely heavily on these detectors to provide high-resolution imaging with low noise and enhanced contrast sensitivity for a variety of clinical applications.

5.3. The Ideal X-ray Photoconductor

A material that effectively transforms incident X-ray photons into electrical signals with high sensitivity, stability, and spatial resolution while reducing noise and radiation dose is the perfect X-ray photoconductor. The physical characteristics of the material, such as its atomic number, density, bandgap energy, mobility, and stability, as well as its suitability for fabrication into thin-film structures compatible with digital radiography systems, must be carefully taken into account to achieve these characteristics.

Amorphous selenium (a-Se), a semiconductor with a high atomic number (Z=34), high X-ray absorption efficiency, and an appropriate bandgap energy for X-ray photon absorption, is one of the most promising materials for X-ray photoconductors. Since a-Se doesn't have a hexagonal lattice structure like crystalline selenium does, it's better suited for thin-film deposition on materials like glass or plastic. Because of its amorphous structure, large-area detectors with consistent X-ray sensitivity can be produced with more design and fabrication flexibility.

The main method by which a-Se transforms X-ray photons into electrical signals is the photoelectric effect. Through the ejection of inner-shell electrons, an X-ray photon's interaction with a-Se creates electron-hole pairs inside the material. The X-ray photon flux can be directly measured thanks to these electron-hole pairs, which produce an electrical current that is proportional to the incident X-ray energy. The energy of the incident X-ray photons, the thickness of the detector layer, and the X-ray absorption coefficient of a-Se are some of the variables that affect how efficient this process is.

To precisely capture minute details in X-ray images, the perfect X-ray photoconductor must have outstanding spatial resolution in addition to high sensitivity. The size of the detector pixels, the a-Se layer's thickness, and the material's capacity to transfer charge carriers without diffusion or recombination are some of the variables that affect spatial resolution. Thin-film transistor (TFT) arrays are frequently used in a-Se detectors for pixel-level readout and signal processing to achieve high spatial resolution. With the help of these TFT arrays, each detector element's electrical signal can be precisely controlled, resulting in high-resolution imaging with little distortion or blur.

For X-ray photoconductors, stability and dependability are crucial factors, especially in clinical settings where reliable performance is necessary for precise diagnosis. Under normal operating conditions, amorphous selenium shows good stability with low dark current and little degradation over time. But to guarantee dependability in practical applications, a-Se detectors' long-term performance can be impacted by variables like temperature, humidity, and radiation exposure. For this reason, careful design and strong encapsulation techniques are required. Noise is an important factor to consider when it comes to X-ray imaging systems. It can have a negative impact on image quality and the accuracy of diagnoses. Common sources of noise in a-Se detectors are electronic, thermal, and quantum noise caused by the randomized nature of X-ray photon interactions. To reduce noise, a-Se detectors use methods like signal averaging, noise filtering, and advanced image processing algorithms to enhance the signal-to-noise ratio and improve image quality. Amorphous selenium is an ideal X-ray photoconductor material due to its high sensitivity, spatial resolution, stability, and low noise levels, making it suitable for use in digital radiography systems. With its promising characteristics, a-Se is a strong contender for X-ray imaging applications, and ongoing research aims to enhance the performance and reliability of a-Se detectors to meet the ever-changing demands of the medical imaging field.

5.3.1. Intrinsic Resolution of X-ray Photoconductors

The ability of clinicians to accurately detect and diagnose medical conditions is influenced by the clarity and sharpness of X-ray images, which is largely dependent on the intrinsic resolution of X-ray photoconductors. The ability of a photoconductor material to precisely capture and spatially resolve fine details in an X-ray image without noticeably degrading or distorting the image is known as intrinsic resolution. It takes careful consideration of different material properties and device parameters, along with optimization of fabrication processes and imaging system design, to achieve high intrinsic resolution.

A major determinant of the intrinsic resolution of X-ray photoconductors is the physical structure and composition of the material. When it comes to X-ray photoconductors, amorphous selenium (a-Se) is one of the most popular materials because of its high atomic number (Z=34), high absorption efficiency, and appropriate bandgap energy for absorbing X-ray photons. In order to achieve high spatial resolution in X-ray imaging, uniform X-ray sensitivity and efficient charge transport are made possible by the amorphous structure of a-Se, which lacks long-range order.

Intrinsic resolution is also highly dependent on the size and dispersion of the detector elements, also known as pixels. Finer spatial sampling of the X-ray image is made possible by smaller pixel sizes, which improves the visibility of minute anatomical structures and minute abnormalities. However, since smaller pixels may show more noise and less sensitivity to X-ray photons, reducing pixel size must be balanced with factors like the signal-to-noise ratio, detector fill factor, and manufacturing complexity.

Intrinsic resolution is influenced by the thickness of the photoconductor layer in addition to pixel size. More accurate localization of X-ray photon interactions is made possible by thinner detector layers, which also improve spatial resolution and lessen blur. To attain the ideal balance between sensitivity and resolution, the material thickness must be carefully optimized because thinner layers may also show decreased X-ray absorption efficiency and increased noise. Intrinsic resolution is also influenced by the generation and transport of charge carriers that follow the interaction of X-ray photons with the photoconductor material. In a-Se detectors, the main process by which X-ray photons are absorbed and transformed into electrical signals is the photoelectric effect. Because of this process's high efficiency at lower X-ray energies, soft tissue imaging can achieve better spatial resolution. Higher X-ray energies, however, may cause more image blur and decreased resolution due to other interaction mechanisms like Compton scattering and pair production, especially in thicker detector layers. Moreover, intrinsic resolution can be influenced by the electronics used in X-ray photoconductors for readout and signal processing. High-resolution imaging with low noise and distortion is made possible by advanced readout techniques like thin-film transistor (TFT) arrays and charge-coupled devices (CCDs), which enable pixel-level readout and signal processing. In addition, complex image processing algorithms can improve the final image's contrast and sharpness, minimize artifacts, and correct for distortions to further improve intrinsic resolution.

A combination of device design, imaging system integration, and material optimization is needed to achieve high intrinsic resolution in X-ray photoconductors. Through meticulous manipulation of variables like pixel size, layer thickness, material structure, and readout electronics, scientists and engineers can create X-ray photoconductors that generate superior quality images with remarkable spatial resolution, facilitating precise diagnosis and treatment in medical imaging applications. Future improvements in X-ray detector technology could lead to even higher intrinsic resolution and greater potential for digital radiography systems in the medical field.

5.3.2. Absorption, Photoconductor Thickness, and Carrier Schubwegs

Critical parameters that affect the performance of X-ray photoconductors in digital radiography systems are absorption, photoconductor thickness, and carrier Schubwegs (mean free paths). Optimizing image quality, sensitivity, and spatial resolution in medical imaging applications requires an understanding of how these factors interact.

1. **Absorption**: The interaction of X-ray photons with photoconductor material, which results in the transfer of energy to the material's electrons and the creation of electron-hole pairs, is called absorption. High atomic number (Z) elements like selenium have high X-ray absorption coefficients, which make them effective absorbers of X-ray photons in X-ray photoconductors like amorphous selenium (a-Se). The conversion of incident X-ray energy into electrical signals, which are subsequently processed to produce digital X-ray images, depends on this absorption process. The photoconductor material's sensitivity to X-ray photons is directly influenced by its absorption efficiency; higher absorption coefficients result in stronger signals and better image quality.
2. **Photoconductor Thickness**: Sensitivity and spatial resolution of X-ray detectors are highly dependent on the thickness of the photoconductor layer. More accurate localization of X-ray photon interactions is made possible by thinner photoconductor layers, which enhances spatial resolution and produces sharper image details. Less X-ray absorption efficiency, on the other hand, might be seen in thinner layers, which could result in a lower signal-to-noise ratio and less sensitivity to X-ray photons. Conversely, thicker layers of photoconductor improve the efficiency of X-ray absorption, but because of the increased scatter and diffusion of charge carriers, they may cause blur and decrease spatial resolution. Thus, in digital radiography systems, optimizing photoconductor thickness is essential to strike a balance between

sensitivity and spatial resolution.

3. **Carrier Schubwegs (Mean Free Paths)**: The average distance that charge carriers—holes and electrons—travel within the photoconductor material before scattering or recombination is known as a carrier Schubweg, or mean free path. Carrier Schubwegs affect the transport of charge carriers produced by X-ray photon absorption in X-ray photoconductors, which impacts the electrical signal's spatial distribution and collection efficiency. Because charge carriers are less likely to diffuse or scatter over large distances, shorter carrier Schubwegs lead to more localized charge deposition and improved spatial resolution. On the other hand, longer carrier Schubwegs, especially in thicker photoconductor layers, might result in wider charge distribution and a lower spatial resolution. Controlling material purity, defect density, and crystal structure are all part of optimizing carrier Schubwegs, which reduces carrier scattering and improves charge transport efficiency.

The sensitivity, spatial resolution, and image quality of X-ray photoconductors in digital radiography systems are influenced by many interrelated parameters, including absorption, photoconductor thickness, and carrier Schubwegs. To maximize the diagnostic accuracy of medical imaging applications and achieve optimal performance, it is imperative to balance these factors through careful material selection, device design, and fabrication process optimization. Innovations focused on enhancing the effectiveness, resolution, and dependability of digital radiography systems for improved patient care and clinical outcomes are constantly being driven by developments in X-ray detector technology (Kotter and Langer, 2002; Lança, Luís; Silva, Augusto, 2013).

5.3.3. Medical Applications

X-ray photoconductors are used in a broad variety of medical applications, including therapeutic interventions and diagnostic imaging modalities. These applications take advantage of the special qualities of photoconductor materials to meet particular clinical requirements.

These applications include:

1. **Digital Radiography (DR)**: In digital radiography systems, X-ray photoconductors are the main sensing component that transforms X-ray photons into electrical signals for processing and image capture. Compared to conventional film-based radiography, digital radiography (DR) provides several benefits, such as quicker image acquisition times, better image quality, and reduced radiation exposure for patients. For a variety of imaging investigations, such as skeletal imaging, trauma evaluations, and chest X-rays, medical professionals employ DR.
2. **Fluoroscopy**: Fluoroscopy is a diagnostic tool that uses continuous X-ray imaging to show dynamic processes happening in real time inside the body, like cardiac catheterization, GI tract motility, and interventional procedures. High-speed image capture with excellent temporal resolution is made possible by X-ray photoconductors, which makes precise guidance possible for fluoroscopically guided

interventions, angiography, and minimally invasive surgeries.

3. **Computed Tomography (CT)**: Several X-ray projections taken at various angles are acquired during CT imaging to reconstruct intricate cross-sectional pictures of internal organs and structures. To create high-quality CT images, X-ray photoconductors—which capture X-ray photons with high sensitivity and spatial resolution—play a crucial role in CT detectors. CT is frequently used to diagnose vascular diseases, tumors, and fractures.
4. **Mammography**: Mammography is a specialized X-ray imaging technique used for breast cancer screening and diagnosis. X-ray photoconductors with high X-ray absorption efficiency, such as amorphous selenium (a-Se), are well-suited for mammography detectors, enabling the detection of subtle breast lesions with excellent contrast and spatial resolution. Digital mammography offers advantages over film-screen mammography, including improved image quality, faster image retrieval, and digital image storage for remote viewing and archiving.
5. **Dental Radiography**: In dentistry, X-ray photoconductors are employed in intraoral and extraoral dental X-ray systems to visualize dental structures, detect caries, assess bone levels, and plan orthodontic treatments. Digital dental radiography offers enhanced image quality, reduced radiation exposure, and improved workflow efficiency compared to conventional film-based techniques, benefiting both patients and dental practitioners.
6. **Radiation Therapy**: X-ray photoconductors are also utilized in radiation therapy systems for cancer treatment, where high-energy X-ray beams are targeted at tumor sites to destroy cancerous cells while minimizing damage to surrounding healthy tissues. X-ray detectors play a crucial role in verifying treatment delivery accuracy, monitoring patient positioning, and ensuring optimal radiation dose distribution during radiotherapy procedures.
7. **Non-Destructive Testing (NDT)**: X-ray photoconductors are used in non-destructive testing (NDT) of materials and structures in a variety of industries, such as manufacturing, aerospace, and automotive, in addition to medical imaging. Welds, castings, composites, and other components can be inspected for flaws, fractures, and internal anomalies using non-destructive testing (NDT) methods like computed tomography and X-ray radiography without sacrificing their integrity or functionality.

X-ray photoconductors are essential to many medical applications, including materials testing, cancer treatment, and image-guided interventions in addition to diagnostic imaging. Progress in photoconductor materials, detector technologies, and imaging methodologies appears poised to augment the precision, efficacy, and security of X-ray imaging systems utilized in medical and industrial settings (Körner et al, 2007; Grupen, Claus; Buvat, Irène, 2012; Dance et al, 2014).

5.3.5. Chest Radiography

Often referred to as a chest radiograph or X-ray, chest radiography is one of the most widely used and significant imaging modalities in medicine. It involves taking pictures of the chest, including the heart, ribs, lungs, and surrounding structures, using X-ray technology. Chest radiography is an essential tool for healthcare professionals in a variety of clinical settings because it is crucial to the diagnosis, treatment, and surveillance of numerous thoracic conditions and diseases.

5.3.5.1. Indications and Clinical Utility

1. **Diagnostic Evaluation**: Chest radiography is frequently used as a first-line imaging modality for evaluating a variety of respiratory and cardiovascular conditions, including pneumonia, chronic obstructive pulmonary disease (COPD), congestive heart failure, and pulmonary embolism. It helps clinicians identify abnormalities such as lung consolidations, pleural effusions, pulmonary nodules, and cardiomegaly, guiding further diagnostic workup and treatment decisions.
2. **Screening and Surveillance**: Chest radiography is commonly employed for screening and surveillance purposes in asymptomatic individuals at risk for certain diseases, such as lung cancer or tuberculosis. Screening chest X-rays may be recommended for smokers, individuals with occupational exposures to respiratory hazards, or those with a family history of lung disease, allowing for early detection and intervention when indicated.
3. **Trauma Evaluation**: Chest radiography is an essential component of trauma imaging protocols, particularly in patients with suspected thoracic injuries following trauma or accidents. It helps identify fractures, pneumothorax, hemothorax, rib fractures, and other traumatic injuries that may require urgent intervention or surgical management.
4. **Preoperative Assessment**: Chest radiography is routinely performed as part of preoperative assessments to evaluate cardiopulmonary status and identify potential risk factors that may impact surgical outcomes. It helps assess lung function, detect underlying cardiopulmonary diseases, and guide anesthetic management strategies in patients undergoing surgery.

5.3.5.2. Procedure and Interpretation

A radiographic image is obtained by passing X-ray beams through the chest while the patient stands or sits in front of an X-ray detector during a chest radiography procedure. Different tissues in the chest attenuate X-ray beams in different ways, which causes variations in X-ray transmission and the creation of a radiographic image on the detector.

A methodical approach is necessary to evaluate important anatomical structures and spot abnormalities when interpreting a chest X-ray. The thoracic skeleton's integrity, the diaphragmatic contours, the presence of lung fields, the size and shape of the heart, and the pulmonary vasculature are all evaluated by radiologists and medical professionals. To make a diagnosis, abnormal findings like masses, nodules, effusions, infiltrates, opacities, pneumothorax, and consolidations are closely examined and correlated with the patient's symptoms and clinical history.

5.3.5.3. Advantages and Limitations

- **Advantages**: Chest radiography is a vital tool for initial screening and diagnostic evaluation because it is easily accessible, reasonably priced, and produces imaging results quickly. It is simple to use and provides excellent spatial resolution for displaying thoracic anatomy in a variety of clinical contexts, such as intensive care units, emergency rooms, and outpatient clinics.
- **Limitations**: Chest radiography may not be specific enough to differentiate between various pathologies, despite its high sensitivity in identifying some thoracic abnormalities. Additionally, it might overlook minute details or early-stage illnesses that call for more sensitive imaging techniques like magnetic resonance imaging (MRI) or computed tomography (CT). Furthermore, even at low doses, chest X-rays expose patients to ionizing radiation, which raises concerns about radiation risks, especially for pediatric patients and those who need repeat imaging studies.

A key imaging modality in clinical practice, chest radiography provides important diagnostic data for a variety of thoracic diseases and conditions. Even with its drawbacks, chest X-rays are still a vital diagnostic and treatment tool for patients with respiratory, cardiovascular, and traumatic disorders, helping to enhance patient outcomes and care quality.

5.3.6. Mammography

Mammography is a specialized imaging modality used to screen, diagnose, and monitor women for breast cancer. It uses low-dose X-rays to produce fine-grained images of the breast tissue, enabling medical professionals to identify and assess anomalies like calcifications, tumors, and cysts. Early detection of breast cancer can greatly enhance treatment outcomes and lower death rates, and mammography is essential for this.

Finding breast abnormalities early on, when they are most treatable, is the main objective of mammography. As part of routine breast cancer screening programs, screening mammography is advised for asymptomatic women. These programs usually begin at age 40 or earlier for women who have an increased risk of breast cancer because of factors like genetic mutations or family history. The breast is compressed between two flat plates during a screening mammography to minimize image distortion and provide the best possible tissue visualization. Mammograms, or X-ray images, are then taken from various angles to capture various perspectives of the breast tissue.

Women who have abnormal results from screening mammograms or who have breast symptoms like lumps, pain, or nipple discharge are candidates for diagnostic mammography. Diagnostic mammograms use extra imaging views and methods to further assess suspicious areas and give more precise information for diagnosis and treatment planning. Examples of these methods include spot compression, magnification, or specialized imaging modalities like tomosynthesis.

Modern breast imaging centers have mostly transitioned from film-screen mammography to digital mammography because of its many benefits, which include better image quality, quicker image acquisition, and digital image storage for electronic transmission and easy retrieval. X-ray detectors, which are usually based on cesium iodide (CsI) or amorphous selenium (a-Se) scintillator technology, are used in digital mammography systems to convert X-ray photons into electrical signals for image processing and capture. These detectors provide improved clarity and diagnostic accuracy in the detection of subtle breast lesions due to their high spatial resolution and contrast sensitivity.

A sophisticated imaging method called tomosynthesis, sometimes referred to as 3D mammography, creates three-dimensional reconstructions of the breast tissue from several X-ray projections taken at various angles. Compared to traditional mammography, tomosynthesis has some benefits, such as enhanced lesion detection, fewer false positives, and superior visualization of overlapping breast tissue. It is especially helpful for women who have dense breast tissue, as dense fibroglandular tissue may make conventional mammography less sensitive to abnormalities or small tumors.

According to breast cancer screening guidelines, women who are at high risk of developing breast cancer should undergo routine mammography screening in addition to clinical breast examinations and, in certain situations, additional imaging modalities like breast ultrasound or magnetic resonance imaging (MRI). Age recommendations and intervals for mammography screening can change depending on a person's personal preferences, personal risk factors, and professional medical organizations' guidelines. Mammography is still the gold standard for screening for breast cancer, but new developments in science and technology are making it more accurate and useful. Particularly in women with dense breast tissue or high-risk profiles, emerging technologies like contrast-enhanced mammography and molecular breast imaging show promise for improving lesion detection and characterization.

Mammography offers substantial advantages in lowering the morbidity and death linked to the disease, making it an essential tool in the early detection and diagnosis of breast cancer. Mammography continues to be a vital component of breast cancer screening and detection initiatives as breast imaging technologies advance, enabling women and healthcare professionals to take an active role in the battle against breast cancer.

5.3.7. Fluoroscopy

Fluoroscopy is a dynamic imaging method that shows internal organs and structures in the body as moving pictures in real time using X-ray technology. It is essential to many medical treatments and procedures because it gives healthcare professionals real-time, continuous imaging guidance while they perform therapeutic and diagnostic procedures. Fluoroscopy allows for accurate localization, navigation, and real-time procedure monitoring by providing insightful information about anatomical structures, physiological processes, and interventional devices.

5.3.7.1. Principles of Fluoroscopy

Fluoroscopy uses X-ray photons to create images of the internal structures of the body, working on the same fundamental principles as traditional radiography. As opposed to static radiography, which creates single images of anatomical regions, fluoroscopy, on the other hand, creates dynamic, continuous images that record motion and changes in the body in real time. By continuously directing X-ray beams through the patient's body and using a fluoroscopic imaging system to capture the transmitted radiation, this dynamic imaging capability is accomplished.

An X-ray source, a fluoroscopic detector or image intensifier, a patient support table, and a display monitor are the main parts of the fluoroscopic imaging system. A continuous beam of X-ray photons is emitted by the X-ray source, and as it passes through the patient's body, various tissues and structures attenuate the beam of radiation to different degrees. The detector, also known as the image intensifier, then picks up the attenuated X-rays, transforms them into visible light photons, and increases their intensity to create a bright, high-resolution fluoroscopic image that appears on the display monitor in real time.

5.3.7.2. Clinical Applications

Fluoroscopy is utilized in a wide range of medical specialties and procedures, including:

1. **Interventional Radiology**: Fluoroscopy is extensively used in interventional radiology procedures, such as angiography, embolization, stent placement, and percutaneous biopsies. It provides real-time guidance to interventional radiologists, allowing for precise catheter navigation, vessel visualization, and therapeutic interventions without the need for open surgery.
2. **Orthopedics**: Fluoroscopy is commonly employed in orthopedic procedures, including fracture reduction, joint injections, arthrography, and spinal interventions. It enables orthopedic surgeons to visualize bone alignment, joint mobility, and implant positioning during procedures, facilitating accurate placement of hardware and surgical implants.
3. **Gastrointestinal (GI) Imaging**: Fluoroscopy plays a vital role in GI imaging studies, such as barium swallow, upper gastrointestinal series (UGI), small bowel follow-through, and esophagogastroduodenoscopy (EGD). It allows radiologists and gastroenterologists to assess swallowing function, detect anatomical abnormalities, and evaluate GI motility and transit times in real-time.
4. **Cardiology**: In cardiology, fluoroscopy is used for cardiac catheterization procedures, electrophysiology studies, pacemaker implantation, and coronary angiography. It provides cardiologists with dynamic visualization of cardiac anatomy, blood flow patterns, and coronary arteries, guiding diagnostic and therapeutic interventions for heart disease.
5. **Pain Management**: Fluoroscopy-guided pain management techniques, such as epidural steroid injections, nerve blocks, and radiofrequency ablation, are commonly performed to alleviate chronic pain conditions. Fluoroscopic imaging enables pain management specialists to precisely target specific nerves or pain generators, delivering therapeutic agents or thermal energy with high accuracy and efficacy.

5.3.7.3. Advantages and Considerations

Compared to other imaging modalities, fluoroscopy has a number of benefits, such as the capacity to precisely guide minimally invasive procedures and provide real-time visualization and dynamic imaging capabilities. It does, however, bring with it some concerns, including radiation exposure to patients and medical personnel, the requirement for appropriate training and experience in image interpretation and procedural guidance, and the necessity of adhering to radiation safety protocols to reduce radiation risks.

In contemporary medicine, fluoroscopy is a highly adaptable and essential imaging technique that offers dynamic, real-time visualization of internal organs and structures during diagnostic and interventional procedures in a variety of medical specializations. Fluoroscopy systems are developing to include digital imaging technologies, sophisticated image processing algorithms, and dose reduction strategies as a result of ongoing technological advancements, which improves their functionality and safety profile in clinical settings.

5.3.8. Future Trends

Future trends in X-ray detectors are poised to transform medical imaging by improving image quality, reducing radiation dose, enhancing efficiency, and enabling new clinical applications.

Several key trends are shaping the development of X-ray detectors in the coming years:

1. **Advancements in Detector Technology**: To enhance performance and image quality, future X-ray detectors are expected to integrate developments in materials science, electronics, and sensor technology. Novel scintillators and high-Z semiconductors are examples of emerging detector materials that offer improved X-ray absorption efficiency and spatial resolution, allowing for more precise and sensitive imaging. Further advancements in spectral imaging methods and photon-counting detectors could lead to improved contrast enhancement, X-ray imaging artifact reduction, and tissue characterization.
2. **Digital Transformation**: Medical imaging has been completely transformed by the switch from analog film-screen systems to digital X-ray detectors, which provide several benefits like better image quality, quicker image acquisition, and digital data sharing and storage. Future developments in digital X-ray detectors will concentrate on improving dynamic range, resolution, and signal-to-noise ratio in addition to introducing sophisticated image processing algorithms for noise reduction, artifact reduction, and image enhancement.
3. **Dose Reduction and Optimization**: Radiation dose reduction remains a priority in medical imaging to minimize patient exposure to ionizing radiation while maintaining diagnostic image quality. Future X-ray detectors will continue to integrate dose reduction technologies such as iterative reconstruction algorithms, automatic exposure control, and real-time feedback mechanisms to optimize imaging parameters and reduce unnecessary radiation dose. Additionally, innovations in low-dose imaging techniques, such as phase-contrast and dark-field imaging, offer the potential for high-resolution imaging at significantly lower radiation doses.
4. **Multimodal Imaging Integration**:

Multimodal imaging platforms with complementary strengths and capabilities are made possible through the integration of X-ray detectors with other imaging modalities, including computed tomography (CT), magnetic resonance imaging (MRI), ultrasound, and molecular imaging techniques. The development of hybrid imaging systems—which integrate X-ray detectors with other modalities—will be the main focus of future trends. These systems will improve disease characterization, offer comprehensive diagnostic information, and facilitate treatment planning and monitoring for a broad range of clinical applications.

5. **Point-of-Care and Portable Devices**: Compact and lightweight X-ray detectors that are appropriate for use in emergency rooms, ambulatory care settings, and remote healthcare settings are being developed in response to the increasing demand for point-of-care and portable imaging solutions. Portability, usability, and wireless connectivity will be given top priority in X-ray detectors of the future, allowing for quick imaging and real-time diagnosis at the bedside or in the field. Wearable sensors, portable radiography units, and handheld X-ray machines present opportunities for decentralized imaging services and better access to healthcare in underprivileged areas.

6. **Artificial Intelligence and Machine Learning**: Medical imaging could undergo a revolution if artificial intelligence (AI) and machine learning algorithms are integrated with X-ray detectors. This would improve diagnostic accuracy, automate image analysis, and enable predictive analytics. To help radiologists interpret images, identify abnormalities, and forecast patient outcomes, future X-ray detectors will integrate artificial intelligence (AI)-powered image reconstruction techniques, computer-aided detection systems, and decision support tools.

The convergence of clinical requirements, patient safety concerns, and technology breakthroughs will shape future trends in X-ray detectors. X-ray imaging is well-positioned to enhance patient care, boost diagnostic precision, and open up new clinical applications in the healthcare industry by utilizing advancements in detector technology, digital imaging, dose optimization, multimodal integration, portability, and AI-driven analytics (Körner et al, 2007; Grupen, Claus; Buvat, Irène, 2012; Dance et al, 2014).

A Closer Look

Digital Radiography

DR is a major advancement in medical imaging that replaces traditional film-based methods with digital technology. This method utilizes digital detectors to capture images directly, making them immediately available for review on a computer. DR produces high-quality images with lower doses of radiation compared to conventional radiography, making it beneficial for patients needing multiple or frequent imaging studies. Additionally, this technology streamlines the imaging process, resulting in faster acquisition and processing times.

Additionally, the digital format makes it simple to store, retrieve, and share images, which improves patient care and fosters collaboration among healthcare professionals. Furthermore, improved image manipulation and analysis are made possible by the use of software tools, which contribute to more precise diagnosis. DR provides long-term cost savings through lower film, chemical, and storage costs, even with higher initial equipment and setup costs. Its incorporation into healthcare systems highlights the move toward safer, more effective, and efficient diagnostic procedures. Digital radiography is anticipated to include even more sophisticated features as technology develops, reaffirming its position as the mainstay of contemporary medical imaging.

Summary

- These detectors are designed to capture X-ray photons that pass through the patient's body, converting them into electronic signals.
- X-ray detectors are utilized for non-destructive testing (NDT) to inspect the integrity of materials and components without causing damage.
- To obtain an image with any type of image detector the part of the patient to be X-rayed is placed between the X-ray source and the image receptor to produce a shadow of the internal structure of that particular part of the body.
- Typical X-ray film contains silver halide crystal "grains," typically primarily silver bromide. Grain size and composition can be adjusted to affect the film properties, for example to improve resolution in the developed image.
- Phosphor plate radiographyis a method of recording X-rays using photostimulated luminescence (PSL). A photostimulable phosphor plate (PSP) is used in place of the photographic plate.
- X-rays are also used in "real-time" procedures such as angiography or contrast studies of the hollow organs (e.g., barium enema of the small or large intestine) using fluoroscopy.
- Photographic techniques, while much improved upon since the time of Röntgen and still extremely useful for qualitative applications, are not well-suited for more quantitative measurements of X-ray intensities and spectral content.
- A digital X-ray detector is a digital radiographic device used for X-ray inspection of an object that immediately produces a digital image on a computer screen.
- One of the most common image receptor formats is the digital flat-panel detector (FPD), which has largely replaced traditional film-based and computed radiography (CR) systems in modern radiology.
- Spatial resolution in medical imaging refers to the ability of the imaging system to differentiate between small structures or details within an object being imaged.
- The direct and indirect modes of operation are two distinct approaches used in digital radiography (DR) systems to convert X-ray photons into digital signals for image capture and processing.
- The intrinsic resolution of X-ray photoconductors plays a crucial role in determining the clarity and sharpness of X-ray images, influencing the ability of clinicians to detect and diagnose medical conditions accurately.
- Medical applications of X-ray photoconductors encompass a wide range of diagnostic imaging modalities and therapeutic interventions, each leveraging the unique properties of photoconductor materials to address specific clinical needs.

References

1. Benjamin, S. (2010). Phosphor plate radiography: An integral component of the filmless practice. *Dent Today, 29*(11), 89.
2. Dance, D. R., Christofides, S., Maidment, A. D. A., McLean, I. D., & Ng, K. H. (2014). *Diagnostic Radiology Physics: A Handbook for Teachers and Students*. Vienna: International Atomic Energy Agency, Sep 2014; Volume 46.710.
3. Del Sordo, S., Abbene, L., Caroli, E., Mancini, A. M., Zappettini, A., & Ubertini, P. (2009). Progress in the development of CdTe and CdZnTe semiconductor radiation detectors for astrophysical and medical applications. *Sensors, 9*(5), 3491–3526. https://doi.org/10.3390/s90503491.
4. Gonzalez, G. J. (2016). Desarrollo de un detector de Rayos X usando fotodiodos [Development of an X-ray detector using photodiodes]. *INIS, 48*(7), 13.
5. Grupen, C., & Buvat, I. (2012). *Handbook of Particle Detection and Imaging* (p. 443). Springer-Verlag Berlin Heidelberg 2012, DOI 10.1007/978-3-642-13271-1
6. Iniewski, K. (2014). CZT detector technology for medical imaging. *Journal of Instrumentation, 9*(11), C11001. https://doi.org/10.1088/1748-0221/9/11/C11001.
7. Jones, L., Seller, P., Wilson, M., & Hardie, A. (2009). HEXITEC ASIC—a pixelated readout chip for CZT detectors. *Nuclear Instruments and Methods in Physics Research Section A: Accelerators, Spectrometers, Detectors and Associated Equipment, 604*(1–2), 34–37. https://doi.org/10.1016/j.nima.2009.01.036.
8. Körner, M., Weber, C. H., Wirth, S., Pfeifer, K. -J., Reiser, M. F., & Treitl, M. (2007). Advances in digital radiography: Physical principles and system overview. *RadioGraphics, 27*(3), 675–686. https://doi.org/10.1148/rg.273065083.
9. Kotter, E., & Langer, M. (2002). Digital radiography with large-area flat-panel detectors. *European Radiology, 12*(10), 2562–2570. https://doi.org/10.1007/s00330-001-1251-4.
10. Lança, L., & Silva, A. (2013). Digital radiography detectors: A technical overview. In L. Lança & A. Silva (Eds.), *Digital Imaging Systems for Plain Radiography* (pp. 1–22). New York: Springer.
11. Lowe, B. G., & Sareen, R. A. (2013). *Semiconductor X-ray Detectors* (p. 106). Hoboken: Taylor and Francis, CRC Press. https://doi.org/10.1201/b16093
12. Martin, J. E. (2006). *Physics for Radiation Protection: A Handbook* (2nd ed., pp. 707–709). Weinheim: John Wiley & Sons, Medical Physics 33(12):4773-
13. Masebinu, S. O., & Muzenda, E. (2014). Review of silver recovery techniques from radiographic effluent and X-ray film waste. *Proceedings of the World Congress on Engineering and Computer Science, II*, 1–6. San Francisco.
14. Ristić, S. G. (2013). The digital flat-panel X-ray detectors. *Proceedings of the Third Conference on Medical Physics and Biomedical Engineering* (pp. 65–71). Skopje: IAEA.
15. Rowlands, J. A. (2002). The physics of computed radiography. *Physics in Medicine and Biology, 47*(23), R123–R166. https://doi.org/10.1088/0031-9155/47/23/201.
16. Saha, G. B. (2012). Gas-filled detectors. In *Physics and Radiobiology of Nuclear Medicine* (4th ed., pp. 79–90). New York: Springer.

17. Seco, J., Clasie, B., & Partridge, M. (2014). Review on the characteristics of radiation detectors for dosimetry and imaging. *Physics in Medicine and Biology, 59*(20), R303–R347. https://doi.org/10.1088/0031-9155/59/20/R303.

18. Takahashi, T., & Watanabe, S. (2001). Recent progress in CdTe and CdZnTe detectors. *IEEE Transactions on Nuclear Science, 48*(4), 950–959. https://doi.org/10.1109/23.958730.

19. Watt, K. N., Yan, K., DeCrescenzo, G., & Rowlands, J. A. (2005). The physics of computed radiography: Measurements of pulse height spectra of photostimulable phosphor screens using prompt luminescence. *Medical Physics, 32*(12), 3589–3598. https://doi.org/10.1118/1.2135884.

20. Williams, M., & Metcalfe, P. (2011). Radiochromic film dosimetry and its applications in radiotherapy. *AIP Conference Proceedings, 1345*(1), 75–99. https://doi.org/10.1063/1.3576194.

21. Zang, A., Anton, G., Ballabriga, R., Bisello, F., Campbell, M., Celi, J. C., Fauler, A., Fiederle, M., Jensch, M., Kochanski, N., Llopart, X., Michel, N., Mollenhauer, U., Ritter, I., Tennert, F., Wölfel, S., Wong, W., & Michel, T. (2015). The Dosepix detector—An energy-resolving photon-counting pixel detector for spectrometric measurements. *Journal of Instrumentation, 10*(4), C04015. https://doi.org/10.1088/1748-0221/10/04/C04015.

Chapter

DENTAL RADIOGRAPHY

6

Contents

Introduction

Dental radiography, a cornerstone of modern dentistry, encompasses a range of imaging techniques essential for diagnosing and treating various dental conditions. Utilizing X-rays, dental radiography provides invaluable insights into the internal structures of the oral cavity, including teeth, jaws, and surrounding tissues, aiding dentists in making accurate diagnoses and developing effective treatment plans.

Dental radiography serves as a non-invasive diagnostic tool, offering detailed visualizations of dental anatomy, pathology, and treatment outcomes. By capturing images of teeth, roots, bone, and soft tissues, dental radiographs reveal abnormalities such as cavities, fractures, infections, and developmental anomalies that may not be apparent during a clinical examination. This diagnostic capability is particularly valuable for detecting early signs of dental disease, facilitating prompt intervention, and preventing the progression of oral health issues.

The evolution of dental radiography has seen a transition from traditional film-based systems to digital imaging technologies, revolutionizing the way dental professionals acquire, analyze, and store radiographic images. Digital radiography offers numerous advantages over conventional film, including immediate image acquisition, enhanced image quality, reduced radiation exposure, and seamless integration with electronic health records. These advancements have streamlined workflow efficiency, improved diagnostic accuracy, and enhanced patient care in dental practices worldwide.

In addition to diagnostic purposes, dental radiography plays a pivotal role in treatment planning and monitoring. From routine dental examinations to complex surgical procedures, radiographic imaging provides vital information for assessing treatment options, evaluating treatment outcomes, and ensuring the long-term success of dental interventions. Whether it's determining the extent of tooth decay, assessing bone levels for implant placement, or diagnosing temporomandibular joint disorders, dental radiography serves as an indispensable tool for comprehensive dental care.

Moreover, dental radiography is not only confined to intraoral imaging of individual teeth but also encompasses extraoral imaging techniques such as panoramic radiography, cephalometric imaging, and cone beam computed tomography (CBCT). These advanced imaging modalities offer panoramic views of the entire dentition, craniofacial structures, and temporomandibular joints, providing valuable information for orthodontic treatment planning, oral and maxillofacial surgery, and complex dental reconstructions

Orientation and Directional Terms

Term	Definition	Illustration
Cephalometric imaging	Cephalometric X-rays (also called ceph X-rays or radiographs) show a side view of your head, exposing teeth, jaw, and surrounding structures. This technology is considered safe and often useful or necessary to help professionals evaluate and assist patients.	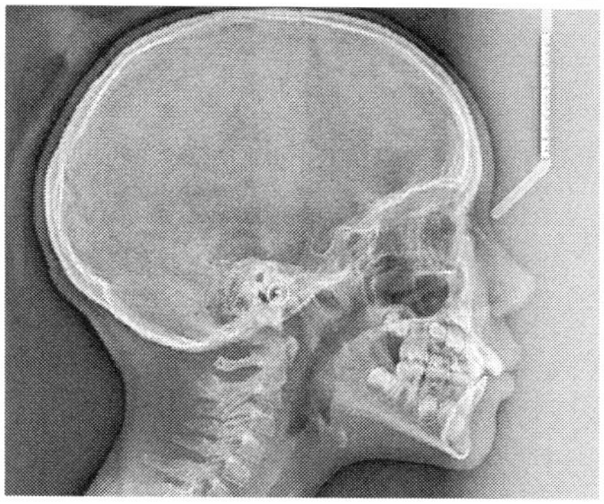
Bitewing X-ray	Bitewings show the upper and lower teeth in one area of your mouth. These dental X-rays help your dentist detect decay between your teeth or any changes that occur just below your gum line. Bitewing X-rays don't usually show the roots of your teeth.	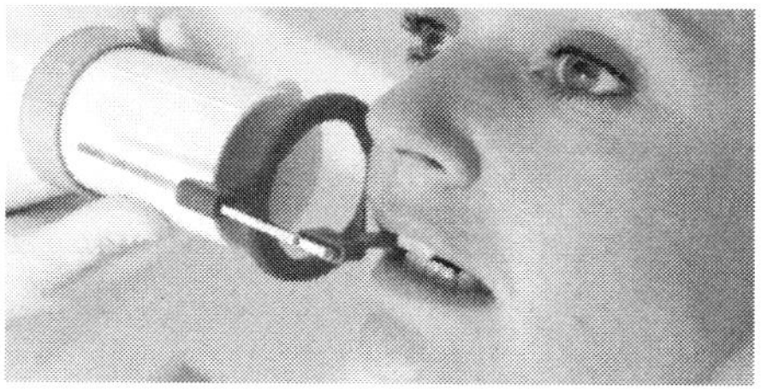
Cone-beam computed tomography systems (CBCT)	Cone-beam computed tomography systems (CBCT) are a variation of traditional computed tomography (CT) systems. The CBCT systems used by dental professionals rotate around the patient, capturing data using a cone-shaped X-ray beam.	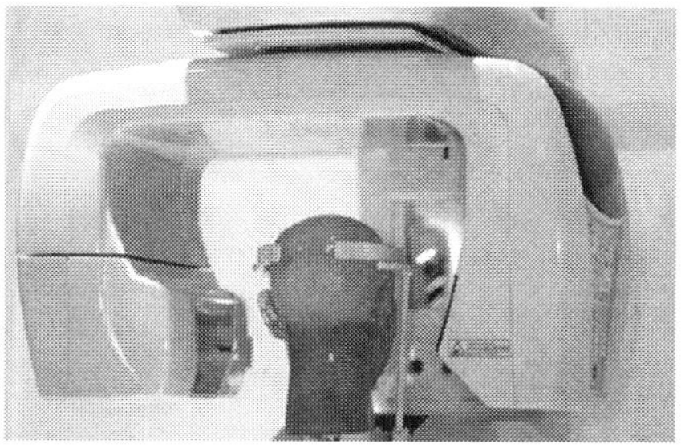
Periapical X-ray	A periapical X-ray shows your entire tooth, from the crown to the root tip. This type of X-ray helps your dentist detect decay, gum disease, bone loss and any other abnormalities of your tooth or surrounding bone.	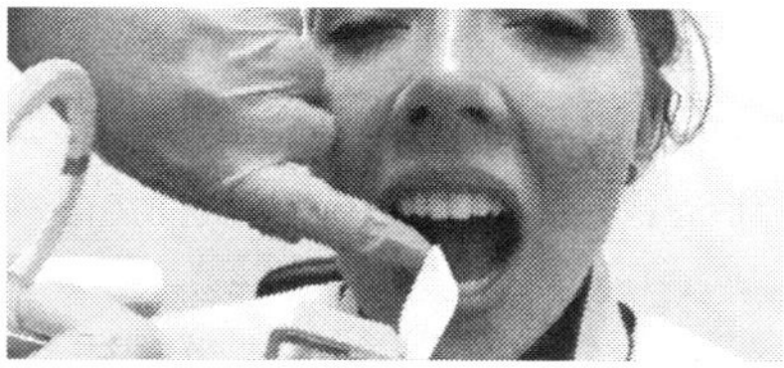
Occlusal X-rays	Occlusal X-rays show the roof or floor of the mouth and are used to find extra teeth, teeth that have not yet broken through the gums, jaw fractures, a cleft palate, cysts, abscesses or growths.	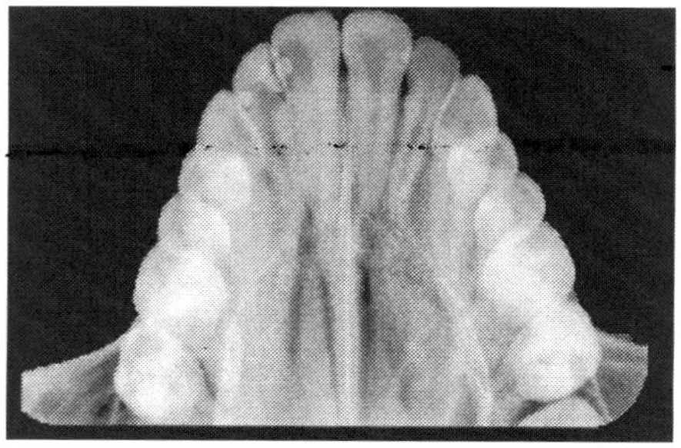

6.1. Dental Radiography Equipment

Dental radiography equipment encompasses a variety of tools and devices used in dental practices to capture images of the oral cavity, teeth, and surrounding structures for diagnostic and treatment planning purposes.

6.1.1. Intraoral X-ray Systems

- **X-ray Generator:** This device produces X-ray radiation used to create images. It typically includes controls for adjusting exposure settings such as kilovoltage (kV) and milliamperage (mA).
- **X-ray Tube:** The X-ray tube emits the X-ray beam toward the patient's mouth. It consists of a cathode and an anode within a vacuum tube, where electrons are accelerated to produce X-rays when they strike the target.
- **Positioning Devices:** Positioning devices such as X-ray cones and aiming devices help align the X-ray tube head accurately and maintain a consistent distance from the patient's mouth, ensuring optimal image quality and radiation safety.
- **X-ray Film Holders or Digital Sensors:** In film-based systems, X-ray film holders hold the film in place during exposure. In digital systems, digital sensors capture X-ray images, converting them into digital data for immediate viewing on a computer monitor.
- **X-ray Film or Digital Sensors:** These devices capture the X-ray image projected through the patient's teeth and surrounding tissues. X-ray film is sensitive to X-rays and produces a latent image that is developed using chemical processing. Digital sensors capture X-ray images electronically and transmit them to a computer for viewing and storage (Wiggs and Lobprise, 1997; Deforge and Colmery, 2000; Pasler and Visser, 2007; Monsour and Dudhia, 2008).

6.1.2. Extraoral X-ray Systems

- **Panoramic X-ray Machines:** Panoramic X-ray machines capture wide-angle views of the entire dental arch, jaws, and surrounding structures in a single image. They are commonly used for orthodontic assessment, dental implant planning, and detecting pathology in the maxillofacial region (Figure 6.1).

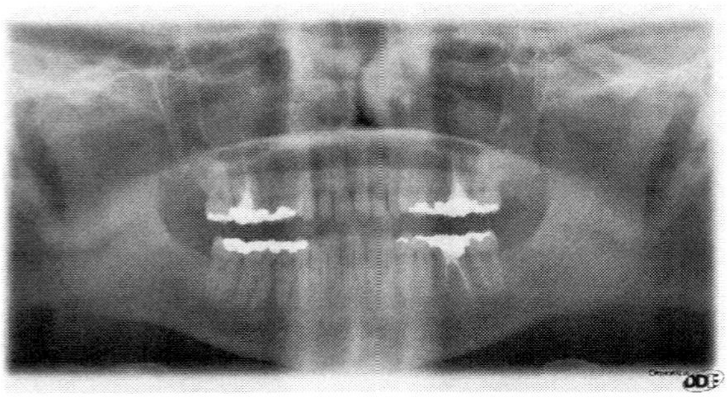

Figure 6.1. *Panoramic X-ray machines.*

Source: Public Domain, https://commons.wikimedia.org/w/index.php?curid=95297205.

- **Cephalometric X-ray Machines:** Cephalometric X-ray machines capture lateral (side) views of the head, providing detailed images of the skull, facial bones, and soft tissues. They are essential for orthodontic diagnosis and treatment planning (Figure 6.2).

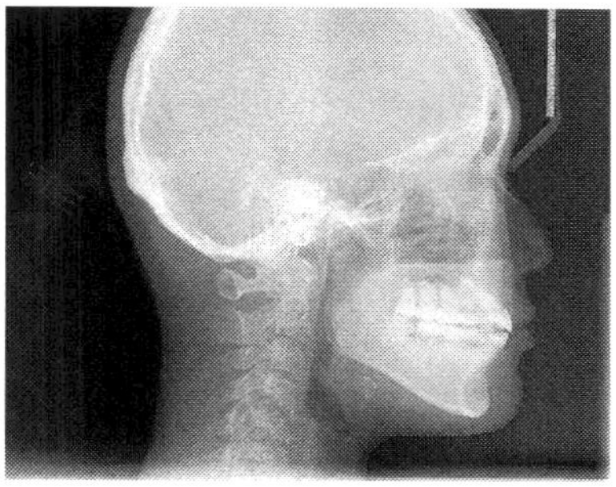

Figure 6.2. *Cephalometric X-rays machine*

Source: By ANUG – Own work, CC BY-SA 4.0, https://commons.wikimedia.org/w/index.php?curid=38139764.

- **Cone Beam Computed Tomography (CBCT) Scanners:** CBCT scanners produce three-dimensional (3D) images of the teeth, jaws, and surrounding structures with high spatial resolution. They offer detailed anatomical information for dental implant planning, oral surgery, orthodontics, and diagnosing complex dental conditions (Figure 6.3).

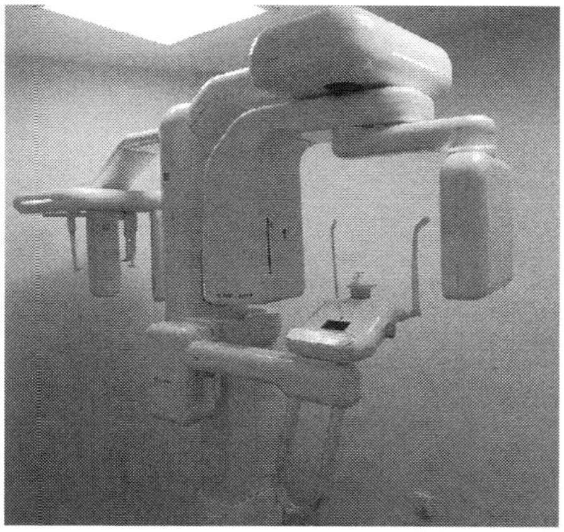

Figure 6.3. *Cone beam CT scanner.*

Source: https://en.wikipedia.org/wiki/Cone_beam_computed_tomography#/media/File:Cone_Beam_CT.jpg.

- **Digital Panoramic and Cephalometric Systems:** Digital panoramic and cephalometric systems use digital sensors to capture X-ray images, providing immediate visualization and electronic storage without the need for film and chemical processing. They offer advantages in terms of image quality, efficiency, and environmental sustainability (Figure 6.4).

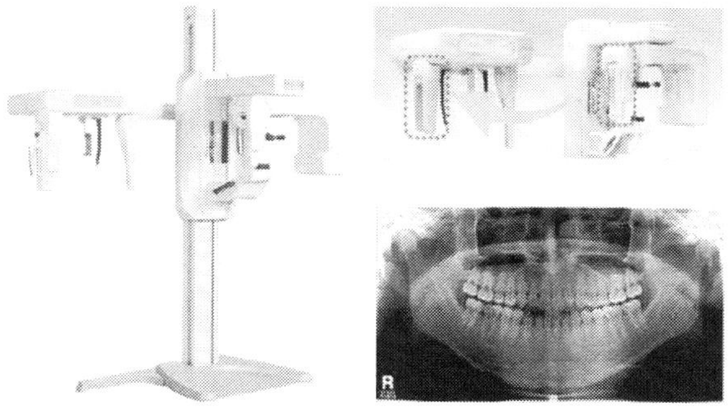

Figure 6.4. *Digital panoramic and cephalometric x-ray.*

Source: https://image.ec21.com/image/vatech/oimg_GC00283648_CA00283719/Digital-Panoramic-Cephalometric-X-ray-System-for-Dental-Use.jpg.

6.1.3. Accessories and Ancillary Equipment

- **Lead Aprons and Thyroid Collars:** These protective garments shield patients from unnecessary radiation exposure during X-ray procedures, reducing the risk of radiation-related health effects.
- **X-ray Positioning Instruments:** Positioning instruments such as bite blocks, aiming devices, and alignment guides help standardize patient positioning and X-ray beam

alignment, ensuring consistent image quality and diagnostic accuracy.

- **Film Processing Equipment:** Film processing equipment includes automatic film processors and manual processing tanks used to develop, fix, wash, and dry X-ray films after exposure.
- **Image Viewing Devices:** Image viewing devices such as light boxes or computer monitors are used to visualize and interpret X-ray images. Digital systems often integrate image viewing software for enhanced image manipulation, analysis, and archiving.
- **Sterilization Equipment:** Infection control measures are essential in dental radiography. Autoclaves and sterilization units are used to sterilize reusable instruments and equipment to prevent cross-contamination between patients.

6.1.4. Mobile and Portable Systems

- **Portable X-ray Units:** Portable X-ray units are compact, lightweight devices that can be easily transported and used in various clinical settings, including hospitals, nursing homes, and emergency situations where traditional X-ray equipment may be impractical.
- **Handheld X-ray Devices:** Handheld X-ray devices offer flexibility and maneuverability for capturing X-ray images in confined spaces or during patient care procedures where mobility is required.

6.1.5. Advanced Features and Technologies

1. **Digital Imaging and PACS (Picture Archiving and Communication Systems)**: Digital radiography systems integrate with PACS for storing, retrieving, and sharing digital X-ray images electronically, enhancing workflow efficiency and collaboration between dental professionals.
2. **Automated Exposure Control**: Some X-ray systems feature automated exposure control algorithms that adjust exposure settings based on patient characteristics, anatomy, and diagnostic requirements, optimizing image quality while minimizing radiation dose.
3. **Image Enhancement and Analysis Software**: Advanced software tools provide image enhancement, measurement, annotation, and analysis capabilities, facilitating accurate diagnosis and treatment planning.
4. **Radiation Dose Monitoring and Management**: Radiation dose monitoring systems track patient radiation exposure over time and provide feedback to clinicians, enabling dose optimization and adherence to radiation safety guidelines (Wiggs and Lobprise, 1997; Deforge and Colmery, 2000; Pasler and Visser, 2007; Monsour and Dudhia, 2008).

6.2. Types Of Dental X-rays

There are several types of dental X-rays, each serving a specific purpose:

6.2.1. Bitewing X-ray

Bitewing X-rays are a type of dental radiograph that provides a detailed view of the upper and lower teeth in a single image. Unlike panoramic X-rays, which offer a broad overview of the entire mouth, bitewing X-rays focus on specific areas, particularly the crowns of the teeth and the surrounding bone levels.

- **When Your Dentist May Recommend Bitewing X-rays**

  You may need a bitewing X-ray if:
- You're experiencing some kind of tooth pain or discomfort
- You want to keep track of the general health and condition of your teeth and gums
- Your dentist suspects you have cavities, gum disease, or periodontal disease.

Generally, your dentist will recommend that you have new bitewing X-rays taken each year as they provide important information about your oral health and the progress of dental decay.

A bitewing X-ray is one of the most important tools your dentist will use to assess the health of your teeth, since it is able to reveal areas that would otherwise be hard for them to see.

- **Purpose and Utility:**
  1. **Detection of Dental Caries (Cavities)**: Bitewing X-rays are particularly adept at revealing cavities between teeth (interproximal cavities) that may not be visible during a clinical examination. Early detection allows for prompt intervention, preventing the progression of decay.
  2. **Assessment of Dental Restorations**: These X-rays help dentists evaluate the integrity and fit of existing dental restorations such as fillings, crowns, and bridges.
  3. **Monitoring Periodontal Health**: Bitewing X-rays can detect signs of gum disease by revealing changes in the bone levels around the teeth, indicating bone loss associated with periodontal conditions.
  4. **Orthodontic Assessment**: In orthodontic treatment planning, bitewing X-rays provide valuable information about tooth alignment, eruption patterns, and potential crowding issues.
  5. **Evaluation of Interdental Spaces**: They aid in assessing the space between adjacent teeth, which is crucial for diagnosing conditions like impacted teeth and planning for orthodontic treatment.
- **Procedure**
  1. **Preparation**: The patient is typically seated in a dental chair, and a lead apron or thyroid collar may be provided for radiation protection.
  2. **Placement of X-ray Film or Sensor**: The dentist or dental assistant positions a small, flat X-ray film or digital sensor inside the patient's mouth, usually between the teeth.
  3. **X-ray Exposure**: The X-ray machine is positioned outside

the mouth, and the X-ray beam is directed towards the film/sensor. The dentist may take multiple bitewing X-rays, capturing images from both sides of the mouth.

4. **Image Development**: In traditional film-based X-rays, the exposed film is developed using chemical processing. In digital systems, the captured images are instantly available on a computer screen for review.

- **Interpretation:** Dentists analyze bitewing X-rays to assess various aspects of dental health and detect potential abnormalities:
  1. **Presence of Cavities**: Dark areas (radiolucencies) on the X-ray indicate areas of decay.
  2. **Integrity of Dental Restorations**: Gaps or irregularities around fillings or crowns may indicate decay or poor restoration fit.
  3. **Bone Levels**: Changes in bone density and height around the teeth may suggest periodontal disease.
  4. **Alignment and Spacing**: Tooth alignment, interdental spacing, and eruption patterns are evaluated for orthodontic purposes.
  5. **Presence of Impacted Teeth**: Bitewing X-rays can reveal impacted teeth that have not erupted properly.
- **Benefits**
  1. **Early Detection**: Bitewing X-rays enable the detection of dental issues at an early stage, facilitating timely intervention and preventing the progression of oral diseases.
  2. **Precision**: These X-rays provide detailed views of specific areas of the mouth, allowing dentists to pinpoint abnormalities with accuracy.
  3. **Treatment Planning**: The information obtained from bitewing X-rays guides treatment planning for conditions such as cavities, gum disease, and orthodontic problems.
  4. **Patient Education**: Visualizing the X-ray images helps patients understand their oral health status and the need for recommended treatments.
  5. **Minimized Radiation Exposure**: Modern digital X-ray systems use lower radiation doses compared to traditional film-based X-rays, ensuring patient safety.
- **Risks and Considerations:** While bitewing X-rays offer numerous benefits, it's essential to consider potential risks and take appropriate precautions:
  1. **Radiation Exposure**: Although the radiation dose from dental X-rays is minimal, repeated exposure over time can accumulate. Dentists follow ALARA (As Low As Reasonably Achievable) principles to minimize radiation exposure.
  2. **Pregnancy**: Pregnant women are advised to avoid unnecessary X-rays, especially during the first trimester, unless the benefits outweigh the risks. In such cases, lead

aprons and thyroid collars provide shielding to protect the fetus.

3. **Patient Comfort**: Some patients may experience discomfort or gagging sensations while biting on the X-ray film or sensor. Dentists should ensure patient comfort and address any concerns before proceeding with the X-ray procedure.

- **Technological Advancements:**
  1. **Digital Imaging**: Digital bitewing X-ray systems have largely replaced traditional film-based methods. Digital sensors capture images more quickly and produce instant results, eliminating the need for chemical processing.
  2. **Computer-Aided Diagnosis (CAD)**: CAD software assists dentists in analyzing X-ray images, highlighting areas of concern and aiding in diagnosis.
  3. **Cone Beam Computed Tomography (CBCT)**: While not typically used for routine bitewing X-rays, CBCT provides detailed 3D images of the teeth and jaws, offering valuable information for complex dental procedures such as implant placement and orthodontic treatment.
  4. **Reduced Radiation Exposure**: Ongoing advancements in X-ray technology continue to reduce radiation doses while maintaining image quality, further enhancing patient safety.

6.2.2. Periapical X-rays

Periapical X-rays, also known as periapical radiographs, are a type of dental radiograph that provides detailed images of specific teeth, including the crown, root, surrounding bone, and supporting structures. They are instrumental in diagnosing various dental conditions and assessing the health of individual teeth.

- **Purpose and Utility:**
  1. **Detection of Dental Pathologies**: Periapical X-rays are primarily used to diagnose dental caries (cavities), infections, abscesses, and other pathologies affecting the teeth and surrounding tissues.
  2. **Assessment of Root Structure**: They provide detailed views of the tooth roots, including the number, length, curvature, and integrity of the roots.
  3. **Evaluation of Periapical Areas**: Periapical X-rays reveal the periapical region, which includes the tooth apex (root tip) and surrounding bone. Changes in bone density or morphology may indicate conditions such as periapical infections or bone loss.
  4. **Endodontic Treatment Planning**: Periapical X-rays are essential for planning and monitoring endodontic (root canal) treatment, allowing dentists to assess the root canal system's shape, fillings, and post placement.
  5. **Assessment of Trauma**: They help evaluate the extent of dental trauma, including fractures, luxations, and

avulsions, aiding in treatment planning and monitoring healing.

- **Procedure**
  1. **Preparation**: The patient is seated in a dental chair, and appropriate protective measures, such as lead aprons, are provided for radiation safety.
  2. **Positioning**: The X-ray film or digital sensor is placed inside the patient's mouth, adjacent to the tooth of interest. The patient is instructed to bite gently on the film/sensor to stabilize it during exposure.
  3. **X-ray Exposure**: The X-ray machine is positioned outside the mouth, and the X-ray beam is directed towards the targeted tooth. The exposure is typically brief, and multiple periapical X-rays may be taken from different angles to capture comprehensive views.
  4. **Image Development**: In traditional film-based X-rays, the exposed film is processed using chemical methods. In digital systems, the captured images are immediately available for review on a computer monitor.
- **Interpretation:** Dentists analyze periapical X-rays to assess various aspects of dental health and diagnose underlying conditions:
  1. **Tooth Structure**: Periapical X-rays reveal the anatomy of the tooth, including the crown, roots, pulp chamber, and root canals.
  2. **Periapical Area**: Changes in the periapical region, such as widening of the periodontal ligament space or periapical lucencies, may indicate inflammation, infection, or other pathologies.
  3. **Bone Levels**: Periapical X-rays help evaluate the level and density of the surrounding alveolar bone, providing insights into periodontal health and bone support.
  4. **Root Canal Morphology**: These X-rays assist in assessing the shape, length, and curvature of the root canals, which is crucial for successful endodontic treatment.
  5. **Presence of Foreign Objects**: Periapical X-rays can detect foreign objects lodged in the tooth or surrounding tissues, such as broken instruments or retained roots.
- **Clinical Applications**
  1. **Diagnosis of Dental Caries**: Periapical X-rays reveal cavities that may not be visible during a clinical examination, especially in areas between teeth or below the gumline.
  2. **Endodontic Treatment**: They guide root canal treatment by providing detailed images of the tooth roots and identifying any abnormalities or areas of concern.
  3. **Periodontal Assessment**: Periapical X-rays help assess the bone levels around individual teeth, aiding in the diagnosis and management of

periodontal diseases.

4. **Implant Planning**: Prior to dental implant placement, periapical X-rays help evaluate the quality and quantity of bone in the implant site and assess neighboring structures to avoid complications.
5. **Monitoring Oral Health**: Regular periapical X-rays allow dentists to monitor changes in dental health over time, track the progression of dental conditions, and evaluate the effectiveness of treatments.

- **Benefits**
  1. **Diagnostic Accuracy**: Periapical X-rays provide detailed, high-resolution images of individual teeth and surrounding structures, allowing for accurate diagnosis of dental conditions.
  2. **Treatment Planning**: The information obtained from periapical X-rays guides treatment planning for various dental procedures, including restorative, endodontic, periodontal, and surgical interventions.
  3. **Early Detection**: By detecting dental pathologies at an early stage, periapical X-rays facilitate timely intervention, preventing the progression of disease and minimizing the need for more extensive treatments.
  4. **Patient Education**: Visualizing periapical X-ray images helps patients understand their dental conditions, treatment options, and the importance of oral health maintenance.
  5. **Customization**: Periapical X-rays can be tailored to focus on specific teeth or regions of interest, providing customized views based on the patient's needs and clinical requirements.
- **Risks and Considerations:** While periapical X-rays offer significant benefits, it's essential to consider potential risks and take appropriate precautions:
  1. **Radiation Exposure**: Although the radiation dose from dental X-rays is minimal, repeated exposure over time can accumulate. Dentists adhere to ALARA (As Low As Reasonably Achievable) principles to minimize radiation exposure while maintaining diagnostic quality.
  2. **Pregnancy**: Pregnant women are advised to avoid unnecessary X-rays, especially during the first trimester, unless the benefits outweigh the risks. In cases where X-rays are deemed necessary, lead aprons and thyroid collars provide shielding to protect the fetus.
  3. **Patient Comfort**: Some patients may experience discomfort or gagging sensations while biting on the X-ray film or sensor. Dentists should ensure patient comfort and address any concerns before proceeding with the X-ray procedure.
- **Technological Advancements**

1. **Digital Imaging**: Digital periapical X-ray systems have largely replaced traditional film-based methods. Digital sensors capture images more quickly and produce instant results, eliminating the need for chemical processing.
2. **Cone Beam Computed Tomography (CBCT)**: While not typically used for routine periapical X-rays, CBCT provides detailed 3D images of the teeth and jaws, offering valuable information for complex dental procedures such as implant placement, orthognathic surgery, and trauma assessment.
3. **Image Enhancement Software**: Advanced software tools enhance periapical X-ray images, improving clarity, contrast, and diagnostic accuracy.
4. **Portable X-ray Systems**: Portable periapical X-ray units offer flexibility and convenience, particularly in settings where traditional X-ray equipment may be impractical or inaccessible (Wiggs and Lobprise, 1997; Deforge and Colmery, 2000; Pasler and Visser, 2007; Monsour and Dudhia, 2008).

6.2.3. Occlusal Radiography

Occlusal radiography refers to intraoral radiography techniques that involve placing a small intraoral cassette or a film packet (5.7 x 7.6 cm) in the occlusal plane using a dental X-ray set.

6.2.3.1. Terminology and Classification

There is a lot of confusion in the terminology used in occlusal radiography. There is a lack of clarity in the definition and distinction between the different occlusal projections in the British Standards Glossary of Dental Terms (BS 4492: 1983). As a result, terminology used in various publications and educational settings still varies somewhat.

The terminology used here is based broadly on the British Standards terms, but they have been modified in an attempt to make them more explicit, straightforward and practical.

Maxillary Occlusal Projections:

- Upper standard (or anterior) occlusal (standard occlusal)
- Upper oblique occlusal (oblique occlusal)
- Vertex occlusal (vertex occlusal) – no longer used.

Mandibular Occlusal Projections:

- Lower 90° occlusal (true occlusal)
- Lower 45° (or anterior) occlusal (standard occlusal)
- Lower oblique occlusal (oblique occlusal).

6.2.3.2. Upper Standard Occlusal

This projection shows the anterior part of the maxilla and the upper anterior teeth.

- **Main Clinical Indications**

The main clinical indications include:

- Periapical assessment of the upper anterior teeth, especially in children but also in adults unable to tolerate periapical films
- Detecting the presence of unerupted

canines, supernumeraries and odontomes

- As the midline view, when using the parallax method for determining the bucco/palatal position of unerupted canines
- Evaluation of the size and extent of lesions such as cysts or tumors in the anterior maxilla
- Assessment of fractures of the anterior teeth and alveolar bone. It is especially useful in children following trauma because film placement is straightforward.
- **Technique and Positioning**

The technique can be summarized as follows:

1. The patient is seated with the head supported and with the occlusal plane horizontal and parallel to the floor and is asked to support a protective thyroid shield.
2. The film packet is pressed flat against the occlusal surfaces of the lower teeth, with the white (pebbly) side facing up. The patient is instructed to gently bite together. In adults, the film packet is positioned in the center of the mouth with its long axis crossways; in children, it is positioned anteroposteriorly.
3. The X-ray tubehead is positioned in the midline above the patient, pointing downward through the nose bridge at a 65°–70° angle with respect to the film packet (refer to Figure 6.5 and 6.6).

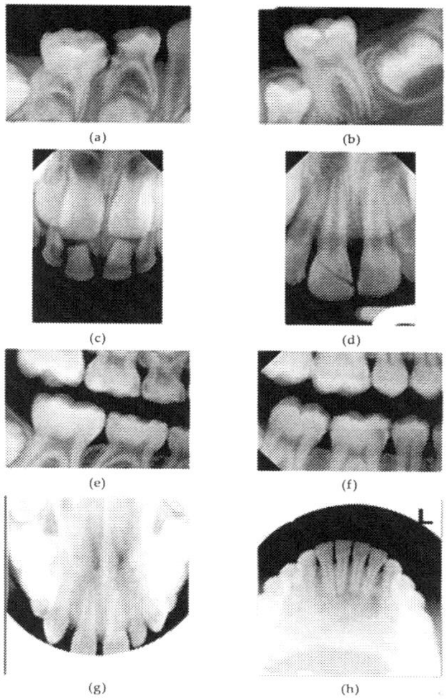

Figure 6.5. *Examples of radiographs: (a) dental radiograph of primary molars for caries and apical diagnostics; (b) dental radiograph of permanent molar for caries progression and apical diagnostics; (c) dental radiograph of primary teeth for trauma diagnostics; (d) dental radiograph of permanent teeth for trauma diagnostics; (e) bitewing radiograph for caries detection in primary molars; (f) bitewing radiographs for caries diagnostics in permanent molars; (g) occlusal radiograph for diagnosis of tooth germ position in the upper jaw; (h) occlusal radiograph for diagnosis of pathology in the lower jaw..*

Source: *Schüler, I. M., Hennig, C.-L., Buschek, R., Scherbaum, R., Jacobs, C., Scheithauer, M., & Mentzel, H.-J. Radiation Exposure and Frequency of Dental, Bitewing and Occlusal Radiographs in Children and Adolescents. Journal of Personalized Medicine. 2023; 13(4), 692. https://doi.org/10.3390/jpm13040692.*

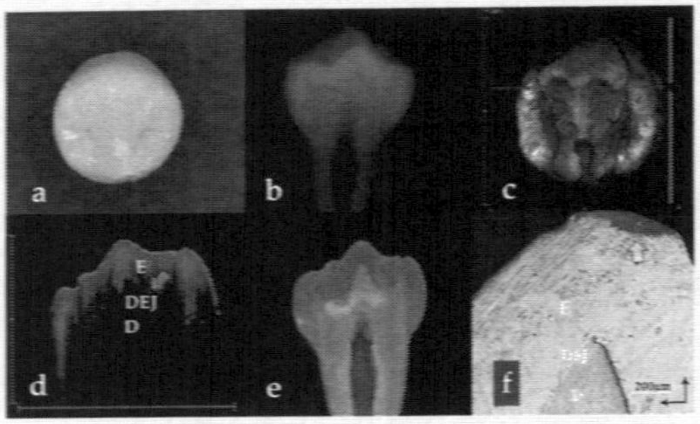

Figure 6.6. *Slight enamel wear (score 1): (a): Occlusal view. Visibly, evidence of occlusal tooth wear was not observed; (b): Digital intraoral radiography; (c): Optical coherence tomography (OCT) en face intensity projection; (d): Swept-source (SS)-OCT image. Occlusal enamel and underlining dentin were distinguished by the dentin enamel junction (DEJ) (arrow); (e): Histological view; (f): Confocal laser scanning microscopy (CLSM) image of histological view. A tip of the cusp was slightly cracked (arrow).*

Source: *Kashiwa, M., Shimada, Y., Sadr, A., Yoshiyama, M., Sumi, Y., & Tagami, J. Diagnosis of Occlusal Tooth Wear Using 3D Imaging of Optical Coherence Tomography Ex Vivo. Sensors. 2020; 20(21), 6016. https://doi.org/10.3390/s20216016.*

6.2.3.3. Upper Oblique Occlusal

This projection shows the posterior part of the maxilla and the upper posterior teeth on one side.

- **Main Clinical Indications**
  - Periapical assessment of the upper posterior teeth, especially in adults unable to tolerate periapical films
  - Evaluation of the size and extent of lesions such as cysts, tumors or osteodystrophies affecting the posterior maxilla
  - Assessment of the condition of the antral floor
  - As an aid to determining the position of roots displaced inadvertently into the antrum during attempted extraction of upper posterior teeth
  - Assessment of fractures of the posterior teeth and associated alveolar bone including the tuberosity.

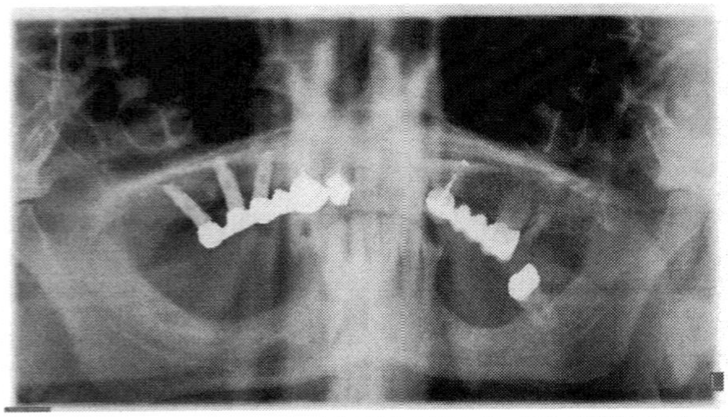

Figure 6.7. *Nodding up. Panoramic radiography. The occlusal plane loses the normal upper concavity and its curve is inverted. Note the radiopaque band overlapping the anterior area of both jaws.*

Source: *Izzetti, R., Nisi, M., Aringhieri, G., Crocetti, L., Graziani, F., & Nardi, C. Basic Knowledge and New Advances in Panoramic Radiography Imaging Techniques: A Narrative Review on What Dentists and Radiologists Should Know. Applied Sciences. 2021; 11(17), 7858. https://doi.org/10.3390/app11177858.*

- **Technique and Positioning**
  1. The patient is seated with the head supported and with the occlusal plane horizontal and parallel to the floor.
  2. The film packet, with the white (pebbly) surface facing uppermost, is inserted into the mouth onto the occlusal surfaces of the lower teeth, with its long axis anteroposteriorly. It is

placed to the side of the mouth under investigation, and the patient is asked to bite together gently.

3. The X-ray tubehead is positioned to the side of the patient's face, aiming downwards through the cheek at an angle of 65°-70° to the film, centering on the region of interest (Figure 6.7 and 6.8).

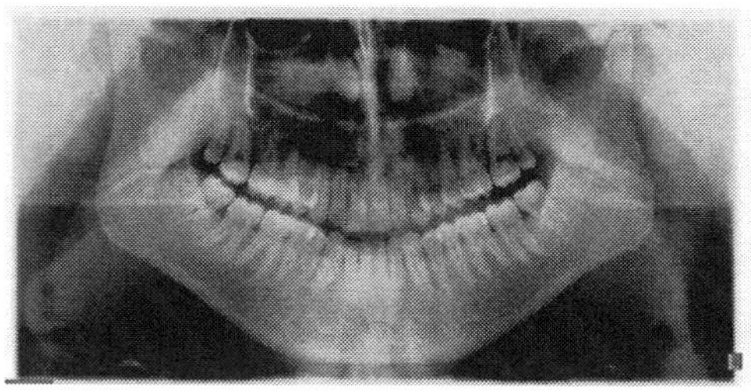

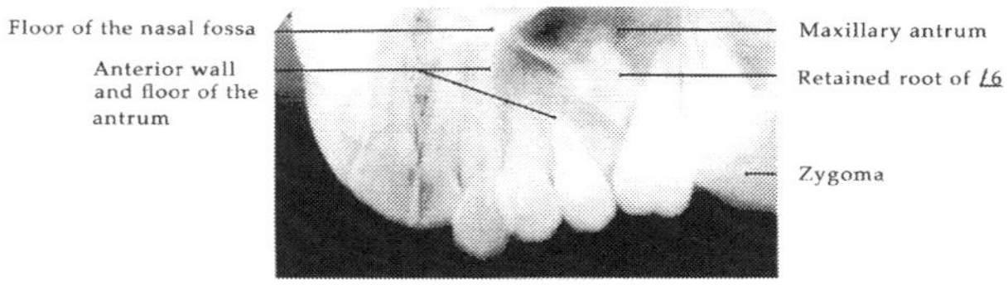

Figure 6.8. *Nodding down. Panoramic radiography. The upper concavity of the occlusal plane is pronounced.*

Source: Izzetti, R., Nisi, M., Aringhieri, G., Crocetti, L., Graziani, F., & Nardi, C. Basic Knowledge and New Advances in Panoramic Radiography Imaging Techniques: A Narrative Review on What Dentists and Radiologists Should Know. Applied Sciences. 2021; 11(17), 7858. https://doi.org/10.3390/app11177858.

6.2.3.4. Vertex Occlusal

This projection displays an overhead plan view of the maxilla's tooth-bearing region. The X-ray beam must travel through a significant amount of tissue in order to get this view, which exposes the patient to a high radiation dosage. To lower the dosage, an intraoral cassette with intensifying screens is used for this projection.

- **Main Clinical Indication**

- Assessment of the bucco/palatal position of unerupted canines.
- **Technique and Positioning**

The technique can be summarized as follows:

1. The patient is seated with the head supported and with the occlusal plane horizontal and parallel to the floor.
2. The cassette is placed inside a small plastic bag to prevent salivary contamination and cross infection.
3. It is then inserted into the mouth on to the occlusal surfaces of the lower teeth, with

its long axis anteroposteriorly and the patient is asked to bite on to it.

4. The X-ray tubehead is positioned above the patient, in the midline, aiming downwards through the vertex of the skull. The main beam is therefore aimed approximately down the long axis of the root canals of the upper incisor teeth (Figure 6.9).

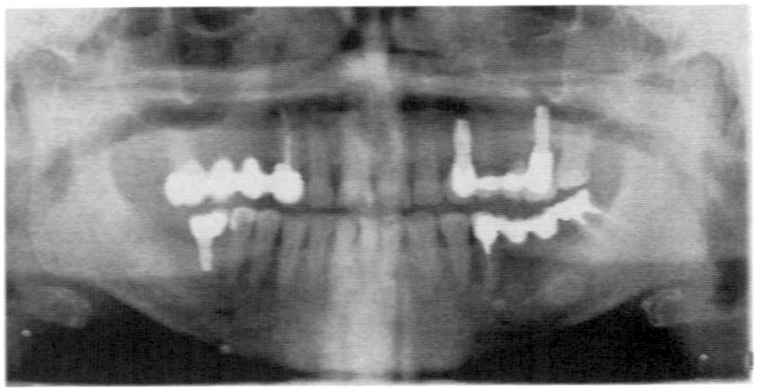

Figure 6.9. *Backward position. Panoramic radiography. Anterior teeth of both arches are placed behind the focal trough, with a consequent increase in their size (incisive teeth seem larger than molar ones). Note the radiopaque band overlapping the mandibular incisive area.*

Source: *Izzetti, R., Nisi, M., Aringhieri, G., Crocetti, L., Graziani, F., & Nardi, C. Basic Knowledge and New Advances in Panoramic Radiography Imaging Techniques: A Narrative Review on What Dentists and Radiologists Should Know. Applied Sciences. 2021; 11(17), 7858. https://doi.org/10.3390/app11177858.*

- **Disadvantages**

  The vertex occlusal projection is not often used because it has several drawbacks and disadvantages:

- There is a lack of detail and contrast on the film because of the intensifying screens, the mass of tissue the X-ray beam has to penetrate and the consequent scatter.
- The primary X-ray beam may be in direct line with the reproductive organs.
- A relatively long exposure time is needed (about 1 second) despite the use of intensifying screens.
- There is direct radiation to the pituitary gland and the lens of the eye.
- If the X-ray beam is positioned too far anteriorly, superimposition of the shadow of the frontal bones may obscure the anterior part of the maxilla (Figure 6.10).

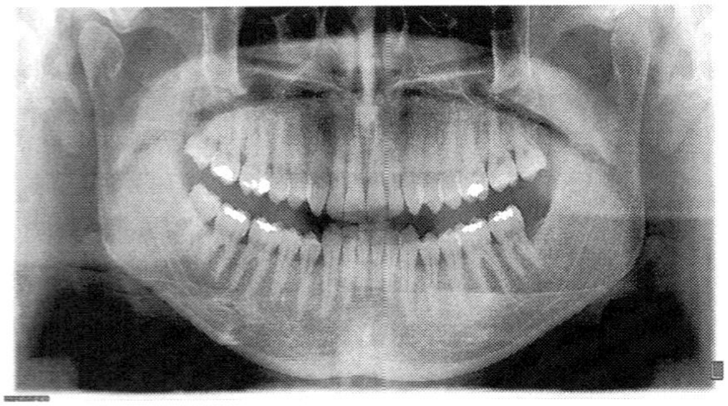

Figure 6.10. *Panoramic radiography carried out perfectly. The dark space between the two dental arches represented by the occlusal plane shows a mild upper concavity, since the Frankfort and occlusal planes tend to converge posteriorly.*

Source: *Izzetti, R., Nisi, M., Aringhieri, G., Crocetti, L., Graziani, F., & Nardi, C. Basic Knowledge and New Advances in Panoramic Radiography Imaging Techniques: A Narrative Review on What Dentists and Radiologists Should Know. Applied Sciences. 2021; 11(17), 7858. https://doi.org/10.3390/app11177858.*

6.2.3.5. Lower 90° Occlusal

This projection shows a planned view of the tooth bearing portion of the mandible and the floor of the mouth. A minor variation of the technique is also used to show unilateral lesions.

- **Main Clinical Indications**
  - Detection of the presence and position of radiopaque calculi in the submandibular salivary ducts
  - Assessment of the Bucco-lingual position of unerupted mandibular teeth
  - Evaluation of the Bucco-lingual expansion of the body of the mandible by cysts, tumors or osteodystrophies
  - Assessment of displacement fractures of the anterior body of the mandible in the horizontal plane.
- **Technique and Positioning**
  - The film packet, with the white (pebbly) surface facing downwards, is placed centrally into the mouth, onto the occlusal surfaces of the lower teeth, with its long axis crossways. The patient is asked to bite together gently.
  - The patient then leans forwards and then tips the head backwards as far as is comfortable, where it is supported.
  - The X-ray tubehead, with circular collimator fitted, is placed below the patient's chin, in the midline, centring on an imaginary line joining the first molars, at an angle of 90° to the film.

6.2.3.6. Lower 45° Occlusal

The anterior portion of the mandible and the lower anterior teeth are visible in this projection. Periapically, the resulting radiograph looks like a large bisected angle technique.

- **Main clinical indications**
  - Periapical assessment of the lower incisor teeth, especially useful in adults and children unable to tolerate periapical films
  - Evaluation of the size and extent of lesions such as cysts or tumors affecting the anterior part of the mandible
  - Assessment of displacement fractures of the anterior mandible in the vertical plane.
- **Technique and Positioning**
  - The patient is seated with the head supported and with the occlusal plane horizontal and parallel to the floor.
  - The film packet, with the white (pebbly) surface facing downwards, is placed centrally into the mouth, on to the occlusal surfaces of the lower teeth, with its long axis anteroposteriorly, and the patient is asked to bite gently together.
  - The X-ray tubehead is positioned in the midline, centring through the chin point, at an angle of 45° to the film ().

6.2.3.7. Lower Oblique Occlusal

The purpose of this projection is to enable the film to display the image of the submandibular salivary gland on the side of interest. Nevertheless, every anatomical tissue visible is deformed due to the oblique nature of the X-ray beam.

- **Main Indications**

The main clinical indications include:

- Detection of radiopaque calculi in a submandibular salivary gland
- Assessment of the Bucco-lingual position of unerupted lower wisdom teeth
- Evaluation of the extent and expansion of cysts, tumors or osteodystrophies in the posterior part of the body and angle of the mandible.

- **Technique and Positioning**

The technique can be summarized as follows:

- The film packet, with the white (pebbly) surface facing downwards, is inserted into the mouth, on to the occlusal surfaces of the lower teeth, over to the side under investigation, with its long axis anteroposteriorly. The patient is asked to bite together gently.
- The patient's head is supported, then rotated away from the side under investigation and the chin is raised. This rotated positioning allows the subsequent positioning of the X-ray tubehead.
- The X-ray tube head with circular collimator is aimed upwards and forwards towards the film, from below and behind the angle of the mandible and parallel to the lingual surface of the mandible (Rondon et al., 2014).

6.2.4. Panoramic Radiography

An extraoral radiography method called panoramic radiography gives two-dimensional data regarding the maxillofacial skeleton and teeth. Because it enables one-time imaging of all teeth, the mandible, portions of the maxilla, including a sizable portion of the maxillary sinus, the hard palate, and the temporomandibular joints (TMJs), it is a useful adjunct for diagnosis and treatment planning. Since tomographic images are prone to errors and artifacts, most patients can get a good-quality radiograph by positioning themselves properly and adhering to standard protocols.

- **Indications**

Indications for panoramic radiography imaging are:

  - Periodontal disease with simultaneous evaluation of all teeth and the extent of periodontal bone defects
  - Orthodontic evaluation, including presence of teeth germs, developmental stage of the dentition and the presence of retained, supernumerary or impacted teeth
  - Impacted third molars
  - Dental age estimation
  - Lesions such as tumors, cysts, and other bone diseases that cannot be entirely imaged by periapical radiographs
  - Mandibular trauma
- Implant planning
- **Materials/Instruments**
  - Lead apron
  - Bite piece
  - Chin support
  - Cotton roll (optional)
  - Single use protective sleeve
  - Disinfectant solution spray
  - Step stool
  - Panoramic machine
  - Camera (optional)

- Ruler (optional for TMJ tomography)

- **Procedure:** The most common extraoral radiography method is panoramic radiography. It is an interpretation of tomographic images of curved structures in two dimensions. For the diagnosis of various physiological and pathological conditions affecting the oral and maxillofacial regions, panoramic radiography is indicated. It makes it easier to image the teeth, mandibular bone, hard palate, portions of the maxilla, including the maxillary sinus, and both TMJs all at once.

The indications and radiation-risk assessment should support the referral for a panoramic radiograph. It shouldn't be interpreted as a standard radiograph. Since it's a tomographic radiograph, only objects inside the trough or focal plane can be seen clearly; objects outside the trough or focal plane are obscured or invisible (Table 6.1).

Table 6.1. Frequency of Indications for Intraoral Radiographs

Indication	Number of Radiographs	Percentage (%)
Apical diagnostics	495	22.7
Endodontics	244	11.2
Focus detection	68	3.1
Caries diagnostics	496	22.7
Orthodontic	15	0.7
Dental surgery	130	6.0
Prosthetics	4	0.2
Trauma	627	28.7
Detection of developing teeth	104	4.8
TOTAL	2138	100.0

Source: *Schüler, I. M., Hennig, C.-L., Buschek, R., Scherbaum, R., Jacobs, C., Scheithauer, M., & Mentzel, H.-J. Radiation Exposure and Frequency of Dental, Bitewing and Occlusal Radiographs in Children and Adolescents. Journal of Personalized Medicine. 2023; 13(4), 692. https://doi.org/10.3390/jpm13040692.*

- **Taking a Panoramic Radiograph:** Synchronized movement of the X-ray tube and the image detector in opposite directions results in an appropriate panoramic radiograph. Due to the application of a robotic C-arm in a panoramic machine, the tomographic movement is performed in a horizontal plane along a curve adjusted to the shape of the dental arches (Fig. 6.19). Its complex projection geometry along with rotational movement results in different shadows in the panoramic radiograph (Table 6.2).
  - Structures located within the focal trough have single shadows
  - Single structures located adjacent to the midline and outside the focal trough have double real shadows
  - Double structures closer to the radiographic edges outside the focal plane have ghost shadows

Table 6.2. Advantages and Disadvantages of Digital Panoramic Radiography

Digital Panoramic Radiography	
Advantages	Disadvantages
Ease of execution	One-time high cost of implementation of the digital system
Significant reduction in time between exposure and ready radiograph	Need for knowledge of computing technology by operators
Image post-processing options	Lack of control over radiographs with too many retaking examinations
Long-lasting archive of images with the easy retrieval of multiple copies	Need to protect sensitive patient data
Teleradiology. Image transfer and reporting via internet	Possibility of tampering with images
Wide dynamic range of X-ray exposures	
Automatic modulation of X-ray beam energy	
Decrease in radiation dose	

Source: Izzetti, R., Nisi, M., Aringhieri, G., Crocetti, L., Graziani, F., & Nardi, C. Basic knowledge and new advances in panoramic radiography imaging techniques: A narrative review on what dentists and radiologists should know. Applied Sciences. 2021; 11(17), 7858. https://doi.org/10.3390/app11177858.

Advances in panoramic radiography depend on:

- Exposure time reduction
- Exposure dose reduction
- Increase in image sharpness
- Registration of several parallel thinner layers within the focal trough
- Automatic image post-processing for selecting best-quality segments within the layers to compile into a high-quality radiograph. An operator can also scroll through the layers and choose images as required.

Obtaining a panoramic radiograph is comparatively simple with proper patient positioning. If the appropriate steps are carefully followed, a good quality radiograph can be obtained in most patients.

- **Steps in Obtaining a Panoramic Radiograph**
    - **Introductory Steps**

§ Read and evaluate the referral prescription to ensure justification of the radiograph.

- § Inform the patient and/or guardian about the radiation risk, and ensure that an informed consent form is signed per applicable regulation.
- § In female patients of child-bearing age, enquire about the possibility of pregnancy. Pregnancy is not an absolute contraindication for radiography but should be delayed until after birth, whenever possible.
- § Generate or open a patient file in a dedicated software. The dental arch shape and exposure settings can be selected based on the software. Entering the patient's gender and birth date leads to default settings that can be adjusted as required. A section of a panoramic radiograph should be selected instead of the whole radiograph if possible.

- **Patient Preparation**
  - § Instruct the patient to remove all metallic objects including removable orthodontic appliances, removable prostheses, piercings, glasses, necklaces, hearing aids and hair pins to prevent artifacts from the radiographed site.
  - § When the local legislation mandates the use of a lead apron during X-ray exposure, a lead apron with the longer side on the patient's back or a two-sided apron is used. If the patient's guardian accompanies the patient during the exposure, he/she should also wear a lead apron.
- **Patient Positioning**
  - § A bite piece is selected according to the patient's dentition.
  - § In case the patient's teeth (anterior or more) are missing or mobile (due to periodontal bone disease) or the patient has sustained a trauma, the use of a chin support is advised.
  - § Use a sterile bite piece or cover the bite piece with a single use protective sleeve. Disinfect the chin support with a disinfectant solution spray.
  - § The level of the C-arm is adjusted to the patient's height using a positioning device.
  - § Instruct the patient to enter the C-arm. Most machines have the ability to select a C-arm position that makes it more convenient for the patient to enter it with minimal risk of colliding with the device elements. If the device has a dedicated seat, ask the patient to sit down. If the machine accommodates standing patients only, technique modification is required. Tall patients will need to sit on a stool with no back rest. A step stool is used for a small child. Patients in a wheelchair can be examined in machines without a seat, only if the wheels do not collide with the machine base. After stabilizing the patient in the machine, adjust the C-arm to the level of the patient's head.

§ Instruct the patient to hold the handles. In standing patients, the patient may have to be asked to take half a step forward to straighten the cervical spine.

§ Ask the patient to rest the chin on a regular chin support or on a special chin support for edentulous patients. The level of chin support should ensure that the patient's neck remains straight.

§ A dentulous patient is instructed to bite on the sterile bite piece by articulating the incisal edges of the upper and lower incisors in the grooves on the bite piece.

§ Patient positioning can be guided by laser lights.

§ Symmetrical positioning of the head depends on the first laser light, which should lie between the upper central incisors. It is essential to keep in mind that facial soft tissues can be asymmetrical, and the dental arch midline may not correlate with midline of the patient's facial structures. In patients with missing anteriors or dental anomalies associated with the anterior teeth, positioning the first laser light can be difficult.

§ A second laser light highlights the Frankfort plane. Proper positioning of the Frankfort plane ensures the horizontal alignment of the occlusal plane, which appears as a flat or a wide, flat 'U.'

§ Cameras are fitted in some panoramic devices to facilitate positioning. In a camera image, the Frankfort plane is highlighted in color. E.g., green for acceptable and red for incorrect positioning.

§ Some panoramic machines also have a third laser light that helps to select the proper focal trough. It should extend between the upper lateral incisor and canine, and should fall on the angle of the mouth in edentulous patients. Verify the line of light in a lateral camera image or while the operator stands at the patient's side.

§ Verify the correct position of the patient.

§ After verifying the position, close the temporal supports by pressing a specific button or by pressing the 'Ready' button on the control panel (Figure 6.11).

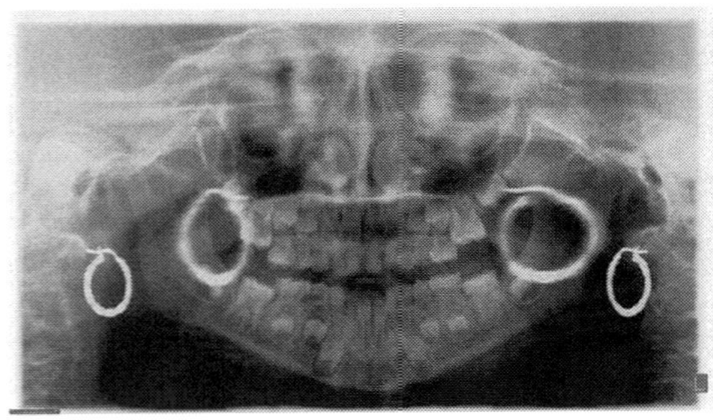

Figure 6.11. *Artefacts by earrings. Note that the shape of each earring is mirror-like and is reflected on the contralateral mandibular ramus/third molar area in the form of an artifact.*

Source: *Izzetti, R., Nisi, M., Aringhieri, G., Crocetti, L., Graziani, F., & Nardi, C. Basic Knowledge and New Advances in Panoramic Radiography Imaging Techniques: A Narrative Review on What Dentists and Radiologists Should Know. Applied Sciences. 2021; 11(17), 7858. https://doi.org/10.3390/app11177858.*

- **Patient Instructions**
  - § Obtaining a high-quality radiograph requires proper fulfillment of instructions by the patient.
- **X-ray Exposure**
  - § Press the 'Ready' button on the control panel.
  - § Per local guidelines, the operator has to exit the X-ray room or protect herself/himself behind a lead screen or a wall. He/she can also step away from the X-ray source to move away from the exposure area.
  - § Press the exposure button and hold it down during the exposure. There is a slight delay in X-ray production after pressing the exposure button. The exposure does not occur if it is just pressed and released. X-ray generation can be detected through audio or visual signals. E.g., yellow light on the machine and the exposure button.
  - § During the exposure, observe the patient through a video camera screen or a lead window.
  - § Patient movement during X-ray exposure will mostly require a retake of the radiograph. Therefore, discontinue the X-ray generation. Certain devices provide a live image preview during exposure to cross-check for motion artifacts in the radiograph due to patient movement. Some panoramic devices can also apply patient movement compensation in a limited range of up to 1.5 cm and does not help in case of severe, sharp movements.
- **After Exposure**
  - § Allow the patient to exit the patient positioning area safely.
  - § Whenever applicable, remove their protective lead apron.
  - § Save the radiograph in the database.
  - § Prepare the panoramic device for the next patient by changing the single-use protective sleeve over the bite piece and disinfecting the parts of the machine touched by the patient using a disinfectant spray.
- **Limitations and Difficulties in Panoramic Radiography**
  - § In some patients, it is challenging to take a good diagnostic radiograph because of anatomic or pathologic variations or uncooperativeness in spite of technological advances like positioning devices and image registration.
  - § Artefacts and errors can occur at any stage of obtaining a panoramic radiograph.
  - § Panoramic radiographs cannot be obtained in unconscious patients, neonates and patients who cannot maintain a straight cervical spinal position even while sitting.
  - § Obtaining a proper panoramic radiograph requires that the patient follows staff

instructions and to remain motionless during the exposure. Panoramic radiography is not advised in young children due to lack of justified indications at their age. Few countries also have a strict age limit (5 years), below which panoramic radiography is contraindicated as per local legal provisions.

§ Involuntary movements such as tremors, jerks, tics and myoclonic seizures can lead to poor quality radiographs or ending of the exposure. In patients with movement disorders like Parkinson's disease, panoramic radiographs must be taken in devices applying patient movement compensation.

§ In patients with cognitive limitations or elderly patients with dementia, obtaining a panoramic radiograph can be difficult due to lack of comprehension of staff instructions and difficulty in standing or remaining still during the X-ray exposure.

§ In patients with severe Class II or Class III malocclusion, placement of upper and lower incisors in the grooves of the bite piece is almost impossible. Therefore, only one jaw will be seen clearly in the resultant radiograph depending on whether the upper or lower teeth were placed within the focal trough. In such patients, systems that permit one-time registration of multiple thin layers within the focal trough are preferred.

§ Severe facial skeletal asymmetry results in difficulty in positioning the left and right side of the face within the focal trough leading to only one side being seen clearly on the radiograph.

§ Patients with advanced periodontal bone disease and tooth mobility may be unable to bite in the groove of the bite piece as mobile teeth tend to tilt while closing the mouth. In such scenarios, it is recommended to use a chin support with a cotton roll to separate the upper and lower incisors.

§ Patients with lockjaw, swelling or injuries of the tongue or lips following trauma may require the use of a chin support with a cotton roll.

- **Tomographic Radiographs of the TMJs:** The majority of panoramic machines also allow the recording of tomographic images of the TMJ in open and closed mouth positions. Machine and patient preparation are the same as for a panoramic radiograph. The TMJ imaging mode should be selected on the control panel or the screen. In case the patient has a prior axial skull radiograph, the angulation of the long axis of the condylar heads in relation to the coronal plane can be measured from the radiograph. These values should be entered into the software or control panel. Default values (17°) are applied when the angulation is unknown.

A dedicated positioning device that provides stable support for the nose and also allows adequate mouth opening is used (Figure 6.12).

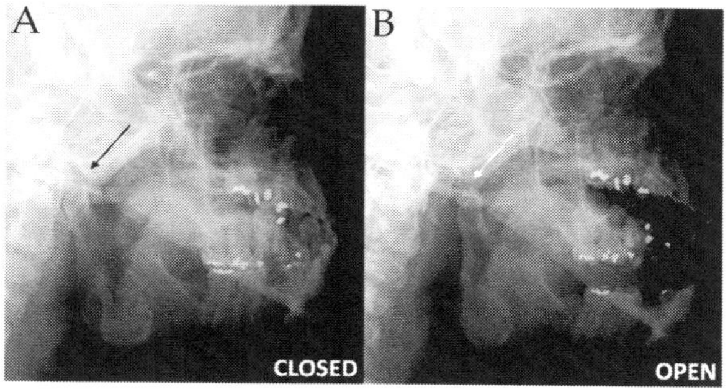

Figure 6.12. *TMJ tomographic imaging.*

Source: Gharavi, S. M., Qiao, Y., Faghihimehr, A., & Vossen, J. Imaging of the Temporomandibular Joint. Diagnostics. 2022; 12(4), 1006. https://doi.org/10.3390/diagnostics12041006.

Steps for Taking a Tomographic Radiograph of the TMJs

- The radiograph has two stages, first with the mouth closed, and the second with the mouth open. This sequence can be the opposite in other machines.
- In the first part, the mouth is closed with the teeth in complete intercuspation.
- The head is symmetrically positioned in the sagittal plane using the first laser light.
- Caudal tilting of the Frankfort plane to 5° is performed (second laser light).
- The distance between the condylar head and the third laser light is measured with a ruler. This value is entered on the screen or control panel.
- Verify the head position, close the temporal supports and begin with the first stage of X-ray exposure.
- After the first exposure, instruct the patient to open her/his mouth wide without changing the head position.
- The value set for the distance should be reduced by 10 mm because the condylar heads shift out of the articular fossae in the open mouth position.
- Verify the head position and begin the second stage of exposure.

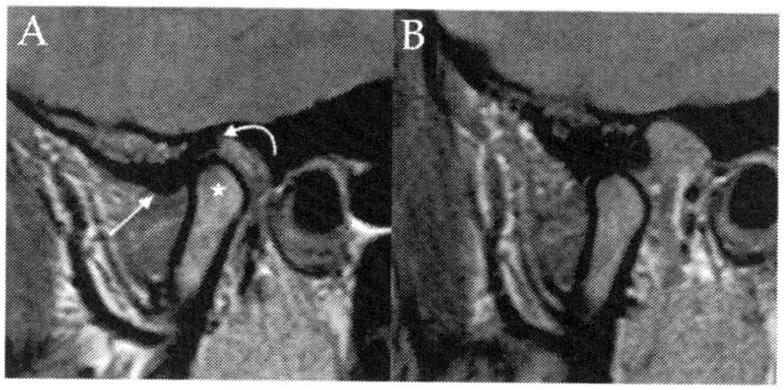

Figure 6.13. *Normal temporomandibular joint MRI. Proton density sagittal image of the TMJ in closed mouth (A) position shows normal location and bow-tie appearance of the articular disc with anterior (straight arrow) and posterior bands (curved arrow). The mandibular condyle (star) is in an anatomic location within the mandibular fossa. On open mouth images (B), normal condylar rotation and anterior translation are noted.*

Source: Gharavi, S. M., Qiao, Y., Faghihimehr, A., & Vossen, J. Imaging of the Temporomandibular Joint. Diagnostics. 2022; 12(4), 1006. https://doi.org/10.3390/diagnostics12041006.

- **Limitations of Tomographic Images of TMJs**
  - § With the advent of CBCT, TMJ tomographic imaging has now become obsolete.
  - § The quality of resultant radiograph is compromised by

movement, lack of cooperation, inability to stand or sit still during exposure and inability to maintain a stable, straight neck position.

§ Lockjaw

§ The result is based on the TMJ anatomy as parasagittal slices are not always at right angles to the long axis of the condylar head, particularly without a prior axial skull radiograph (Wiggs and Lobprise, 1997; Deforge and Colmery, 2000; Pasler and Visser, 2007; Monsour and Dudhia, 2008).

A Closer Look

Uses of Cephalometric X-ray Machines

Cephalometric X-ray machines represent a specialized category of dental radiography equipment designed to capture lateral (side) views of the skull, facial bones, and dentition. These machines play a critical role in orthodontic diagnosis, treatment planning, and monitoring by providing detailed anatomical information essential for evaluating skeletal relationships, facial growth patterns, and dental occlusion.

One of the primary applications of cephalometric X-ray machines is in orthodontics, where they serve as invaluable tools for assessing craniofacial structures and identifying abnormalities that may contribute to malocclusions and dentofacial deformities. By capturing lateral views of the patient's head and neck, cephalometric X-rays enable orthodontists to analyze the position, size, and shape of the jaws, teeth, and surrounding soft tissues, facilitating the development of customized treatment plans tailored to each patient's unique anatomical characteristics.

Cephalometric X-ray machines operate by emitting a controlled beam of X-rays that passes through the patient's head, producing an image receptor on the opposite side. The resulting cephalometric radiograph provides a two-dimensional representation of the patient's craniofacial anatomy, including the maxilla, mandible, nasal structures, temporomandibular joints (TMJs), and surrounding soft tissues. Orthodontists use these images to assess skeletal growth patterns, identify dental anomalies, and predict the outcome of orthodontic treatment, such as tooth movement and facial esthetics.

In addition to orthodontics, cephalometric X-ray machines find applications in oral and maxillofacial surgery, prosthodontics, and facial reconstructive surgery. They aid surgeons in planning and executing complex procedures, such as orthognathic surgery for correcting skeletal discrepancies, dental implant placement, and facial trauma reconstruction. By providing detailed anatomical information with minimal distortion, cephalometric X-rays enhance surgical precision, optimize treatment outcomes, and improve patient satisfaction.

Recent advancements in cephalometric X-ray technology have led to the development of digital cephalometric systems, which offer several advantages over traditional film-based imaging, including enhanced image quality, lower radiation doses, and improved workflow efficiency. Digital cephalometric X-ray machines integrate with computerized imaging software, allowing for image manipulation, measurement, and analysis, as well as electronic storage and retrieval of patient records. These capabilities facilitate interdisciplinary collaboration, enable more accurate treatment planning, and enhance communication between dental professionals and patients.

Summary

- Dental X-rays, also known as dental radiographs, are a type of imaging technique that uses low levels of radiation to capture images of the interior of the teeth and gums. This might seem simple, but it's a game-changer in the field of dentistry.
- Dental X-rays offer a detailed image of your patient's teeth, bones and supporting tissues of the mouth. This invaluable information allows you to spot early signs of dental issues that might be invisible to the naked eye, such as hidden decay, infections, tumors, or impactions.
- Operating dental X-ray machines might seem like a complex task, but with proper training and adherence to safety protocols, it becomes a routine part of dental practice. Whether you're using a traditional wall-mounted unit or a portable handheld device, the fundamentals remain the same. Position the X-ray machine correctly, ensure the patient is adequately protected from unnecessary radiation, and capture high-quality images for accurate diagnosis and treatment planning.
- Bitewing X-rays are incredibly common and are often taken for preventative purposes because they are a great way to see any decay between teeth or below the gumline. The term bitewing comes from how patients must bite down on the X-ray film. These types of X-rays can be taken right in the dental chair.
- Occlusal X-rays are designed to capture what goes on inside the roof or floor of the mouth, which helps the dentist see full tooth development and placement. This may be used to find out why teeth haven't erupted yet or to spot supernumerary (extra) teeth, which can damage healthy permanent teeth.
- A panoramic X-ray uses a special machine that takes one image of your entire upper and lower teeth. The result is a 2-D image of your 3-D mouth. If you suffer from frequent complications or have had major dental work in the past, your dentist may recommend a panoramic X-ray every now and then to make sure nothing is brewing.

References

1. Cheng, S., Butler, J. E., Gandevia, S. C., & Bilston, L. E. (2008). Movement of the tongue during normal breathing in awake healthy humans. *Journal of Physiology, 586*(Pt 17), 4283–4294. https://doi.org/10.1113/jphysiol.2008.155275.
2. Choi, J. W. (2011). Assessment of panoramic radiography as a national oral examination tool: Review of the literature. *Imaging Science in Dentistry, 41*(1), 1–6. https://doi.org/10.5624/isd.2011.41.1.1.
3. Cordesmeyer, R., Engelke, W., Sömmer, C., & Kauffmann, P. (2016). Can tongue shadow in panoramic radiographs be avoided by using the tongue repositioning maneuver? *Oral Surgery, Oral Medicine, Oral Pathology, Oral Radiology, 121*(2), e175–e180. https://doi.org/10.1016/j.oooo.2015.10.007.
4. Engelke, W. (2003). A maneuver for repositioning of the tongue at the palate. *Sprache - Stimme - Gehor, 27*(4), 171–175.

5. Farhat-McHayleh, N., Harfouche, A., & Souaid, P. (2009). Techniques for managing behavior in pediatric dentistry: Comparative study of live modeling and tell-show-do based on children's heart rates during treatment. *Journal of the Canadian Dental Association, 75*(4), 283.

6. Loughlin, A., Drage, N., Greenall, C., & Farnell, D. J. J. (2017). An investigation into the impact of acquisition location on error type and rate when undertaking panoramic radiography. *Radiography, 23*(4), 305–309. https://doi.org/10.1016/j.radi.2017.05.003.

7. Monsour, P. A., & Dudhia, R. (2008). Implant radiography and radiology. *Australian Dental Journal, 53*(Suppl 1), S11–S25. https://doi.org/10.1111/j.1834-7819.2008.00040.x.

8. Rondon, R. H., Pereira, Y. C., & do Nascimento, G. C. (2014). Common positioning errors in panoramic radiography: A review. *Imaging Science in Dentistry, 44*(1), 1–6. https://doi.org/10.5624/isd.2014.44.1.1.

9. Taguchi, A., Asano, A., Ohtsuka, M., et al. (2008). Observer performance in diagnosing osteoporosis by dental panoramic radiographs: Results from the osteoporosis screening project in dentistry (OSPD). *Bone, 43*(2), 209–213. https://doi.org/10.1016/j.bone.2008.04.001.

10. Wiggs, R. B., & Lobprise, H. B. (1997). Veterinary Dentistry - Dental and Oral Radiology. In *Veterinary Dentistry* (pp. 140–166). Philadelphia: Lippincott.

Chapter

7

ULTRASOUND IMAGING

Contents

Introduction

In medicine, ultrasound refers to the process of creating images of internal body structures using high-frequency sound waves, also known as ultrasonic waves. Sound waves that fall outside of the human hearing range are known as ultrasonic waves. A specific region of the body can be targeted by ultrasonic waves, which are created by electrically stimulating a piezoelectric crystal. The waves are reflected back as they pass through the body's tissues at any location where there is a shift in the density of the tissue, such as the boundary separating two organs. An electronic device that receives the reflected echoes and measures its intensity as well as the location of the tissue producing the echoes. The images that are created in this way can be shown static or, by employing quick, repeated audio scans, they can actually create a moving image of the inside of the body.

The fact that ultrasonography sound waves pose less of a risk to human tissue than X-rays or other ionizing radiations contributes to its usefulness. Although there are potential risks to the tissues due to the invasive nature of the procedure, there have been no documented cases of tissue damage resulting from conventional ultrasound imaging. The most common application of ultrasound technology is examining fetuses in utero to determine their size, position, and any anomalies. Images of the heart, liver, kidneys, gallbladder, breasts, eyes, and major blood vessels can also be obtained via ultrasound. Additionally, it can be used to guide certain procedures like intrauterine corrective surgery, drainage tube insertion, and needle biopsies for tumor diagnosis.

The precision of images obtained through computerized axial tomography (CAT) or magnetic resonance imaging (MRI) is higher than that of ultrasound. Nonetheless, ultrasound is widely utilized in medical procedures due to its speed, affordability, and lack of known biological hazards when utilized within the diagnostic range.

Studies have suggested that ultrasonography can be employed as a therapeutic modality. For instance, certain kinds of bone fractures, such as stress fractures and delayed union fractures (fractures that heal abnormally slowly), can be aided in healing by low-intensity pulsed ultrasonography.

The advent of ultrasound in obstetrics and gynecology has had a profound effect on patient care because it made it possible to image the internal organs of the mother in gynecology and the fetus and placenta in obstetrics with such clarity that it allowed for advanced diagnosis and guided various life-saving interventions. Comprehending the fundamental principles of ultrasonography is crucial for grasping the fundamentals of instrument control, as well as for comprehending the safety and bioeffects of this technology. This chapter covers the fundamental ideas behind the physical principles of ultrasonography, clarifies key terms, examines safety and bioeffects, and summarizes national and international organizations' statements regarding ultrasonography.

Orientation and Directional Terms

Term	Definition	Illustration
Ultrasound	Ultrasound is a non-invasive diagnostic technique that uses high-frequency sound waves to create images of internal body structures.	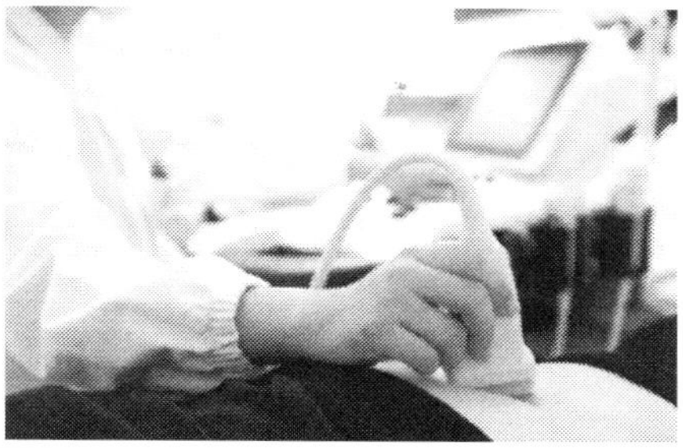
Bladder scan	A bladder scan, also known as a radionuclide cystogram, is a noninvasive test that uses ultrasonic reflections and a liquid with radioactive material to diagnose, manage, and treat urinary outflow dysfunction.	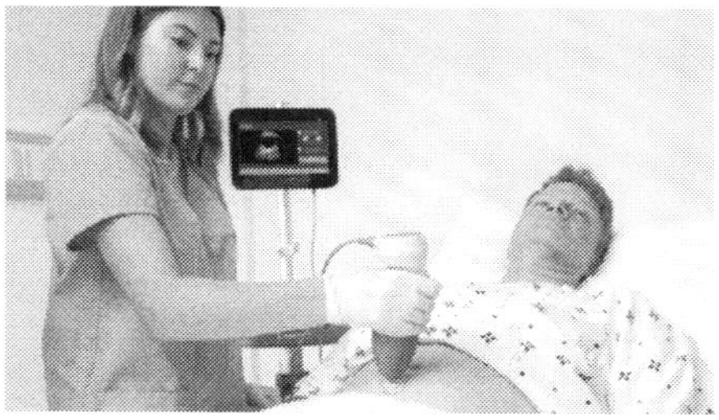
Doppler ultrasound	Doppler ultrasonography is medical ultrasonography that employs the Doppler effect to perform imaging of the movement of tissues and body fluids, and their relative velocity to the probe.	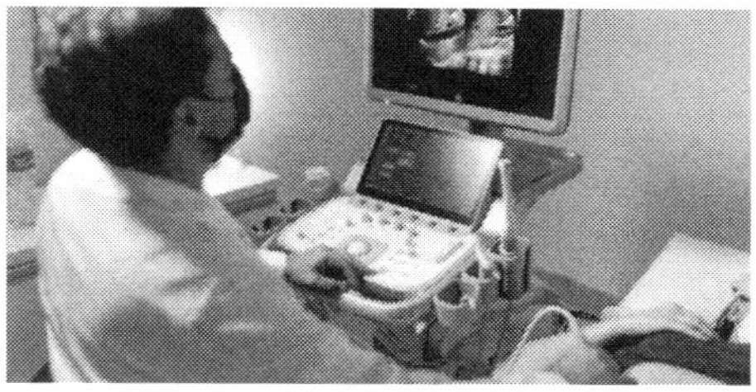
Elastography	Elastography is a medical imaging technique that measures the stiffness and elastic properties of soft tissue. It can provide diagnostic information about disease presence or status, as the type of tissue determines whether it's hard or soft.	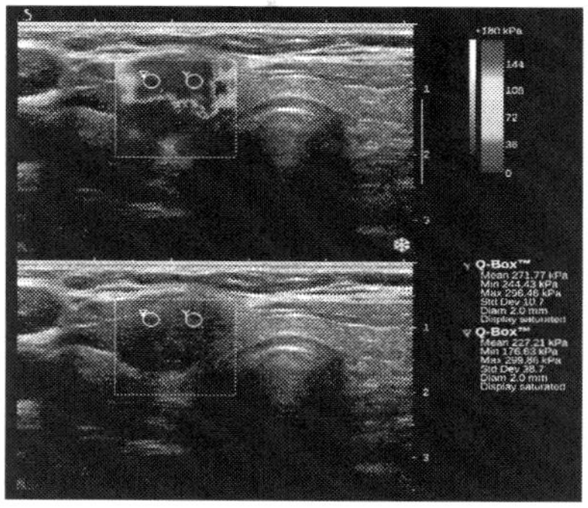
Sonography	Sonography is a type of allied healthcare that uses ultrasonic imaging devices to create diagnostic images, scans, videos, or 3D volumes of anatomy and diagnostic data.	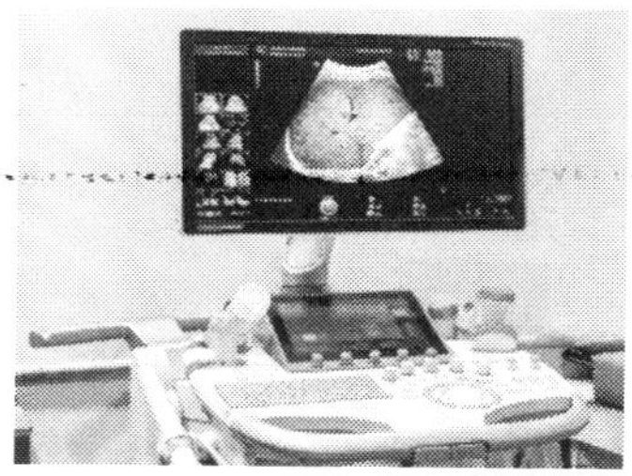

7.1. Medical Ultrasound

Medical ultrasound falls into two distinct categories: diagnostic and therapeutic. A non-invasive diagnostic method for imaging inside the body is diagnostic ultrasound. Transducers, also known as ultrasound probes, generate sound waves with frequencies above the 20 kHz threshold for human hearing; however, the majority of transducers in use today operate at frequencies much higher than this, in the megahertz (MHz) range. The majority of diagnostic ultrasound probes are applied topically. Nonetheless, probes may be inserted into the body through the vagina, gastrointestinal tract, or blood vessels to maximize image quality. Additionally, a sterile probe is occasionally inserted into the surgical site to use ultrasound technology during the procedure.

Anatomical and functional ultrasound are two more subcategories of diagnostic ultrasound. Images of internal organs or other structures can be obtained through anatomical ultrasound. Functional ultrasound creates "information maps" by fusing anatomical images with data about the softness and hardness of tissue, blood flow and velocity, and other physical attributes. These maps aid medical professionals in seeing modifications or variations in an organ's or structure's function. Although it does not create images, therapeutic ultrasonography employs sound waves that are higher than the range of human hearing. Its goal is to cause changes or destruction to bodily tissues through interaction. Modifications include pushing or moving tissue, heating tissue, breaking up blood clots, and administering medications to particular parts of the body. Extremely high-intensity beams that can destroy diseased or abnormal tissues like tumors enable these destructive, or ablative, functions. One benefit of ultrasound therapies is that they are typically non-invasive. There is no need to make any skin incisions or cuts, so there won't be any wounds or scars.

7.1.1. How Does It Work?

A transducer generates ultrasound waves by being able to detect ultrasonic echoes that are reflected back in addition to emitting ultrasound waves. Ultrasonic transducers' active elements are typically composed of unique ceramic crystal materials known as piezoelectrics. When an electric field is applied to these materials, they can produce sound waves; conversely, when a sound wave strikes them, they can produce an electric field.

The transducer emits a beam of sound waves into the body when it is utilized in an ultrasound scanner. Boundaries between tissues in the beam's path reflect sound waves to the transducer (e.g., the line separating bone or soft tissue from fluid. The transducer receives electrical signals from these echoes, and the ultrasound scanner receives those signals. The scanner determines how far away the tissue boundary is from the transducer by measuring the sound speed and the duration of each echo's return. The two-dimensional pictures of tissues and organs are then created using these distances (Figure 7.1).

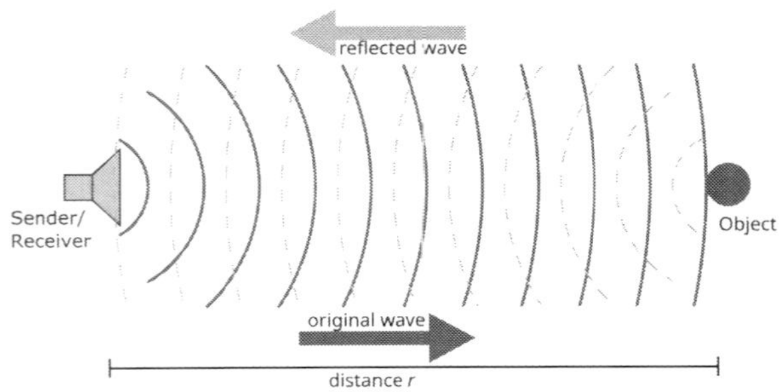

Figure 7.1. *Working of ultrasound.*

Source. By Georg Wiora (Dr. Schorsch) – Self drawn with Inkscape, CC BY-SA 3.0, https://commons.wikimedia.org/w/index.php?curid=353362.

The ultrasonography technician will apply a gel to the patient's skin. By doing this, air pockets that could prevent ultrasound waves from entering the body from forming between the transducer and the skin are prevented.

7.1.2. Using of Ultrasound

Diagnostic ultrasound. Internal organs within the body can be imaged non-invasively using diagnostic ultrasound. On the other hand, it is not suitable for imaging bones or any air-containing tissues, such as the lungs. When the lungs are fully or partially filled with fluid, ultrasound can image the lining surrounding the lungs, the bones (such as in a fetus or small baby), or both. There are numerous applications for ultrasound, including imaging the heart, blood vessels, eyes, thyroid, brain, breast, abdominal organs, skin, and muscles. One of the most popular uses of ultrasound is to track the growth and development of the fetus during pregnancy. The three image formats for ultrasounds are 2D, 3D, and 4D, or 3D in motion (Figure 7.2).

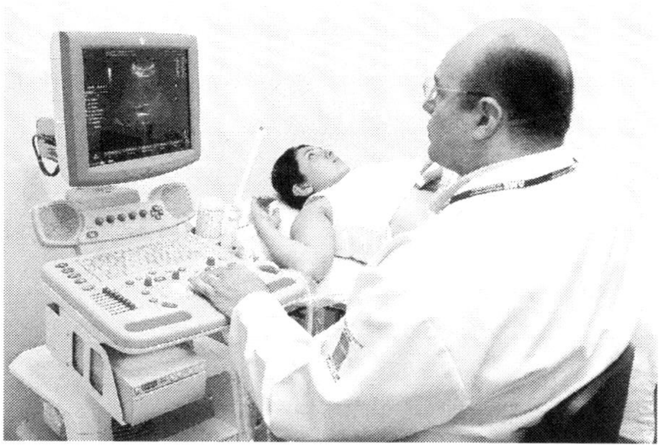

Figure 7.2. *The ultrasound probe (transducer) is placed at the site and analyzed.*

Source. By Leval – Own work, Public Domain, https://commons.wikimedia.org/w/index.php?curid=3349818.

- **Functional Ultrasound:** Doppler and color Doppler ultrasonography are two functional ultrasound applications that are used to measure and visualize blood flow in body or heart vessels. It is also capable of measuring the direction and velocity of blood flow. Color Doppler imaging, which uses color-coded maps, is used for this. To ascertain whether plaque accumulation inside the carotid arteries is obstructing blood flow to the brain, Doppler ultrasonography is frequently employed.

Elasticography, a technique for determining and displaying the relative stiffness of tissues, is another useful application of ultrasound that helps distinguish between tumors and healthy tissue. Color-coded maps of the relative stiffness, black-and-white maps showing high-contrast tumor images in comparison to anatomical images, or color-coded maps superimposed on the anatomical image are some possible ways to present this information. Tests for liver fibrosis, a disorder in which the liver develops an excessive amount of scar tissue as a result of inflammation, can be performed using elastography.

Another crucial technique for imaging interventions inside the body is ultrasound. For instance, ultrasound-guided needle biopsy enables doctors to view the needle's location as it is guided toward a particular target, like a breast tumor or mass. Moreover, ultrasound is used to image in real time where a catheter tip is as it is inserted into a blood vessel and moved along its length. With real-time images of the inside of the body, it can also be used to guide the surgeon during minimally invasive surgery.

- **Therapeutic or Interventional Ultrasound:** To heat, ablate, or break up tissue, therapeutic ultrasound generates high levels of acoustic output that can be targeted to particular targets. High Intensity Focussed Ultrasound (HIFU) is a type of therapeutic ultrasound that employs highly targeted, high-intensity sound beams. HIFU is being researched as a potential technique to alter or eliminate abnormal or diseased tissues within the body (e.g., tumors) without requiring skin tearing, opening, or harming surrounding tissue. The tissue to be treated is identified and targeted using either MRI or ultrasound, which is also used to guide and control the treatment in real-time and verify its efficacy. As of right now, HIFU has FDA approval for the ablation of prostate tissue, the treatment of uterine fibroids, and the relief of pain from bone metastases. Additionally, HIFU is being researched as a means of dissolving blood clots in blood vessels, sealing wounds to stop bleeding, and momentarily opening the blood-brain barrier to allow medication to pass through.

Compared to X-rays, diagnostic ultrasound is generally thought to be safe and does not emit ionizing radiation. Still, in certain situations and environments, ultrasound can have some biological effects on the body. Because of this, the FDA mandates that diagnostic ultrasound equipment function within reasonable bounds. Numerous professional societies and the FDA oppose the careless application of ultrasound (e.g., for memento videos) and advise against using it unless there is an actual medical necessity (Dowdey et al, 1990; Shriki, 2014; Frederick and Kremkau, 2015).

7.2. Ultrasound Imaging

High-frequency sound waves are used in ultrasound imaging, also known as sonography, to view inside the body. Ultrasound images can depict blood flowing through blood vessels and the movement of the body's internal organs because they are taken in real-time. Ultrasound imaging does not involve exposure to ionizing radiation, in contrast to X-ray imaging.

A transducer, or probe, is positioned directly on the skin or within a bodily opening during an ultrasound examination. To allow the ultrasonic waves from the transducer to enter the body through the gel, a thin layer of gel is applied to the skin (Figure 7.3).

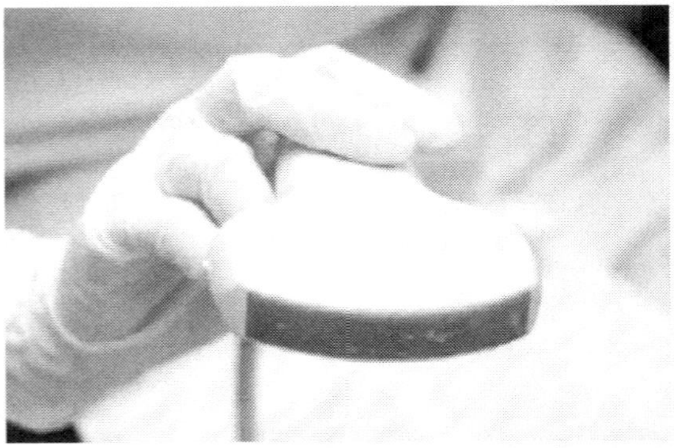

Figure 7.3. *Picture of a transducer (probe) used during an ultrasound exam.*

Source: https://www.fda.gov/files/ultrasound_transducer.jpg.

The ultrasound image is generated through wave reflection from the body structures. An image can be created by using the information provided by the sound signal's strength (amplitude) and the length of time it takes for the wave to pass through the body.

An ultrasound examination, also known as a "sonogram," is a painless diagnostic method that utilizes the body's natural ability to conduct sound waves. Sound waves travel through the body and reflect off organs and tissues in different ways. It is possible to create images of the internal organs using the reflected waves. There is no radiation and the sound waves do not harm the body.

A hospital, an outpatient facility, or the doctor's office can all perform ultrasound imaging. The purpose of the study and the specifics of the case will aid in determining the appropriate location for the test.

Very little work usually needs to be done in advance of an ultrasound exam. On the examination table lies the patient. The area of skin that needs to be examined is covered with a clear, water-based gel. This gel facilitates the body's absorption of sound waves. The next step is to move a hand-held probe, or "transducer," over that area. To perform prostate ultrasound exams, the rectum is probed with a specially made device.

Radiation risk does not exist. After the test, the patient can immediately resume their regular activities. Certain tests, like a bladder scan to check for leftover urine, don't require a lot of experience from the user. Certain exams require the user to have more training or experience, such as ultrasounds of the prostate, testicles, or kidneys.

7.2.1. Uses

Ultrasound imaging is a medical tool that can help a physician evaluate, diagnose and treat medical conditions. Common ultrasound imaging procedures include:

- Abdominal ultrasound (to visualize abdominal tissues and organs)
- Bone sonometry (to assess bone fragility)
- Breast ultrasound (to visualize breast tissue)
- Doppler fetal heart rate monitors (to listen to the fetal heart beat)
- Doppler ultrasound (to visualize blood flow through a blood vessel, organs, or other structures)
- Echocardiogram (to view the heart)
- Fetal ultrasound (to view the fetus in pregnancy)
- Ultrasound-guided biopsies (to collect a sample of tissue)
- Ophthalmic ultrasound (to visualize ocular structures
- Ultrasound-guided needle placement (in blood vessels or other tissues of interest)

7.2.2. Benefits/Risks

With more than 20 years of use, ultrasound imaging has a stellar safety record. It does not carry the same risks as X-rays or other imaging systems that use ionizing radiation because it is based on non-ionizing radiation.

Ultrasound radiation can have biological effects on the body, even though it is generally thought to be safe when used carefully by medical professionals with the necessary training. The tissues may get somewhat heated by ultrasound waves. It may also occasionally result in cavitation, or tiny pockets of gas in bodily fluids or tissues. It's still unclear what these effects will mean in the long run. Organizations like the American Institute of Ultrasound in Medicine External Link Disclaimer have promoted the cautious use of ultrasound imaging during pregnancy due to the special concern for effects on the fetus. Moreover, it is not advised to use ultrasound for non-medical purposes alone, such as creating "keepsake" videos of fetuses. If the photos or videos are taken during a medically necessary examination and no further exposure is needed, then they are reasonable keepsakes.

7.2.3. Information for Patients Including Expectant Mothers

The FDA advises patients to discuss all medical imaging procedures with their healthcare provider so they are aware of the purpose of the test, the medical information that will be obtained, any possible risks, and how the results will be used to manage the ailment or pregnancy. Ultrasonography is especially helpful for women who are pregnant or nursing when CT or other imaging techniques would expose them to radiation because it does not use ionizing radiation.

7.2.3.1. Expectant Mothers

The most popular medical imaging technique for seeing the fetus during pregnancy is ultrasound. The purpose of routine exams is to evaluate and track the mother's and fetus's health. Ultrasound examinations offer parents a priceless chance to see and hear the fetus's heartbeat, form a bond with the unborn child, and take pictures to send to loved ones.

Three-dimensional (3D) ultrasonography makes it possible to see some of the fetus's facial features as well as potentially other parts like its fingers and toes. Ultrasound in four dimensions (4D) is essentially 3D ultrasound in motion. Although ultrasonography is usually thought to be safe and has very little risks, there is a chance that things could go wrong if users operate the device incorrectly or expose themselves to ultrasonography energy for an extended time.

Concerns about buying doptones, or over-the-counter fetal heartbeat monitors, should also be known to expectant mothers. When medically necessary, these devices should only be used by qualified healthcare professionals. Untrained users of these devices run the risk of exposing the fetus to dangerously high energy levels for extended periods of time or receiving information that is misinterpreted by the user.

7.2.4. Types of Ultrasounds

Ultrasounds can be used to look at different organs in the body. Below is a list of ultrasounds:

- Bladder Ultrasound
- Kidney (Renal) Ultrasound
- Scrotum/ Testicular Ultrasound
- Prostate Ultrasound (with Biopsy)
- Other Uses

Smooth muscle makes up the organ known as the bladder. Urine is stored there until you need to release it to use the restroom. Urinary tract ultrasounds are most frequently performed to assess bladder emptying. Post-void residual urine is the urine that stays in the bladder after urinating and is measured. If urine remains, there can be a problem like:

- Enlarged prostate
- Urethral stricture (narrowing)
- Bladder dysfunction

Bladder ultrasound can also give information about:

- The bladder wall
- Diverticula (pouches) of the bladder
- Prostate size
- Stones
- Large tumors in the bladder

Bladder ultrasound doesn't check the ovaries, uterus, or colon.

There is no need to fast or prepare your bowels for this test. A full bladder is required if you are not checking for post-void residuals. You might be instructed to consume a large amount of water an hour prior to the test.

You lie on your back on the exam table to complete the exam. To aid in the transmission of the sound waves, a gel is applied to the skin. Your pubic bone and navel are where the transducer is positioned. The image is immediately read and seen on a monitor. You will be asked to void to assess bladder emptying. The bladder will be imaged once more when you get back.

Located on either side of your midsection, the kidneys are two fist-sized organs called the "retroperitoneum." The kidneys produce urine and filter waste from the blood. They also maintain the body's equilibrium of salts, or "electrolytes," like potassium and sodium. The kidneys also produce the hormones that regulate blood pressure and the production of red blood cells.

Renal ultrasound studies can show the size and position of the kidneys. They can also show if there are:

- Blockages
- Stones
- Tumors

Using sound waves reflected from the kidney tissue, an ultrasound of the kidney produces images. Numerous photos are obtained to comprehend kidney issues.

Doppler imaging is used by your doctor to see how blood travels to and from the kidney. Using ultrasound technology, color images of blood flow can be created. It displays how blood moves through the vessels. It offers superior motion information that isn't seen on a typical sonogram. There's no need to have a full bladder, fast, or prepare your bowels. You take the test while lying on your back on the examination table. To aid in the transmission of the sound waves, a gel is applied to the skin. The transducer is placed over both sides of the upper abdomen to image the kidneys.

The scrotum is a muscular sac with skin covering that houses a man's testicles, or testicles. Sperm cells are produced in the testicles for reproduction. Additionally, they produce testosterone, a male hormone. Scrotal ultrasounds are primarily performed to assess for pain or swelling. Additionally, masses in the testes or scrotum are checked with it.

Often, fluid will pool around the testicles. This is not cancerous; it is referred to as a hydrocele. Other things that could be discovered include varicocele, or large veins in the scrotum, and spermatocele, or cysts in the epididymis. Solid masses can also be examined with this study to see if they indicate testicular cancer.

Testicular ultrasound is used to evaluate almost all issues in the scrotum, the sac containing the testicles. It can identify solid, cystic, intratesticular, or extra testicular masses, as well as patterns from cancer. It is used to treat issues with blood flow in the testes and testicular torsion. It can be used to prevent testicular death. For this test, Color-Doppler imaging is used. This high-quality color imaging has made testicular ultrasound an accurate and specific test.

There is no need to prepare for this test. You lie on your back on the examination table and complete it. To help transmit sound waves, the scrotum is raised onto a towel and warm gel is applied. To produce images, the transducer is moved over the region.

Men's prostates are located at the base of their bladders. It forms a ring-like motion around the urethra. A portion of the ejaculatory fluid—which is necessary for reproduction—is produced by the prostate. The bladder may become blocked if the prostate grows large.

Examining men who may be at risk for prostate cancer is the main purpose of a prostate ultrasound, also known as a "transrectal ultrasound." Ultrasound alone is not a reliable way to diagnose early-stage cancer. This is the reason a prostate biopsy, or tissue sample, is also performed.

Your doctor will want to examine your prostate gland and surrounding tissue in order to make a diagnosis of prostate disease. Nearly 70% of prostate cancer malignancies are located near the rectum in the prostate's outer zone.

To aid in treatment planning, prostate ultrasound can quantify the prostate's size or volume. Transrectal ultrasounds are used for this purpose in patients undergoing radioactive seed implantation, or "brachytherapy," to treat prostate cancer. It is employed to determine how many seeds are required and where to plant them. Prostate surgery or other therapies (like thermal therapies) may also be planned using the results of this test. The prostate-specific antigen density can be measured by the study.

You might be asked to use an enema before this test. You will lie on your side or back on the examination table throughout the test. To view the prostate, the ultrasonography transducer probe is placed inside the rectum. Through the rectum's wall and into the prostate gland, the probe transmits and receives sound waves. These acoustic waves produce diagnostic images. Urologist searching for prostate cancer symptoms. A tiny tissue sample may be obtained concurrently for a biopsy.

A biopsy may or may not involve the use of local anesthesia. A specialized needle is inserted through a transducer channel to perform a biopsy. A speedy biopsy is performed. Many biopsy "cores" are removed so that a pathologist can examine them.

This test carries comparatively few risks. You might have mild discomfort following a biopsy. Receiving the results of the biopsy can take several days. Your urologist will discuss available treatment options if cancer is discovered. If the biopsy reveals no cancer, you and your urologist will discuss your follow-up options.

- **Evaluation of Infertility:** Transrectal ultrasonography can occasionally help identify prostate and seminal vesicle anomalies. The testes can also be examined with it.
- **Evaluation of the Female Urethra:** A urethral diverticulum can be located using transvaginal ultrasound. Urinary tract infections and urethral pain can both be brought on by a urethral diverticulum.
- **Pediatric Urology:** Because ultrasound is painless and performed outside of the body, it is perfect for use with young patients. Furthermore, the outcomes are immediately apparent. Excellent images of the kidneys and bladder can be obtained with ultrasound. It is helpful in the diagnosis and treatment of urinary tract infections as well as problems related to voiding.
- **Evaluation of Blood Flow:** The flow of blood through the urological organs can be observed using a kind of ultrasound known as Doppler ultrasound. The kidneys and testes benefit from this (Dowdey et al, 1990; Shriki, 2014; Frederick and Kremkau, 2015).

7.3. Physical Characteristics of Sound

Sound is a mechanical wave that moves straight and longitudinally through a medium. The molecules of a medium undergo alternate compression (squeezing) and stretching (rarefaction) when sound travels through it. Since sound is a mechanical energy that is transferred from one molecule to another, it cannot travel in a vacuum and needs a medium to do so. It is significant to note that the molecules oscillate back and forth, creating zones of compression and rarefaction in the medium, rather than moving when the sound wave passes through them. A sound wave's properties are described by seven acoustic parameters. Table 7.1 enumerates these attributes.

Table 7.1. Characteristics of Sound Waves

Characteristic	Symbols
Sound pressure	*p*, SPL, L_{PA}
Particle velocity	*v*, SVL
Particle displacement	*Δ*
Sound intensity	*I*, SIL
Sound power	*P*, SWL, L_{WA}
Sound energy	*W*
Sound energy density	*W*
Sound exposure	*E*, SEL
Acoustic impedance	*Z*
Audio frequency	AF
Transmission loss	TL

Source. https://en.wikipedia.org/wiki/Sound.

The number of cycles that a sound wave goes through in a second is its frequency. Hertz is measured in cycles per second. Since frequency influences both sound penetration and image quality, frequency is a crucial aspect of sound in ultrasonic imaging. The duration of a sound wave's oscillation is directly proportional to its frequency, meaning that the two are correlated. A sound wave with a frequency of 10 Hertz, for example, will have a duration of 1/10 second. Three wave properties—amplitude, power, and intensity—relate to how strong a sound wave is. The difference between the wave's maximum or minimum peaks and average values is known as its amplitude. The zone of compression is represented by the peak, or crest, and the zone of rarefaction by the trough. In clinical imaging, amplitudes are expressed in million Pascals (MPa) and pressure parameters (Pascals). The amplitude of a sound wave decreases as it travels through the body. Power, which is measured in Watts, is the rate at which energy is transmitted through a sound wave. A sound wave's power is directly proportional to its squared amplitude. One of the ultrasound machine's controls allows you to adjust the power level. Since intensity is the concentration of energy in a sound wave, it is influenced by the power and the sound beam's cross-sectional area. The power of a sound beam (Watts) divided by its cross-sectional area (cm2) yields the intensity of the beam, which is then expressed in W/cm^2 units. The wavelength of a sound wave is its length and is defined as the distance of a full cycle. It is denoted by the symbol lambda (λ), can be calculated by dividing the wave's velocity by its frequency ($\lambda = v/f$), and is expressed in millimeters in clinical settings. The distance a sound wave travels through a given medium in one second is known as its propagation speed (Figures 7.4, 7.5, and 7.6) (Table 7.2).

The ultrasonic machine or transducer, as the source of sound, controls the sound's frequency, duration, amplitude, power, and intensity. The propagation speed is solely dependent on the medium, while the wavelength is influenced by the sound source. In soft tissue, sound travels at a constant speed of 1,540 m/s (Dowdey et al, 1990; Shriki, 2014; Frederick and Kremkau, 2015).

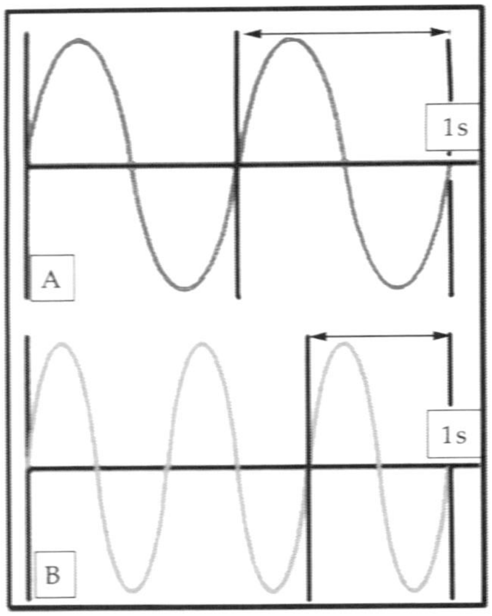

Figure 7.4. *Frequency of sound is the number of cycles per second (s) and is expressed in Hertz (1 cycle/sec). In Wave A, the frequency is 2 cycles per sec or 2 Hertz and in wave B the frequency is 3 cycles per sec or 3 Hertz. The double arrows denote sound wavelengths.*

Source. https://www.glowm.com/pdf/Ultrasound_in_obstetrics_and_gynecology-chapter1.pdf.

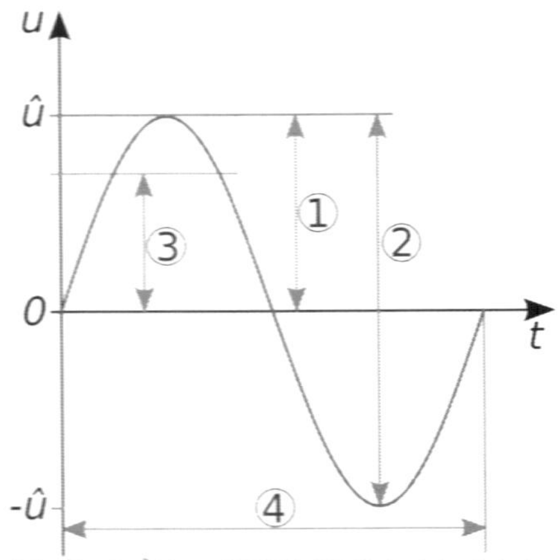

Figure 7.5. *Amplitude (A) is defined by the difference between the peak (maximum) or trough (minimum) of the wave and the average value. Units of amplitude are expressed in million Pascals (MPa).*

Source. By Matthias Krüger – This file was derived from: Sinus-spannung.gif(GIF⍰SVG), Public Domain, https://commons.wikimedia.org/w/index.php?curid=3490976.

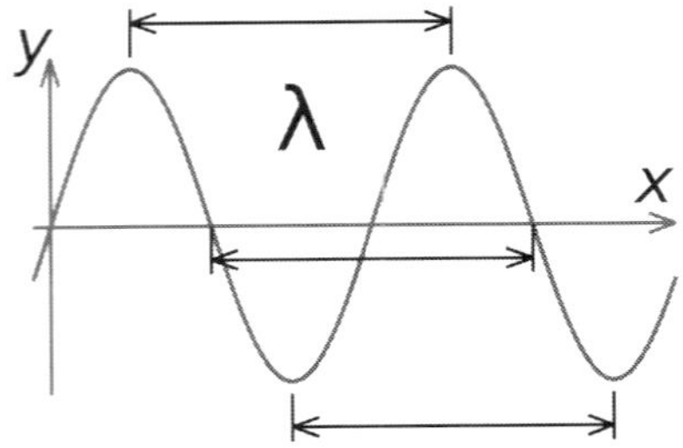

Figure 7.6. *The wavelength of a sound wave is the length of a wave and is defined as the distance of a complete cycle. It is designated by the symbol lambda (λ), and is expressed in mm.*

Source. By Dicklyon (Richard F. Lyon) – Own work, CC BY-SA 3.0, https://commons.wikimedia.org/w/index.php?curid=7184592.

Table 7.2. Speed of Sound in Different Substances or Organs

Material	Speed (m/s)
Air	331
Fat	1450/1465
Water (50°C)	1540
Human soft tissue	1540
Liver	1549
Kidney	1561
Blood	1570/1584
Muscle	1585
Non-fatty tissue	1575
Cortical bone	3635
Amniotic fluid	1535

Source: *Moyano, D. B., Paraiso, D. A., & González-Lezcano, R. A. Possible Effects on Health of Ultrasound Exposure, Risk Factors in the Work Environment and Occupational Safety Review. Healthcare. 2022, 10(3), 423. https://doi.org/10.3390/healthcare10030423.*

7.4. Ultrasound

The classification of sound is determined by the acoustic capacity of the human ear. Audible sound, defined as sounds detected by young, healthy adult human ears, is defined as falling between 20 and 20,000 cycles per second, or Hertz, or 20 KHz (Kilo Hertz). An audible frequency of less than 20 Hz is considered infrasonic, or infrasound, and is unheard by humans. Table 7.3 states that sound frequencies higher than 20 KHz are considered ultrasonic or ultrasound since they are inaudible to humans. In medical ultrasound, typical frequencies range from 2 to 10 MHz (megahertz). In obstetrics and gynecology, ultrasound frequencies that are frequently utilized range from 3 to 10 MHz.

Table 7.3. Frequency Spectrum

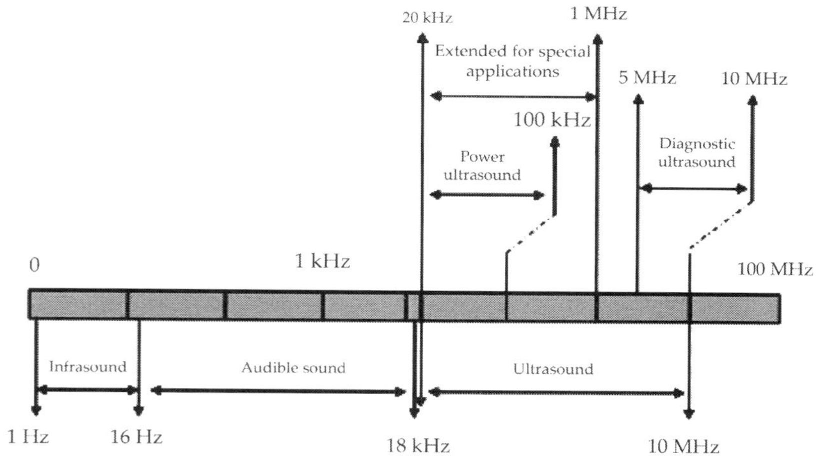

Source. By Arkrishna – Own work, CC BY-SA 3.0, https://commons.wikimedia.org/w/index.php?curid=29899326.

7.4.1. How Is Ultrasound Generated?

The ultrasonic transducers contain tiny piezoelectric crystals that produce ultrasound waves. These crystals contract and expand in response to an alternate current applied to them at the same frequency that the current changes polarity, producing an ultrasound beam. At the same frequency that is generated, the ultrasonic beam passes through the body. On the other hand, these crystals undergo a slight shape change when the ultrasound beam returns to the transducer. This slight change in shape results in a tiny electric current, which the ultrasound machine amplifies to produce an ultrasound image on the monitor. Thus, electric energy is converted into mechanical energy (ultrasound) and vice versa by the piezoelectric crystals inside the transducer. In order to generate an ultrasound beam for clinical imaging, one crystal is insufficient, so contemporary transducers feature many crystals arranged in parallel rows. Nevertheless, each crystal can be stimulated separately. The rubber covering that protects the crystals aids in lowering the impedance—

the resistance—to sound transmission from the crystals to the body. Because transducers produce high frequency sounds that are not well transmitted through air, a watery gel is applied to the patient's skin to couple the transducer to the skin and allow sound waves to periodically reverberate. Thus, tiny crystals that transform electric current into ultrasound and return ultrasound beams from the body into electric currents produce ultrasound inside transducers. Crystals of synthetic plumbium zirconium titanate (PZT) are used in modern transducers (Figure 7.7).

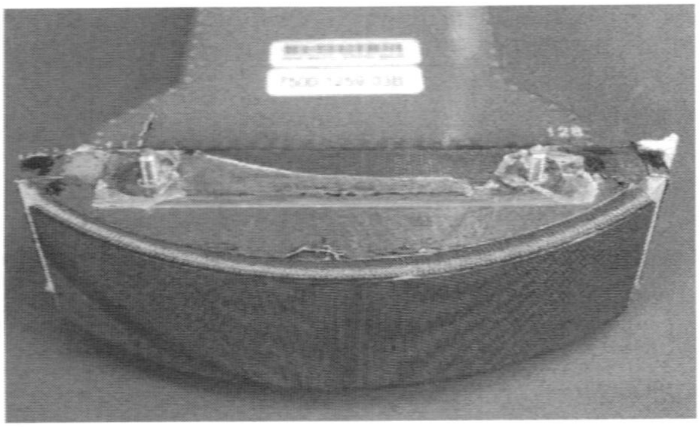

Figure 7.7. *Piezoelectric crystals are present in a transducer.*

Source. By Binarysequence – Own work, CC BY-SA 4.0, https://commons.wikimedia.org/w/index.php?curid=92723746.

7.4.2. An Ultrasound Image Formed

By directing multiple sound pulses from the transducer in slightly different directions and analyzing the return echoes that the crystals receive, modern ultrasound equipment creates an ultrasound image. The specifics of this procedure are outside the purview of this book, but it's crucial to understand that tissues like air or bone, which strongly reflect ultrasound beams, will cause the piezoelectric crystals to generate a strong electric current, which will appear as a hyperechoic image on the monitor.

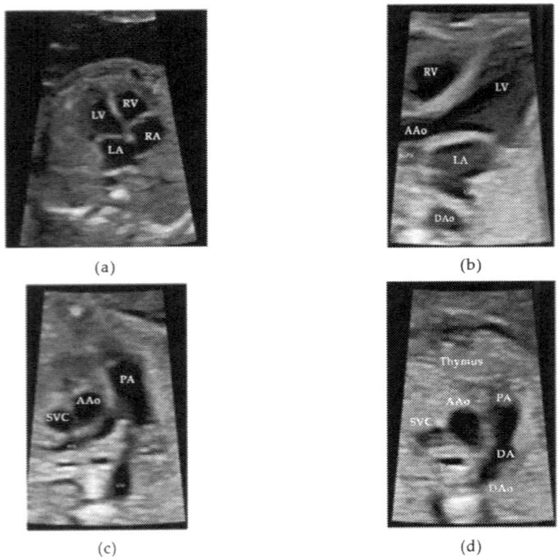

Figure 7.8. *High-resolution ultrasonography of the fetal heart at 20 weeks' gestation showing (**a**) a four-chamber view showing right atrium (RA), left atrium (LA), right ventricle (RV), and left ventricle (LV), (**b**) five-chamber view showing ascending aorta (AAo) arising from the left ventricle, the right and left superior pulmonary veins (RSPV, LSPV) enter the left atrium (LA), and descending aorta (DAo) behind the LA (**c**) Three-vessel view showing the PA dividing into the left (LPA) and right (RPA) PA, AAo, and the superior vena cava (SVC), (**d**) three-vessel and trachea view showing PA with the ductal branch (DA) joining the DAo, AAo, SVC, and trachea (T); Thymus is anterior to the three vessels.*

Source. Leung, K.-Y. Applications of Advanced Ultrasound Technology in Obstetrics. Diagnostics. 2021; 11(7), 1217. https://doi.org/10.3390/diagnostics11071217.

Conversely, weak ultrasonic beam reflectors, like fluid or soft tissue, will produce a weak current, which will show up on the monitor as a hypoechoic or anechoic image. Thus, an intricate analysis of the returning echoes in a grayscale format produces the ultrasound image. As the ultrasonic beam travels in a longitudinal format, it is best to keep its angle of incidence perpendicular to the object of interest in order to obtain the best possible image, since the angle of incidence equals the angle of reflection (Figures 7.8 and 7.9).

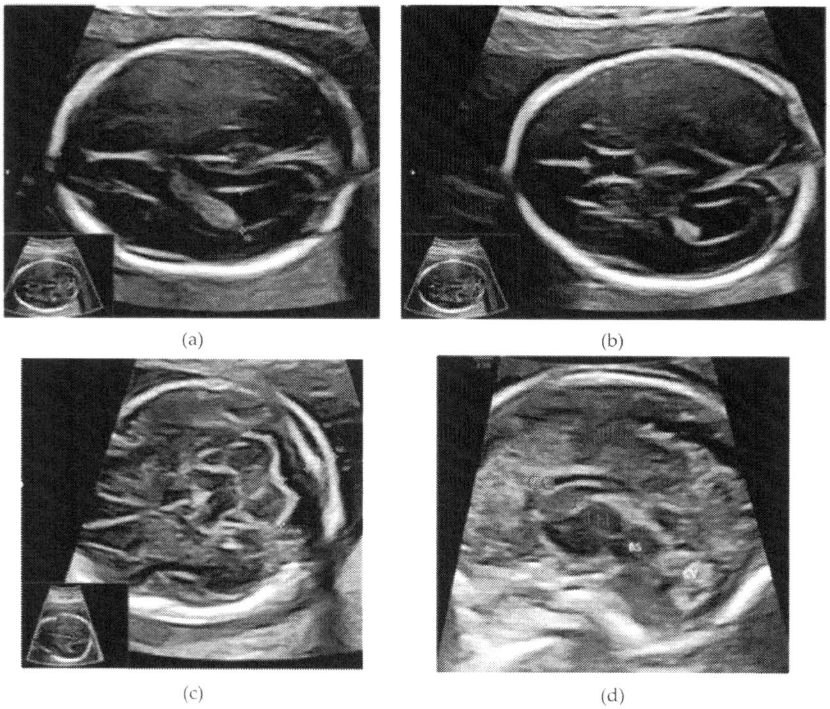

Figure 7.9. *High-resolution ultrasonography of the fetal brain at 20 weeks' gestation: transverse views showing (a) posterior horn of the lateral ventricle (Vp), (b) cavum septi pellucidi (C.S.P.), (c) cerebellum (Cereb), Cisterna magna (CM), nuchal fold (NF), and sagittal view showing (d) corpus callosum (CC), thalamus (TH), brain stem (BS), and cerebellar vermis (CV).*

Source. Leung, K.-Y. Applications of Advanced Ultrasound Technology in Obstetrics. Diagnostics. 2021; 11(7), 1217. https://doi.org/10.3390/diagnostics11071217.

7.5. Different Types of Ultrasound Modes

The "Amplitude mode," or "A-mode," served as the foundation for contemporary ultrasound imaging but is no longer utilized in clinical obstetric and gynecologic ultrasound imaging. Returning ultrasonic echoes are displayed in an A-mode display as a graph, where the y-axis indicates the amplitude of the returning beam and the x-axis indicates the depth of the tissues. Biparietal diameters were previously measured in obstetrics using A-mode ultrasound. The term "Brightness mode," also referred to as "two-dimensional imaging," or "B-mode display," is frequently used to refer to any type of grayscale ultrasound image display. The ultrasound image is formed by the intensity of the reflected ultrasonic beam, which is reflected in a range of grayscale tones. It is crucial to remember that one crucial and essential aspect of ultrasonic imaging is the real-time acquisition of B-mode. The varied echogenicity of normal fetal tissue is displayed in Table 7.4 (Figure 7.10 and 7.11).

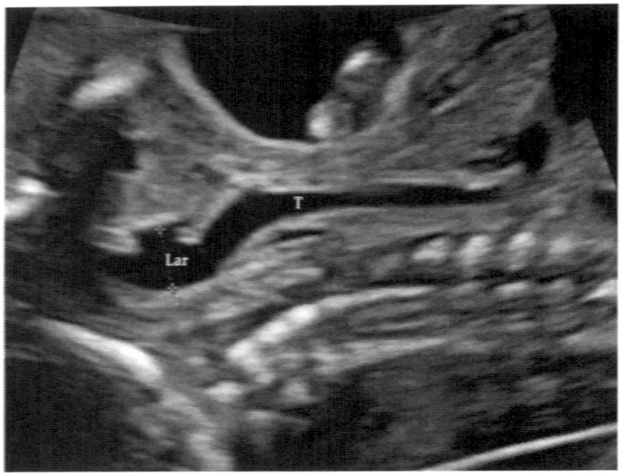

Figure 7.10. *High-resolution ultrasonography of the fetal face at 20 weeks' gestation: (a) mid-sagittal view showing facial profile, (b) coronal view showing both lens (Le), (c) coronal view showing the upper lip (UL) and two nostrils (No), and (d) sagittal view showing the ear.*

Source. Leung, K.-Y. Applications of advanced ultrasound technology in obstetrics. Diagnostics. 2021; 11(7), 1217. https://doi.org/10.3390/diagnostics11071217.

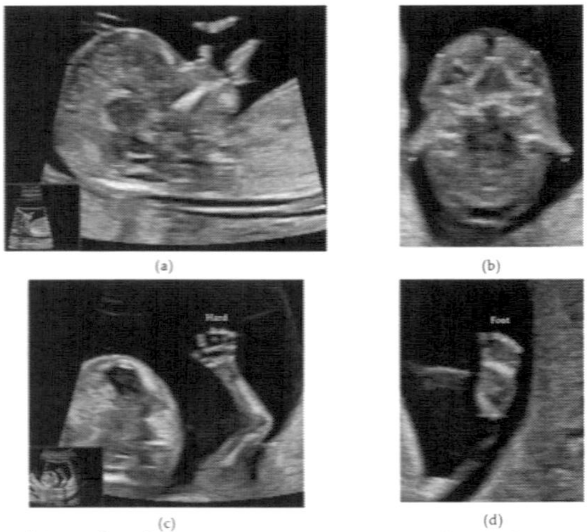

Figure 7.11. *High-resolution ultrasonography of the fetus at 13 weeks' gestation: (**a**) mid-sagittal view showing head, neck, and facial profile, (**b**) coronal view showing both eyes and ears, (**c**) the hand with five fingers, and (**d**) foot.*

Source. Leung, K.-Y. Applications of Advanced Ultrasound Technology in Obstetrics. Diagnostics. 2021; 11(7), 1217. https://doi.org/10.3390/diagnostics11071217.

Table 7.4. Commonly Used Scanning Mode, Volume Acquisition, and Analysis for Three-/Four-Dimensional (3D/4D) Ultrasound Examinations

Mode	Volume Acquisition	3D/4D Analysis
Gray scale	3D: different modes	Multiplanar
Color flow	4D	Multislice
Power doppler	STIC [1]	Rendered view: different modes
High-density power imaging	Matrix probe	Cine loop
B-flow		Semi-automatic analysis
		Volume measurement
		Power Doppler measurements

[1] Spatiotemporal image correlation.

Source: Leung, K.-Y. Applications of Advanced Ultrasound Technology in Obstetrics. Diagnostics. 2021; 11(7), 1217. https://doi.org/10.3390/diagnostics11071217

M-mode, short for "Motion mode," is a display technique that is not commonly utilized in modern ultrasound imaging. However, it is notably used to evaluate the movement of fetal cardiac chambers and valves to document fetal viability, as well as to assess specific fetal cardiac conditions like arrhythmias and congenital heart disease. The M-mode is generated by a single beam penetrating the body at a high pulse repetition frequency. The resulting display on the monitor represents the time of the M-mode display on the x-axis and the depth on the y-axis

(American Institute of Ultrasound in Medicine official statement, 2012) (Figure 7.12).

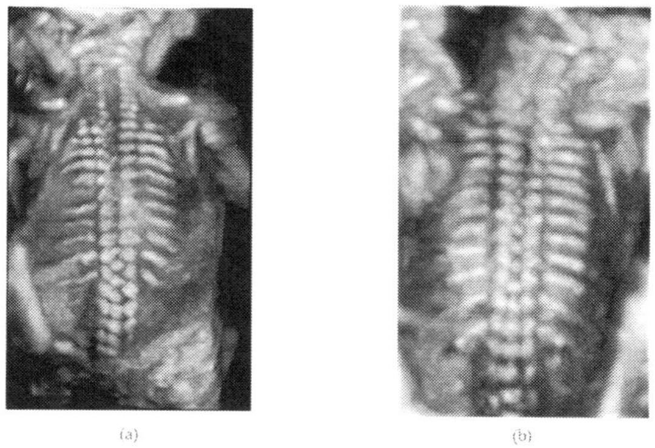

Figure 7.12. *Three-dimensional rendered views of fetal spine at 20 weeks' gestation after a volume acquisition with skeletal mode: (a) usual mode, and (b) X-ray mode.*

Source. Leung, K.-Y. Applications of Advanced Ultrasound Technology in Obstetrics. Diagnostics. 2021; 11(7), 1217. https://doi.org/10.3390/diagnostics11071217.

The Doppler principle (effect) governs color and spectral (pulsed) Doppler modes. The apparent change in frequency of a light or sound wave as it moves toward or away from its source in relation to an observer is described by the Doppler principle. The typical illustration used to explain this physical phenomenon is the apparent shift in train sound level as it approaches and then leaves a station. As the train gets closer to the station, the sound seems louder, and as it leaves the station, the sound seems quieter. The speed at which the sound-emitting source—in this case, the train—moves is proportional to the apparent change in sound pitch, also known as the frequency shift. It is crucial to remember that the train's actual sound is not changing; rather, the "Doppler effect" is determined by how a stationary observer perceives a change in sound. When a specific blood vessel is insonated using ultrasound at a given frequency (fo) in a clinical setting, the reflected frequency (fd) or frequency shift is directly proportional to the blood flow velocity (the speed at which blood moves through the vessel).

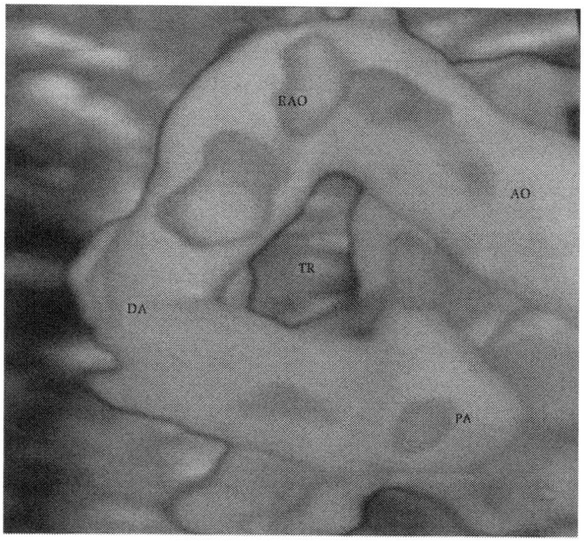

Figure 7.13. *Glass-body rendering mode with high-definition doppler showing a fetus with right aortic arch at 36 weeks' gestation. Noted that the trachea (TR) is surrounded by Aorta (AO), right aortic arch (RAO), pulmonary artery (PA) and ductus arteriosus (DA).*

Source: *Leung, K.-Y. Application of Color Doppler with 3- and 4-Dimensional Ultrasonography in the Prenatal Evaluation of Fetal Extracardiac and Placental Abnormalities. Healthcare. 2023; 11(4):488. https://doi.org/10.3390/healthcare11040488.*

A time-dependent plot represents this returning signal's frequency shift graphically. The horizontal axis in this display shows the temporal change of the frequency shift as it relates to the cardiac cycle's events, while the vertical axis represents the frequency shift. This frequency shift peaks in systole, the fastest phase of the peripheral blood circulation, and troughs end diastole, the slowest phase. The frequency shift thus yields information on the downstream impedance to flow of the vascular bed under study, since the downstream impedance to flow in a given vascular bed is inversely proportional to the velocity of flow in that vascular bed.

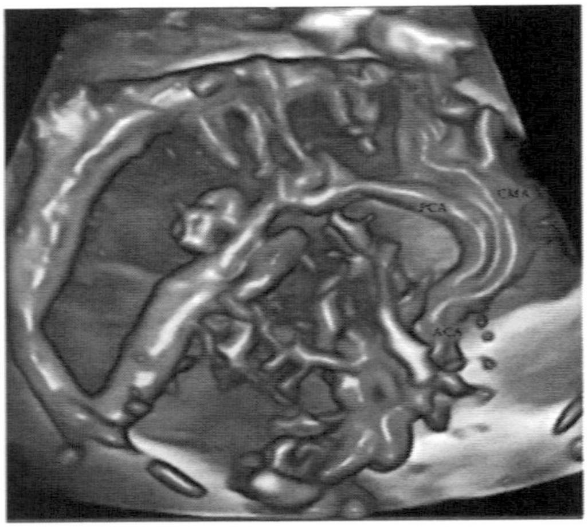

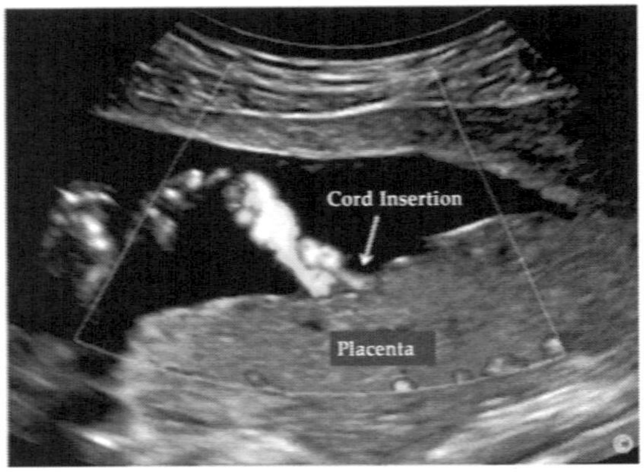

Figure 7.14. *Glass-body rendering mode with high-definition Doppler showing the normal course of pericallosal artery (PCA) and its main branch, and callosomarginal artery (CMA) in a fetus with severe fetal growth restriction at 31 weeks' gestation. ACA, anterior cerebral artery.*

Source. Leung, K.-Y. Application of Color Doppler with 3- and 4-Dimensional Ultrasonography in the Prenatal Evaluation of Fetal Extracardiac and Placental Abnormalities. Healthcare. 2023; 11(4):488. https://doi.org/10.3390/healthcare11040488.

The cosine of the angle formed by the ultrasound beam with the targeted blood vessel affects the frequency shift as well. Since it is challenging to measure the insonating angle (angle of incidence) in clinical practice, Doppler waveforms were quantitated using indices based on ratios of frequency shifts. These Doppler indices are thus unaffected by the ultrasonic beam's insonating angle since they depend only on ratios of frequency shifts. The Doppler indices displayed in are frequently used in obstetric and gynecologic practice (Dowdey et al, 1990; Shriki, 2014; Frederick and Kremkau, 2015) (Figure 7.13 and 7.14).

A mode that is superimposed on the live Bmode image is called color flow mode or color doppler mode. This mode is employed to ascertain whether vascular flow is present in the tissue that is being insonated. As a rule, the flow is colored blue when it is moving away from the transducer and red when it is moving towards it. The velocity scale or pulse repetition frequency (PRF), wall filter, area size within the B-mode field, and angle of incidence of the ultrasound beam with respect to blood flow direction are just a few of the parameters of the color Doppler that the operator can adjust. High velocity scales and filters are set aside for high impedance circulation, such as cardiac outflow tracts, and low velocity scales and filters are reserved for low impedance vascular beds, such as ovarian flow in gynecology. The angle of insonation should be as parallel to the direction of blood flow as feasible to maximize the color Doppler display. The "Doppler effect" depends on the cosine of the angle of insonation, and since the cosine of 90 degrees is equal to zero, no color flow will be seen if the angle of insonation gets close to that value (Table 7.5).

Table 7.5. Use of Color Doppler Flow Imaging (CDFI)/High-Definition Flow Imaging (HDFI) with 3-Dimensional Ultrasonography (3DUS)/Spatiotemporal Image Correlation (STIC) in the Prenatal evaluation of Fetal Cardiac and Placental Abnormalities

Fetus/Placenta	CDFI/HDFI	3DUS/ STIC	Examples of Abormalities
Heart/chest	High flow (CDFI) Small/low flow (HDFI)	GBM	Abnormal outflow tracts Course of trachea in right aortic arch Pulmonary vessels in lung dysplasia Liver vessels in diaphragmatic hernia Esophageal pouch in esophageal atresia
Brain	Pericallosal artery (HDFI)	GBM	Altered callosum development in FGR
Abdomen	Precordial veins (HDFI)	GBM TUI	Anomalies of the precoridal venous system Persistent right umbilical vein Abnormal venous returns to the right atrium
Umbilical cord	Cord vessels and insertion site (HDFI)	GBM TUI	Velamentous or marginal cord insertion, vasa previa, cord round neck, single umbilical artery, umbilical cord knot, abnormal thickening
Placenta	High flow (CDFI) Chorionic and decidual vessels, Spiral artery jets (HDFI)	GBM	Different intraplacental vascularization in PAS, FGR, and PET
Twin	Placental vascular anastomoses (HDFI) Intraplacental branches of umbilical artery (HDFI)	GBM TUI	Placental anastomoses in TTTS Different intraplacental vascularization in selective FGR TRAP, Cord entanglement in monoamniotic twin

Fetal growth restriction (FGR), Glass-body mode (GBM), placental accreta spectrum disorders (PAS), pre-eclampsia (PET), tomographic ultrasound imaging (TUI), twin reversed arterial perfusion (TRAP), twin-twin transfusion syndrome (TTTS).

Source. Leung, K.-Y. Application of Color Doppler with 3- and 4-Dimensional Ultrasonography in the Prenatal Evaluation of Fetal Extracardiac and Placental Abnormalities. Healthcare. 2023; 11(4):488. https://doi.org/10.3390/healthcare11040488.

By putting a sample volume or the gate inside the blood vessel, one can obtain a quantitative assessment of vascular flow in the spectral Doppler mode, also known as the pulsed Doppler mode. The operator regulates the velocity scale, wall filter, and angle of incidence, much like in color Doppler. Above the baseline is the flow toward the transducer, and below the baseline is the flow away from the transducer. Spectral Doppler mode usually only requires one crystal, which alternates between transmitting and receiving ultrasound pulses.

Some high-end ultrasound equipment has Doppler mode, also known as Energy mode, High Definition Doppler mode, or Doppler mode, which is a sensitive mode that helps detect low velocity flow. The primary processing parameter is the reflected signal's strength, or amplitude. Compared to conventional color or spectral Doppler, the angle of insonation has less of an impact on the power Doppler mode.

7.6. The Bioeffects of Ultrasound

As a mechanical energy, ultrasound has different outputs depending on the mode that is used. Generally speaking, pulsed Doppler has the highest energy, while B-mode has the lowest. The advantages for the patient must always exceed the risks, considering the theoretical and potential harm associated with ultrasound. When contrasted with other imaging modalities that use ionizing radiation, such as computed tomography (CT) and X-rays, ultrasound is generally thought to be a safe imaging technique. There are two key indices for quantifying the bioeffects of ultrasonography: the Mechanical Index (MI) and the Thermal Index (TI). The Thermal Index, which is defined as the ratio of power used to power required to produce a 1°C temperature rise, is a predictor of maximum temperature increase under clinically relevant conditions. Thermal index (TI) can be reported in three different ways: Thermal index soft tissue (TIS) indicates that sound is assumed to be traveling through soft tissue; Thermal index bone (TIB) indicates that sound is at or near bone; and Thermal index cranial (TIC) indicates that the cranial bone is in the near field of the sound beam. The cavitation effect of ultrasonography, which arises from sound waves interacting with tiny, stabilized gas bubbles in the tissues, is estimated by the Mechanical Index (MI). The physical (shock wave) and chemical (free radical release) effects of ultrasound on tissue are also included in this category.

In 1992, all diagnostic ultrasound devices had to comply with the Output Display Standard (ODS). In order to inform the user of the bioeffects of the ultrasound examination, the manufacturers of this ODS are mandated to display the TI and the MI in real time on the ultrasound screen. It is the user's responsibility to monitor power output and ensure that appropriate levels are maintained. Although there aren't any scientific studies proving that exposure to diagnostic ultrasound causes harmful bioeffects, one should still weigh the potential benefits and risks of the test and always abide by the ALARA principle. For the purpose of minimizing risk when adjusting the controls of the ultrasound equipment, the acronym ALARA stands for as low as reasonably achievable. During obstetrical ultrasound imaging, it is important to consistently monitor the TI and MI values on the screen, ensuring that the TI is less than 1 and the MI is less than 1 (Dowdey et al, 1990; Shriki, 2014; Frederick and Kremkau, 2015).

7.7. Some Relevant Official Statements from Ultrasound Societies

Official statements regarding the use of medical ultrasound in obstetrics and gynecology have been released by a number of national and international societies. This chapter contains a compilation of some pertinent official statements and an Internet link to their original source. Official societal statements are subject to periodic revisions, so readers are advised to check the society's website for the most recent version.

7.7.1. International Society of Ultrasound in Obstetrics and Gynecology (ISUOG)

1. ISUOG- Statement on the Safe Use of Doppler in the 11 to 13+6-Week Fetal Ultrasound Examination
    i. Pulsed Doppler (spectral, power and color flow imaging) ultrasound should not be used routinely.
    ii. Pulsed Doppler ultrasound may be used for clinical indications such as to refine risks for trisomies.
    iii. When performing Doppler ultrasound, the displayed thermal index (TI) should be ≤1.0 and exposure time should be kept as short as possible (usually no longer than 5–10 min) and should not exceed 60 min.
    iv. When using Doppler ultrasound for research, teaching and training purposes, the displayed TI should be ≤1.0 and exposure time should be kept as short as possible (usually no longer than 5–10 min) and should not exceed 60 min. Informed consent should be obtained.
    v. In educational settings, discussion of first-trimester pulsed or color Doppler should be accompanied by information on safety and bioeffects (e.g., TI, exposure times and how to reduce output power)
    vi. When scanning maternal uterine arteries in the first trimester, there are unlikely to be any fetal safety implications as long as the embryo/fetus lies outside the Doppler ultrasound beam.
2. **ISUOG- Safety Statement, 2000 (Reconfirmed 2003):** Although the mechanical index (MI) and the thermal index (TI) are not perfect measures of the risks associated with thermal and nonthermal bioeffects, they should currently be acknowledged as the most useful and comprehensible approaches to assessing the likelihood of such risks.
    i. **B-mode and M-mode:** Generally speaking, acoustic outputs are not loud enough to have negative effects. Therefore, it seems safe to use them during any stage of pregnancy.
    ii. **Doppler Ultrasound:** Spectral Doppler mode can cause a significant increase in temperature, especially near bone. This shouldn't stop the user from using this mode when it's clinically necessary, as long as they are familiar enough with the instrument's acoustic output and have access to the necessary TI. Since color Doppler mode has the highest potential for

bioeffects, caution is advised when using it with a very small region of interest. There is no reason not to use scanners that have been approved by the Food and Drug Administration in tissues that do not contain detectable gas bodies when ultrasound examination is clinically indicated. Because ultrasonic contrast agents are primarily gas-carriers, there is an increased risk of inducing and maintaining inertial cavitation when these agents are used.

iii **Pregnancy:** It is not contraindicated to use real-time B-mode imaging for routine clinical scanning of all pregnant women, according to the available evidence. In the first trimester, there is an increased risk of teratogenic agents harming the developing fetus. When utilizing the transvaginal approach, it is important to keep in mind that heat is produced at the transducer surface. High intensities may be produced by spectral and color Doppler, so routine use of this modality for examination during the embryonic stage is rarely recommended. Furthermore, one must consider the possibility of heating nearby tissues due to the high acoustic absorption of bone. Exposure duration and sound output ought to be restricted to medically necessary procedures and maintained at the lowest levels compatible with gathering diagnostic data, as opposed to being used only for amusement.

iv. **Education:** Since the manufacturers, who should guarantee the accuracy of the output display, and users now share responsibility for the safe use of ultrasound devices, training ultrasonographers is crucial.

3. **ISUOG-Statement on the Non-medical use of Ultrasound (2009):** The World Federation of Ultrasound in Medicine and Biology (WFUMB) and the International Society of Ultrasound in Obstetrics and Gynecology (ISUOG) oppose the use of ultrasound to obtain fetus images only for keepsakes. After more than 40 years of widespread use of medically indicated and supervised diagnostic ultrasound, there have been no documented cases of human fetal harm. However, because ultrasound exposes users to energy, there is a chance that biological effects could be initiated. In some cases, some of these effects could be harmful to the developing fetus. Therefore, it is best to avoid using ultrasound uncontrollably if there is no medical benefit. Additionally, only medical professionals who have received up-to-date training in the clinical application and bioeffects of ultrasound should use it.

7.7.2. American Institute of Ultrasound in Medicine (AIUM)

1. **AIUM-as Low as Reasonably Achievable (ALARA) Principle (2008):** Each examination's possible

advantages and disadvantages should be taken into account. When adjusting controls that impact the acoustical output, the ALARA (As Low as Reasonably Achievable) Principle should be followed, as well as transducer dwell times. You can find more information about ALARA in the AIUM publication "Medical Ultrasound Safety."

2. **AIUM-Conclusions Regarding Epidemiology for Obstetric Ultrasound (2010):** Given the available epidemiologic data and our current understanding of interactive mechanisms, there is not enough evidence to draw the conclusion that diagnostic ultrasonography causes the known negative effects in humans. Pregnancy-related effects of diagnostic ultrasound exposure include dyslexia, low birth weight, delayed speech, and non-right-handedness, according to certain studies. Such effects have not been shown in other studies. The majority of the epidemiologic evidence is based on exposure circumstances that existed before 1992, when ultrasound machines' acoustic limits were significantly raised for fetal and obstetric applications.

3. **AIUM-Prudent Use and Clinical Safety (2012):** Since the late 1950s, diagnostic ultrasound has been in use. The American Institute of Ultrasound in Medicine discusses the clinical safety of this use below in light of its established advantages and proven effectiveness for medical diagnosis, including use during human pregnancy.

   In the absence of contrast agents, no independently verified negative effects related to exposure from current diagnostic ultrasound equipment have been documented in human patients. Mammalian systems have shown biological effects (e.g., localized pulmonary bleeding) at diagnostically relevant exposures; however, the clinical significance of these effects remains unclear. Only licensed medical professionals should use ultrasound to benefit patients medically. Examinees should be exposed to as little ultrasound as is practical (ALARA).

4. **AIUM-Prudent Use in Pregnancy:** The AIUM strongly opposes the non-medical use of ultrasonography for entertainment purposes and supports the responsible use of ultrasonography for diagnostic purposes. It is improper and against responsible medical practice to use ultrasound without a medical indication in order to view the fetus, take pictures of the fetus, or ascertain the gender of the fetus. Only licensed medical professionals should use ultrasound to benefit patients medically.

5. **AIUM-Statement on Measurement**

of Fetal Heart Rate (2011): AIUM advises starting with M-mode when attempting to obtain fetal heart rate using a diagnostic ultrasound system. This is because M-mode delivers a lower time-averaged acoustic intensity to the fetus than spectral Doppler. If this doesn't work, spectral Doppler ultrasound can be used, but only under certain conditions. For example, use it sparingly (e.g., 4–5 heartbeats) and maintain the lowest feasible temperature (TIB for bones in the second and third trimesters, and TIS for soft tissues in the first trimester) in compliance with the ALARA principle, ideally less than 1 (International Society of Ultrasound in Obstetrics and Gynecology official statement, 2011).

7.8. Ultrasonography

A surgeon working in a setting with limited resources may find it advantageous to be proficient in ultrasonography. Surgeon-performed ultrasounds can provide a wealth of information about the patient's condition, particularly when more sophisticated imaging tests like CT or MRI are delayed. The fundamentals of ultrasonography as they apply to you are discussed, along with some basic instructions for doing ultrasounds and analyzing the pictures.

7.8.1. Physics: The Piezoelectric Effect

Quartz is a solid composed of molecules of silicon and oxygen arranged in a highly ordered pattern. There is a quartz crystal in ultrasound transducers. According to the piezoelectric effect, a crystal vibrates when electricity flows through it. On the other hand, electricity is released when a crystal is made to vibrate. The vibration frequency is determined by the characteristics of the crystal (Figure 7.15).

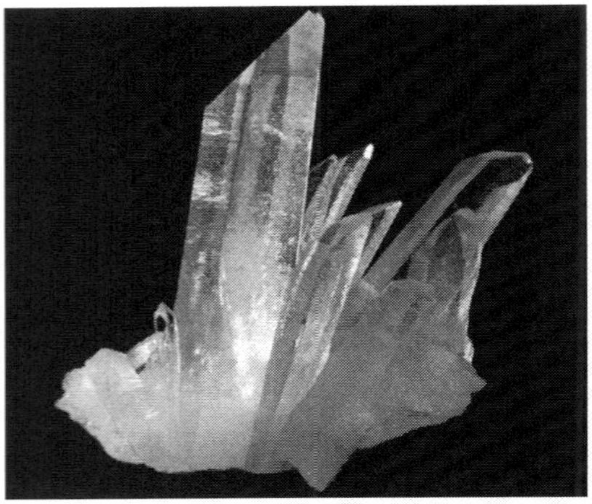

Figure 7.15. *A piece of quartz crystal.*

Source: Harrison, J. J. (https://www.jjharrison.com.au/) – Own work, CC BY-SA 2.5, https://commons.wikimedia.org/w/index.php?curid=6023737.

Both variations of the piezoelectric effect take place inside the transducer. The process of creating ultrasonic waves begins with applying electrical energy to a crystal, which transforms it into high-frequency sound waves that penetrate the tissue beneath the transducer. Depending on the properties of the tissue, these soundwaves interact with it and are reflected back towards the transducer at various frequencies. These sound waves interact with the same crystal when they reappear. Once more, mechanical energy is transformed into electrical energy, and this time, the electrical energy contains data about the tissue from which it has been reflected. An image is subsequently created using this energy.

The crystal emits sound waves with a frequency range of 2 to 10 megahertz (mHz, or millions of cycles per second). Human hearing, in contrast, operates between 20Hz and 20kHz.

Depending on its properties, the tissue beneath the probe reflects the sound waves in different ways. A tissue appears more "bright" on the screen the denser it is. As a result, the image displayed on the screen reflects both the sound wave's strength and duration, or how long it takes for the wave to return to the transducer (deepness of the structure).

7.8.2. Anatomy

7.8.2.1. Acoustic Shadowing

Certain tissues completely block the passage of sound. Since no sound waves reflect off of the tissue below that point, this creates a "acoustic shadow" deep within the tissue. The simplest illustration of this is that if there is insufficient gel between the skin and the probe, the entire image will appear as an acoustic shadow.

The ribs create acoustic shadows when scanning the chest cavity. Rotating the transducer to completely fit inside the area between the ribs is the best method to counteract this effect. Therefore, wherever the transducer is being used, the operator needs to be aware of the rib orientation (Table 7.6).

Table 7.6. Ultrasound Equipment Used to Carry Out Ultrasound Scans Groups

Group	Characteristics
Sectorial	Provide a triangular or fan-shaped image format with a small echo emission start base. Used for cardiac and abdominal explorations since they facilitate a costal approach, and to view deep structures. Usual working frequency between 3.5 and 5 MHz.
Convex	Waves have a curved shape and provide a trapezoid-shaped image format. Used in abdominal and obstetrical to view deep structures. Usual working frequency between 3.5 and 5 MHz.
Linear	Provide a rectangular image format. Used for the study of more superficial structures, such as muscles, tendons, breasts, thyroid, vessels, etc. Usual working frequency between 7.5 and 13 MHz, although some go up to 20 MHz.
Intra-cavity	Linear or convex. Used for intrarectal or intravaginal examinations. Usual working frequency between 5 and 7.5 MHz

Source: Moyano, D. B., Paraiso, D. A., & González-Lezcano, R. A. Possible Effects on Health of Ultrasound Exposure, Risk Factors in the Work Environment and Occupational Safety Review. Healthcare. 2022, 10(3), 423. https://doi.org/10.3390/healthcare10030423.

The detection of calculi, such as gallstones, is another outcome of acoustic shadowing. Even though kidney, bladder, or gallbladder calculi are frequently not visible directly on ultrasonography, their acoustic shadows can be observed. Any stone that is not completely calcified is an exception;

these will reflect some sound waves and could be perceived as "masses" or "sludge" inside the gallbladder.

7.8.2.2. Setup and Orientation

Try to position your portable device so that the patient is on the other side of you. The images are then directly in front of you while you conduct the study or carry out any interventions. You are forced to awkwardly turn your neck or torso to view the images as you obtain them when the machine is on the same side as you (Table 7.7).

Table 7.7. International Regulations Related to the Medical Use of Ultrasound

Name of Regulation
IEC60601-2-37 Edition 2. 2007
IEC61157 Edition 2.0. 2007
IEC61161 Edition 2.0. 2006
IEC62127-1 Edition 1.0. 2007
IEC62359 Edition 2.0. 2010.

Source: *Moyano, D. B., Paraiso, D. A., & González-Lezcano, R. A. Possible Effects on Health of Ultrasound Exposure, Risk Factors in the Work Environment and Occupational Safety Review. Healthcare. 2022, 10(3), 423. https://doi.org/10.3390/healthcare10030423.*

Each transducer has visible or tactile external markings that are visible when the probe is enclosed in a sterile cover. These enable you to line up the transducer with the marker-equipped image on the screen. In most cases, the screen marker is a blue dot. The image on the screen correlates with the anatomy being examined when the transducer and screen markers are aligned, and the images move in the same direction as you move the transducer.

7.8.2.3. Transducers and Settings

If you are fortunate enough to have a selection of transducers, it is beneficial to comprehend the various varieties and their intended functions. The ideal application for a transducer depends on its shape and frequency. Transducers come in two different shapes: curved and linear. For superficial work like vascular studies, vascular access, and breast assessment and biopsy, linear array transducers will be more appropriate. These will be more detailed due to their higher frequency of 5–7 point 5 mHz, but they won't pierce tissue as deeply.

Curved array transducers are more ideal for conducting abdominal or pelvic examinations due to their lower frequency range of 2–3mHz, allowing for deeper penetration of tissue.

The user can adjust the depth at which each transducer sees. This will show up on the right side of the screen as a column of numbers. Depending on what purpose it is intended for, each transducer has a preset depth beyond which it will not operate. A linear array (vascular transducer) typically has a field of vision of up to 6 cm. To see the most detail, set the depth to 3 cm if you are attempting to examine a vessel that is only 2 cm deep. Similarly, set the depth to about 13 cm when inspecting the entire liver with a curved transducer. Adjust the depth of the probe to about

8 cm once you have decided to biopsy a tumor that is 6 cm deep. This gives you a closer look at the tumor.

The gain amplifies the image so the surgeon can work with it. The image will be overly dark if it is not sufficiently amplified. It will be too light if it is amplified excessively. The ideal configuration will change depending on the image's depth as well. As a result, the majority of ultrasound devices let the user change the gain at different depths. Two dials may be present on portable devices, but console machines usually have eight or more sliding dials that correspond to the image's gain at eight or more distinct depths.

As previously mentioned, if you are not getting a useful image, you should consider if you are using the appropriate probe—one that is made to see at the depth you are attempting to see. Then determine how much gel there is. Gel is beneficial to have in large quantities because it allows sound waves to travel more easily, particularly over uneven surfaces like a cachectic person's chest. There should be enough gel between the transducer and the sterile transducer cover if you're using one (or a sterile glove). To get rid of any bubbles between the transducer surface and the sterile cover, run your finger over it. In "Ultrasound-Guided Interventions," we go over how to quickly and easily create a sterile ultrasound transducer cover. If the image still doesn't satisfy you after you have enough gel and there are no bubbles, try adjusting the gain.

7.8.3. Principles

It is challenging to evaluate a patient just with the ultrasound machine. Even with the appropriate transducer and by following all of the previously discussed principles, the images remain difficult to understand.

First, the liver in the abdomen. You should be able to see the hepatic tissue in one of the right lower intercostal spaces if you have the right probe positioned at the correct depth, enough gel, and the gain adjusted correctly. After you've done that, look for the kidney, which is located deep below the liver. Proceed to examine the liver by moving caudally and medially towards the abdomen, inserting the probe beneath the costal margin and pressing upwards. Locate the vena cava and the vein branches that enter the liver by moving medially. In relation to the liver, the aorta, a pulsatile vascular structure located further to the left, is also easily located. Locate the bladder first when doing a pelvic examination, then look at the surrounding structures. By inserting the probe into the abdomen and pushing downward, you can locate a woman's uterus and ovaries by pushing the bowels out of the way.

Start by positioning the linear probe transversely across the bottom third of the sternocleidomastoid muscle in the neck. The larger jugular vein, which collapses with inspiration, and the smaller, pulsatile common carotid artery will both be visible. Since ultrasound waves cannot travel through air, they must pass medially to reveal the thyroid gland and the trachea, a spherical structure that casts a shadow in the middle. Proceed cranially, following the vessels as they ascend to the submandibular gland (Dowdey et al, 1990; Shriki, 2014; Frederick and Kremkau, 2015) (Table 7.8).

Table 7.8. The Absorption of Ultrasound Energy Produces the Following Effects

Effects	Mechanism
Vasodilation	Release of tissue stimulants. Reduction in muscle tone.
Muscle relaxation	Elimination of tissue stimulants. Post-excitatory depression orthosympathetic.
Increased membrane permeability	Forcing the tissue fluid through. pH less acidic.
Increased tissue regeneration	Mechanical effect.
Thermal effect	Can block conduction. Nervous tissue possesses special sensitivity to ultrasound.
Decrease in pain	Normalization of muscle tone. Decrease in pH.

Source: *Moyano, D. B., Paraiso, D. A., & González-Lezcano, R. A. Possible Effects on Health of Ultrasound Exposure, Risk Factors in the Work Environment and Occupational Safety Review. Healthcare. 2022, 10(3), 423. https://doi.org/10.3390/healthcare10030423.*

A Closer Look

Ultrasound Scanner

An ultrasound scanner is a vital medical imaging tool that employs high-frequency sound waves to produce real-time images of internal bodily structures. It operates on the principle of echolocation, where sound waves emitted by a transducer penetrate the body, bounce off tissues, and return to the transducer, which then converts them into images displayed on a monitor. This imaging modality is widely used across medical specialties due to its non-invasiveness, safety, and versatility. Ultrasound scanners come in various types, including 2D, 3D, and 4D ultrasound, each offering unique advantages for different clinical applications. In obstetrics and gynecology, ultrasound scanning is crucial for monitoring fetal development during pregnancy and diagnosing gynecological conditions. Additionally, ultrasound is extensively utilized in radiology for imaging abdominal organs, guiding interventional procedures, and diagnosing musculoskeletal and cardiovascular conditions. Despite its many advantages, ultrasound does have limitations, such as reduced penetration through bone and air and dependence on operator skill for image interpretation. Nonetheless, ultrasound scanners remain indispensable tools in modern medicine, providing valuable diagnostic information without the need for ionizing radiation or invasive procedures.

Ultrasound scanners utilize the principle of echolocation, similar to sonar used in submarines, to create images of internal organs and tissues. A transducer emits high-frequency sound waves into the body, which then bounce off different tissues and organs. The returning sound waves are captured by the transducer and converted into images by a computer.

Ultrasound scanning is non-invasive, painless, and does not involve ionizing radiation, making it safe for patients of all ages, including pregnant women and infants. It provides real-time imaging, allowing for immediate visualization of anatomical structures and dynamic processes.

While ultrasound is valuable for many applications, it has limitations, including limited penetration through bone and air, reduced image quality in obese patients or those with bowel gas, and operator dependence, as image interpretation requires skill and experience.

Summary

- Diagnostic ultrasound is a non-invasive diagnostic technique used to image inside the body.
- Therapeutic ultrasound also uses sound waves above the range of human hearing but does not produce images. Its purpose is to interact with tissues in the body such that they are either modified or destroyed.
- During an ultrasound exam, the technician will apply a gel to the skin. This keeps air pockets from forming between the transducer and the skin, which can block ultrasound waves from passing into the body.
- Functional ultrasound applications include Doppler and color Doppler ultrasound for measuring and visualizing blood flow in vessels within the body or in the heart. It can also measure the speed of the blood flow and direction of movement.
- Ultrasound imaging (sonography) uses high-frequency sound waves to view inside the body. Because ultrasound images are captured in real-time, they can also show movement of the body's internal organs as well as blood flowing through the blood vessels.
- Ultrasound is the most widely used medical imaging method for viewing the fetus during pregnancy. Routine examinations are performed to assess and monitor the health status of the fetus and mother.
- Ultrasound frequencies that are commonly used in obstetrics and gynecology are between 3 and 10 MHz.
- A-mode, which stands for "Amplitude mode," is no longer used in clinical obstetric and gynecologic ultrasound imaging but was the basis of modern ultrasound imaging.
- Color Doppler mode or Color flow mode is a mode that is superimposed on the real-time Bmode image. This mode is used to detect the presence of vascular flow within the tissue being insonated.
- Ultrasound is a form of mechanical energy and its output varies based upon the mode applied. In general B-mode has the lowest energy and pulsed Doppler has the highest energy.

References

1. A Shung KK. Ultrasound: past, present and future. In: Van TV, Khoa TQD, eds. The Third International Conference on the Development of Biomedical Engineering in Vietnam, *IFMBE Proceedings*. Berlin, Heidelberg: Springer; 2010;27:10–13.
2. Goldberg BB, Gramiak R, Freimanis AK. Early history of diagnostic ultrasound: the role of American radiologists. *AJR Am J Roentgenol*. 1993;160:189–194.
3. Graziano, M., Biondino, D., & Fioretto, I. (2023). Carotid-Cavernous Fistulas: The Utility of Ocular Echography in Their Differentiation [Letter]. *Clinical Ophthalmology, 17*, 1421–1422. https://doi.org/10.2147/OPTH.S420582.
4. International Society of Ultrasound in Obstetrics and Gynecology. (2011). Official statement

on the safe use of Doppler in the 11 to 13+6 week fetal ultrasound examination. *Ultrasound in Obstetrics & Gynecology, 37*(6), 628.

5. International Society of Ultrasound in Obstetrics and Gynecology. (2003). Official statement on safety. *Ultrasound in Obstetrics & Gynecology, 21*(1), 100.
6. International Society of Ultrasound in Obstetrics and Gynecology. (2009). Official statement on non-medical use of ultrasound. *Ultrasound in Obstetrics & Gynecology, 33*(5), 617.
7. Mills DM, Smith SW. Multi-layered PZT/polymer composites to increase signal-to-noise ratio and resolution for medical ultrasound transducers part II: thick film technology. *IEEE Trans Ultrason Ferroelectr Freq Control*. 2002;49:1005–1014.
8. Ophir, J., & Maklad, N. (1979). Digital scan converters in diagnostic ultrasound imaging. *Proceedings of the IEEE, 67*(4), 654–664. https://doi.org/10.1109/PROC.1979.11289.
9. Shriki, J. (2014). Ultrasound physics. *Critical Care Clinics, 30*(1), 1–24. https://doi.org/10.1016/j.ccc.2013.08.004.
10. Singh S, Goyal A. The origin of echocardiography: a tribute to Inge Edler. *Tex Heart Inst J*. 2007;34:431–438.
11. Uddin, S., Komatsu, D., Motyka, T., & Petterson, S. (2021). Low-intensity continuous ultrasound therapies—A systematic review of current state-of-the-art and future perspectives. *Journal of Clinical Medicine, 10*(12), 2698. https://doi.org/10.3390/jcm10122698.
12. Wang S, Hossack J, Klibanov A. From anatomy to functional and molecular biomarker imaging, and therapy: ultrasound is safe, ultrafast, portable, and inexpensive. *Invest Radiol*. 2020;55:559–572.

Chapter 8

DIGITAL RADIOGRAPHY

Contents

Introduction

Since WC Roentgen discovered the X-ray in 1895, film-screen radiographic imaging has been the mainstay of radiology. Film-screen radiography is no longer in use today; digital radiography, or simply digital radiography, has taken its place. Digital image processing, display, storage, and image communication are all included in the technologies used in digital radiography, in addition to digital image acquisition methods. Computed radiography, flatpanel digital radiography, digital mammography, and digital fluoroscopy for routine gastrointestinal fluoroscopy and vascular imaging are among the specific digital image acquisition modalities. Information technology also includes the other technologies of image processing, display, storage, and computer-based image communication. Medical imaging informatics is a field of study and practice that has emerged as a result of the use of information technology in digital radiography. At least six significant topics that have drawn more attention in the literature and are crucial for everyone involved in medical imaging and radiation sciences are part of the next era in medical imaging informatics. These include artificial intelligence, cloud computing, big data, enterprise imaging, and machine and deep learning.

An overview of the components of digital radiography (DR) is given in this chapter. The definition of digital radiography is given first, and then the fundamental ideas of film-screen radiography (F-SR), along with some of its drawbacks, are briefly reviewed. Second, a quick summary of the main elements of digital radiography imaging systems is provided. Digital imaging modalities, including computed radiography (CR), flat-panel digital radiography (FPDR), digital fluoroscopy, and digital mammography, were thoroughly explained in the third topic. Additionally, quality control, communication systems, and picture archiving components are introduced. The chapter ends with an overview of subjects that are thought to represent the next wave of imaging informatics, including artificial intelligence, cloud computing, Big Data, machine learning, deep learning, and enterprise imaging.

Orientation and Directional Terms

Term	Definition	Illustration
Computed radiography	Computed radiography (CR) is a digital imaging technique that uses a special X-ray sensitive plate to capture images.	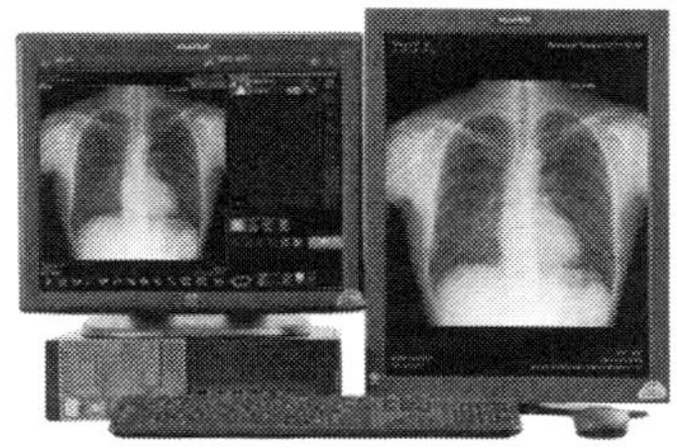
Diagnostic imaging	Diagnostic imaging describes various techniques of viewing the inside of the body to help figure out the causes of an illness or injury and confirm a diagnosis.	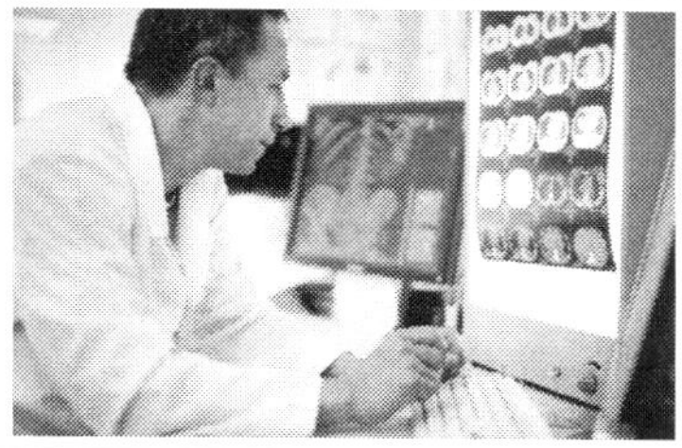
Digital imaging	Digital imaging offers some distinct advantages over film, but like any emerging technology, it presents new and different challenges for the practitioner to overcome.	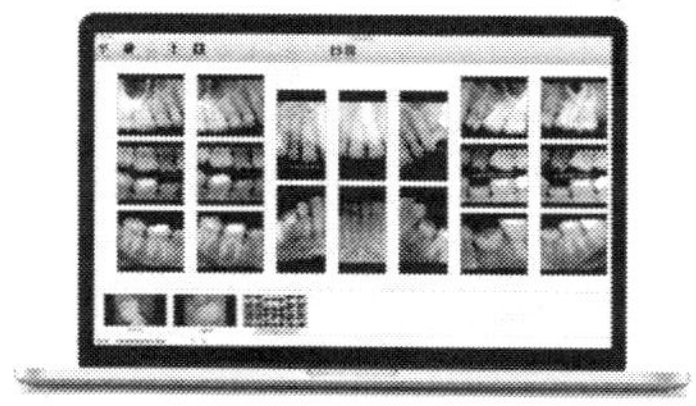
Mammography	Mammography is an X-ray imaging method used to examine the breast for the early detection of cancer and other breast diseases. It is used as both a diagnostic and screening tool.	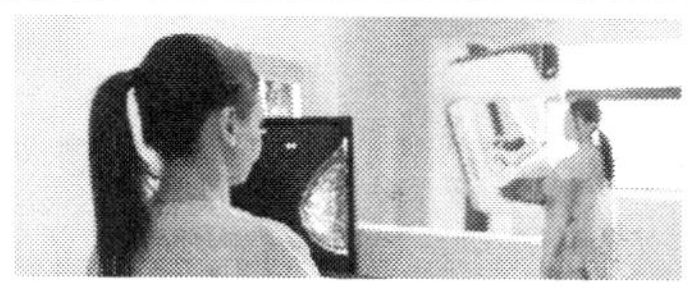
Radiography	Radiography is a technique that uses X-rays or other ionizing radiation to create images of the inside of an object.	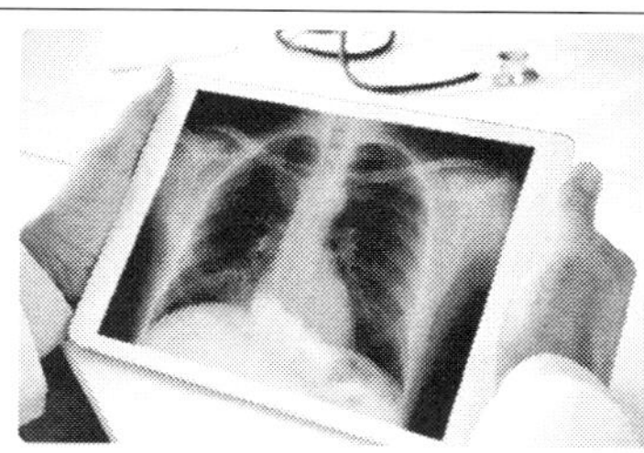
Ultrasound	An ultrasound is a non-invasive imaging test that uses sound waves to create pictures of organs, tissues, and other internal body structures.	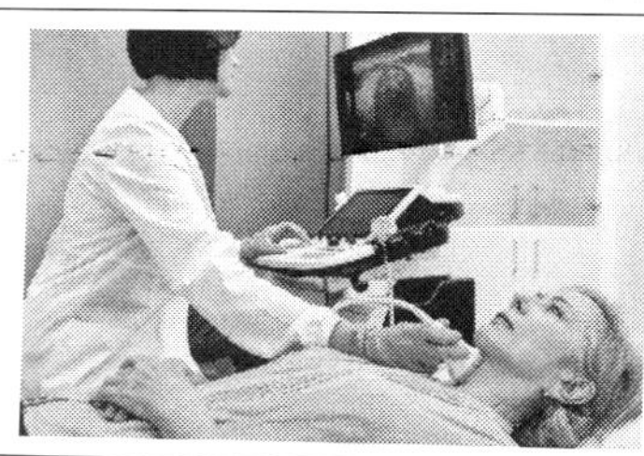

8.1. Digital Radiography: An Overview

Film has been the main medium for recording, displaying, and storing radiographic images ever since X-rays were discovered in 1895. In terms of technique and interpretation, dental practitioners are the most experienced and at ease with this technology. The dental community is gradually embracing digital radiography, the most recent development in dental imaging. Computer technology is used in digital imaging to capture, display, enhance, and store direct radiography images. Compared to film, digital imaging has a few clear advantages, but as with any new technology, there are always new obstacles for photographers to overcome.

Digital radiography is another name for direct digital radiography. The distinction between modern digital cameras and outdated cameras that require darkroom development for film development can be drawn from the differences between digital and conventional radiography. Filmless digital radiography enables instantaneous film acquisition, erasure, editing, and transfer to a computer system, which produces the image nearly instantly.

There is little difference between digital and film radiography in terms of physical principles. Digital radiography creates a digital image using digital detectors, which is then stored independently on a digital medium, in place of using film for image data detection and storage. Digital radiography involves four stages: creating images, processing them, archiving them, and presenting them (Seeram, 2011; Bushberg et al, 2012; Seeram, 2016; Bushong, 2018).

8.1.1. Digital Radiography: A Definition

According to the American Association of Physicists in Medicine (AAPM), digital radiography is defined as "radiographic imaging technology producing digital projection images, such as those using metal oxide semiconductor-field effect transistor (MOSFET) technology, amorphous silicon, amorphous selenium, or photostimulable storage phosphor (computed radiography, or CR)." Comparing these technologies to film-screen radiography, a greater variety of exposure techniques can result in acceptable image quality.

Digital detectors are used to record and transform patient X-ray attenuation data into electronic signals, also known as analog signals. These signals are then transformed into digital data so that a digital computer can process them. Processing leaves a digital image that needs to be transformed into one that an observer can see on a computer monitor. Figure 8.1 shows the key elements of the system as well as the necessary procedures for producing digital images. To improve the interpretation of diagnostic radiology images, various digital image processing techniques can be applied to the displayed image.

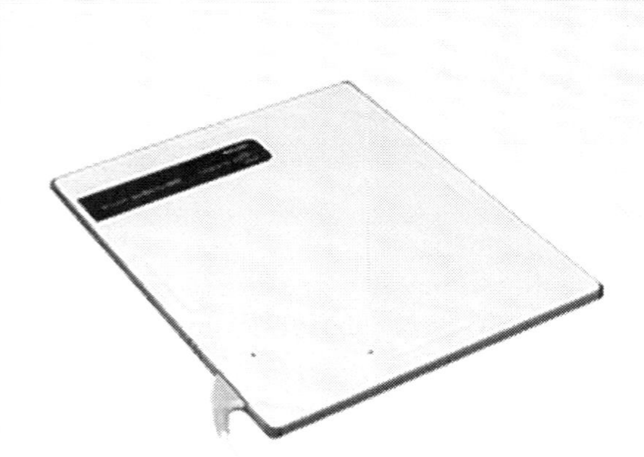

Figure 8.1. *Flat panel detector used.*

Source: *By Mcapdevila – http://histo.cat/1/Flat_panel_detector.jpg, CC BY-SA 3.0,* https://commons.wikimedia.org/w/index.php?curid=21851200.

8.1.2. Image Acquisition and Processing

Digital detection works by converting X-ray energy that is absorbed into electrical charge. This electrical charge needs to be digitally represented in grayscale images to display the amount of X-ray energy that was absorbed at each location in the digital image. Processing software is used to create the final image. Reducing noise, removing artifacts, and, if needed, boosting contrast are all steps in the process of improving image quality.

8.1.3. Image Archiving and Presentation

To view the final images on a computer, they are digitally stored on storage media. The images can be windowed, panned, measured for distance and angle, and zoomed in while being viewed. Pictures can be connected to digital record systems for better retrieval and diagnosis, or they can be sent to other computers for remote viewing.

Therefore, the fundamental idea is to detect X-rays and then, either directly or indirectly (via conversion to light as a first step by phosphors or scintillators), convert the X-rays to charge. Digital processing and viewing are used for these photos. There is no need for a cassette, and the process takes 10 seconds or less.

8.1.4. Flat Panel Detectors

A flat panel detector is one kind of detector plate used in digital radiography. These come in two varieties: flat panel detectors with direct and indirect conversion. When necessary, the entire imaging field is covered by tiled arrays of detectors.

Three layers make up indirect conversion flat panel detectors. Cesium or gadolinium, scintillators (phosphors) that convert incident X-rays to visible light, make up the outermost layer. Amorphous silicon photodiode detectors make up the middle layer, while thin film transistor (TFT) arrays comprise the outermost layer.

The size of the TFT arrays corresponds to the area that needs to be imaged. The TFTs' job is to convert light from the photodiodes into an electrical signal, which is then amplified and stored as an electrical charge. The charge is released from the TFT by applying a high potential difference. The potential that initiates the charge is connected to each row of detectors in the transistor separately. Based on the timing of the signal, the row-by-row application of the potential enables the signal detection to pinpoint the origin pixel's location.

The phrase "indirect conversion" refers to the subsequent conversion of the light generated by this reaction to charge.

The way that direct conversion flat panel detectors work is that they coat a TFT array—which gathers and stores electrical charge—with a light-conductive material, typically selenium. The electrodes that make up the outermost layer have a high voltage bias. Compared to traditional X-rays, these detectors have a lower radiation dosage and a better spatial resolution. Furthermore, the quality of the image is not affected by either overexposure or underexposure.

CCD detectors are another kind of detector used in direct digital radiography. Similar to camera sensors, these indirect conversion flat panel detectors are light-sensitive. The problem with these devices is that they can only be as small as 5 cm^2. Additionally, these are coupled with a phosphor to transform X-rays into light, which can be directed toward the CCD and transformed into an electrical charge. The final data is sent to a TFT array for output.

8.1.5. Advantages of Digital Radiography

The exceptionally high image quality of digital radiography is a key benefit. Most facilities that use digital radiography have very high patient imaging workflows. There is also a significant increase in the speed of diagnosis and processing. Not only is remote viewing an option, but digital image storage allows the patient to take the images with them if they so choose.

The efficiency of X-ray detector systems is determined by the degree of photon detection accuracy and the amount of noise introduced into the detected signal. The detective quantum efficiency, or DQE, is used to quantify this. When the DQE is 100%, all X-ray photons have been detected and there is no noise. Unlike computerized radiography, which typically achieves DQEs of 30%, a digital radiography system can achieve DQEs of up to 65%. The ability to use lower radiation doses without increasing quantum noise is a practical advantage.

8.1.6. Disadvantages of Digital Radiography

The expense of digital radiography is a drawback because two distinct detector plates—one for each Bucky position—are needed. These detectors come at a very high cost. Furthermore, they cannot be angled awkwardly for imaging. New designs have been created as a result to improve this technique's flexibility.

Additional crucial concerns include the requirement for high luminance and high-resolution monitors to view finished digital images, as well as the organization of substantial amounts of digital storage on suitable media. In order to archive these high-resolution images, digital radiography also depends entirely on having a picture archiving and communication system (PACS) with a large bandwidth (Seeram, 2011; Bushberg et al, 2012; Seeram, 2016; Bushong, 2018).

8.2. Film-Based Radiography

The steps involved in film-based imaging are the interaction of X-rays with the film emulsion's electrons, the creation of a latent image, and the chemical processing that turns the latent image into a visible one.

8.2.1. Basic Steps in the Production of a Radiograph

Figure 8.2 illustrates the various steps involved in producing a film-based radiographic image. A latent image is created when X-rays travel through the patient and land on the film. A radiologist can then view and interpret the latent image by having it exposed on a light viewbox after it has undergone chemical processing to make it visible. Because different parts of the anatomy transmit different amounts of exposure, the film image appears with varying degrees of blackening. Figure 8.3 clearly illustrates that while more exposure results in more blackening, less exposure results in less blackening. Furthermore, the term "film contrast" refers to the difference in densities in the image, whereas "blackening" is referred to as "film density." As a result, the film creates film contrast from the radiation that the different kinds of tissues (known as tissue contrast) transmit.

The radiologist who interprets an image sees light transmitted into their eyes when it is displayed on a light view box. This transmitted light is known as the optical density (OD), which is defined as the log of the ratio of the view box's original intensity to the transmitted light's intensity. It can be measured with a densitometer. The amount of blackening of film caused by radiation exposure is expressed by the OD.

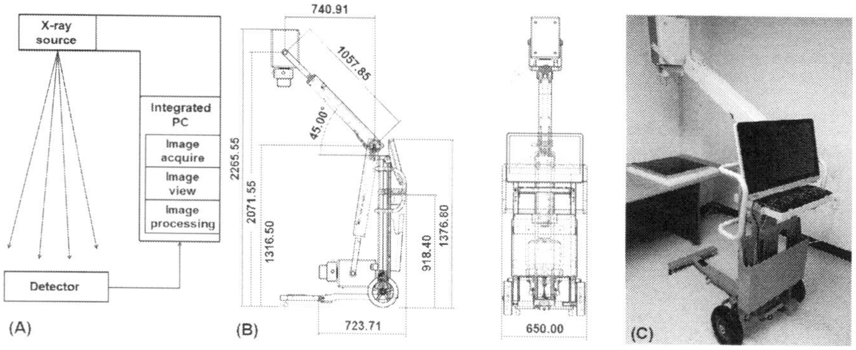

Figure 8.2. A simple diagram of portable digital radiography (PDR) (A), the detailed drawing of PDR structure (B) and developed PDR system (C). Source: Kim, T-H., Heo, D-W., Jeong, C-W., Ryu, J-H., Jun, H. Y., Han, S-J., Ha, T., & Yoon, K-H. Development of portable digital radiography system with a device for monitoring x-ray source-detector angle and its application in chest imaging. Sensors. 2017; 17(3), 531. https://doi.org/10.3390/s17030531.

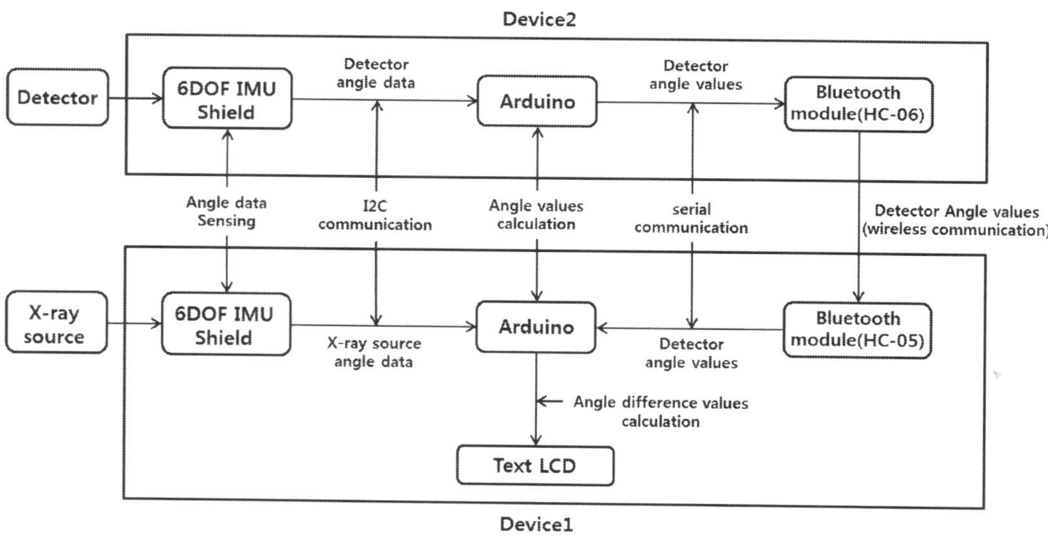

Figure 8.3. An example flowchart.

Source: Kim, T-H., Heo, D-W., Jeong, C-W., Ryu, J-H., Jun, H. Y., Han, S-J., Ha, T., & Yoon, K-H. Development of portable digital radiography system with a device for monitoring x-ray source-detector angle and its application in chest imaging. Sensors. 2017; 17(3), 531. https://doi.org/10.3390/s17030531.

8.2.2. The Film Characteristic Curve

The Hurter-Driffield (H and D) curve, also referred to as the film characteristic curve, is a common way to describe the film contrast. The curve represents the relationship between the radiation exposure and optical density (OD)—or, more precisely, the logarithm of the relative exposure—used in the imaging procedure. The curve's objective is to show the range of exposures that a film can handle to display a given level of contrast or density. Figure 8.4 illustrates an idealized characteristic curve for film-screen radiography that is divided into three main segments: the shoulder, the slope (or straight line portion), and the toe.

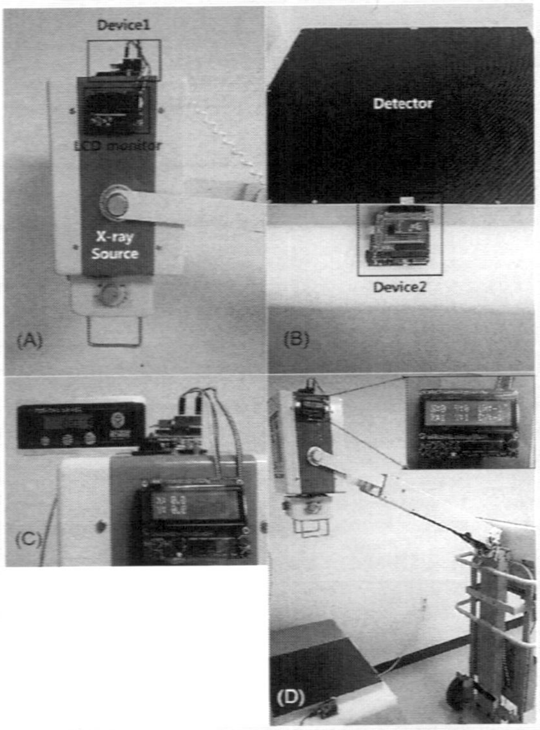

Figure 8.4. *An example device: an X-ray source (A) and a detector (B). Photography showed the initial setting for obtaining the angle degree using the SDA device and digital angle meter (C). The '0.0°' value on the SDA device was accordant with a '0.0°' reference value on the digital angle meter. The measured angle degree using PDR with SDA device displayed on a LCD monitor (D).*

Source: *Kim, T-H., Heo, D-W., Jeong, C-W., Ryu, J-H., Jun, H. Y., Han, S-J., Ha, T., & Yoon, K-H. Development of Portable Digital Radiography System with a Device for Monitoring X-ray Source-Detector Angle and Its Application in Chest Imaging. Sensors. 2017; 17(3), 531. https://doi.org/10.3390/s17030531.*

The slope denotes the useful part of the curve and shows acceptable exposure or the range of useful densities, whereas the toe and shoulder indicate underexposure and overexposure, respectively. This essentially indicates that an image will be light and generally meaningless if an exposure falls in the toe region (OD = 0.12–0.20). An image will be black and useless for diagnosing if the exposure occurs in the shoulder region of the curve (OD = about 3.2). The image contrast (density) will be acceptable if the exposure is within the slope of the curve (OD = 0.3–2.2), and this area of the curve includes the useful range of exposures.

The characteristic curve can also be used to characterize four additional factors. These consist of the film latitude, film gamma, average gradient, and film speed. Any standard text on radiography physics should be consulted by the interested reader for a more detailed explanation of the other terms.

The film speed is as below (E is the exposure)

$$\text{Films peed} = 1/E$$

This implies that faster films—also known as fast films—need less exposure than slower ones. In contrast, the range of exposures that would result in useful densities (contrast) is described by the film latitude. Films with narrow exposure latitude can only react to a limited range of exposures, whereas wide exposure latitude films can respond to a wide range of exposures. In the latter case, the technologist must choose the exposure technique factors carefully to protect the anatomical part being studied. The primary reason for this is the nonlinear reaction of the film emulsion to chemical processing.

8.2.3. Exposure Technique Factors

The amount and quality of the X-ray beam that emerges from the X-ray tube during the examination are influenced by exposure technique factors. These parameters, which the technologist sets on the console, are the tube current or milliamperage (mA), the exposure time in seconds (s), and the kilovolt peak (kVp). They are specifically chosen for the patient size and type of examination. The mA regulates the X-ray beam quantity, or the number of photons in the beam, while the kV controls the X-ray beam quality, or the penetrating power of the X-ray beam. On the other hand, the duration of the X-ray beam's exposure to the patient is determined by the exposure time. In the same way that mA and s used independently produce the mAs, which regulates the X-ray beam quantity, so do mA and s combined.

8.2.4. Automatic Exposure Control

Poor exposures can occasionally be caused by manually selecting exposure technique factors, which ultimately affects the film's image quality. The issue is resolved by using automatic exposure control (AEC), which measures and automatically ends the radiation exposure when a predetermined optical density (or degree of blackening in the case of film) or signal-to-noise ratio (SNR) is reached in the case of a digital detector.

8.2.5. Image Quality Factors

Creating the best possible image quality is the main objective of radiographic imaging. The features of a movie that define its quality are artifacts, noise, distortion, resolution, and contrast.

A feature of a film that makes it possible for viewers to distinguish between different objects is called resolution. Resolution comes in two flavors: contrast resolution and spatial resolution. The latter refers to the variations in tissue contrast that are visible on the film, whereas the former refers to the sharpness or visibility of detail.

Detail is referred to as spatial resolution, and it is expressed in terms of line pairs per millimeter (lp/mm). The amount of detail visible in a film increases with its lp/mm ratio. Several variables, including the focal spot size, the patient's motion, and the features of the image receptor design, influence detail. When using small focal spots, keeping the patient still during the exposure, and using detail cassettes, detail is maximized.

One important aspect of image quality is contrast. It is the variations in density on a radiography picture. Areas of high density (dark) and low density (light) define a high-contrast image. A radiography image's contrast is influenced by various elements, such as the subject, beam energy, scattered radiation, film, grids, and so forth.

However, kVp is the primary controlling factor for image contrast. When low kVp techniques are applied, the greatest contrast is achieved. Through the absorption of scattered radiation before it reaches the film, a grid enhances radiographic contrast.

Images with noise on them appear grainy and mottle (also known as quantum mottle). Since mAs is the primary factor regulating the number of photons from the X-ray tube, this happens when few photons are used to create an image on the X-ray film. More noise will be produced by low mAs techniques than by high mAs techniques. In addition, there are additional variables like the kVp that influence noise. For the same mA settings, higher kVp techniques result in less noise. Therefore, in order to achieve the best possible image quality, the technologist needs to choose the best factors.

8.2.6. Radiation Dose Considerations

Many variables, such as exposure technique factors, filtration, collimation and field size, scattered radiation grids, image receptors (detectors), and source-to-image receptor distance (SID), influence the radiation dose in film-screen radiography. Although the dose is directly proportional to the mAs, which means that doubling the mAs doubles the dose, the dose is also proportional to the square of the kVp change. The patient will absorb less of the dose when using higher kVp techniques.

8.2.7. Limitations of Film-Screen Radiography

Despite being successfully used for over a century and still being used in many departments today, film-based radiography has been the mainstay of radiology since the discovery of X-rays in 1895. One of the main issues with the radiographic imaging process is poor image quality if the initial radiation exposure has not been accurately determined. For instance, the radiologist cannot diagnose from an image if the radiation exposure is too high, the film is overexposed, and the processed image looks too dark. A low radiation exposure can result in a processed image that is too light and unhelpful to the radiologist. It would be necessary to take new pictures in each of these cases to achieve the appropriate image density and contrast for a diagnosis. Repeated exposures would also result in higher radiation exposures for the patient.

There are other problems associated with film-based radiography. For example:

1. As a radiation detector, film-screen cannot show differences in tissue contrast less than 10%. This means that film-based imaging is limited in its contrast resolution. For example, while the contrast resolution (mm at 0.5% difference) for film-screen radiography is 10, it is 20 for nuclear medicine, 10 for ultrasound, 4 for computed tomography, and 1 for magnetic resonance imaging. The spatial resolution (line pairs/mm) for radiography, however, is the highest of all the other imaging modalities and can range of 5–15 line pairs/mm. This is the main reason why radiography has been so popular through the years.
2. As a display medium, the optical range and contrast for film are fixed and limited. Film can only display once, the optical range and contrast determined by the exposure technique factors used to produce the image. In order to change the image display (optical range and contrast), another set of exposure technique factors would have to be used, thus increasing the dose to the patient by virtue of a repeat exposure.
3. As an archive medium, film is usually stored in envelopes and housed in a large room. It thus requires manual handling for archiving and retrieval by an individual.

These problems can be overcome by a digital radiography imaging system (Seeram, 2011; Bushberg et al, 2012; Seeram, 2016; Bushong, 2018).

8.3. Major Components of a Digital Radiography Imaging System

The data acquisition, computer data processing, image display and post-processing, image storage, image and data communications, and image and information management are the main technical elements of a digital radiography system. Each of these will now be described briefly (Figure 8.5).

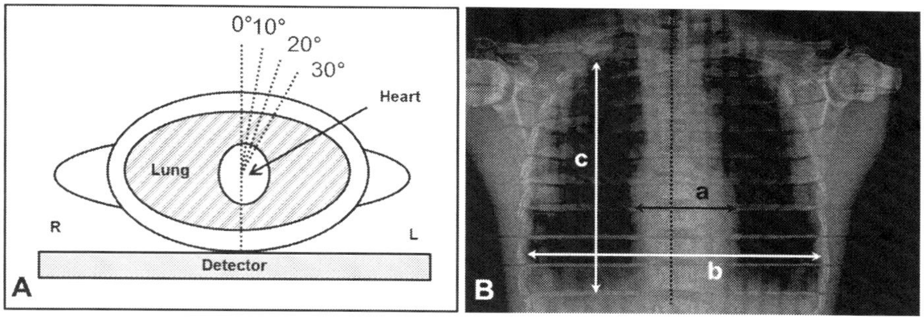

Figure 8.5. *An example measurement.*

Source: *Kim, T-H., Heo, D-W., Jeong, C-W., Ryu, J-H., Jun, H. Y., Han, S-J., Ha, T., & Yoon, K-H. Development of portable digital radiography system with a device for monitoring x-ray source-detector angle and its application in chest imaging. Sensors. 2017; 17(3), 531. https://doi.org/10.3390/s17030531.*

8.3.1. Data Acquisition

The collection of X-rays transmitted through the patient is referred to as data acquisition. It is the initial stage of creating the image. In digital radiography, the X-ray film cassette used in film-based radiography is replaced with specialized electronic detectors known as digital detectors. There are various kinds of these detectors that use technologies to transform X-rays into electrical signals, or analog signals. For instance, one kind of detector will first convert X-rays into light, which will then instantly be converted into electrical signals. However, another kind of digital detector will convert X-rays straight into electrical signals, skipping the light-to-electricity conversion step. To be processed by a digital computer, the analog signals must be transformed into digital data. The analog-to-digital converter's (ADC) function is to convert analog signals.

8.3.2. Computer Data Processing

Digital data is sent by the ADC to a digital computer for processing. The computer builds up digital images using the binary number system through the use of special software. Computers use the binary number system (which operates with base 2, that is, 0 or 1), while humans use the decimal number system (which operates with base 10, that is, 10 different numbers; 0,1,2,3,4,5,6,7,8,9). We refer to these two numbers as binary digits, or bits. Bits are discrete units rather than continuous ones. Binary numbers, or 0s and 1s, are discrete units used by computers that can be processed and changed into different discrete units. The word Euclid would need to be transformed into digital data (binary representation) in order to be processed. The word Euclid has the binary representation 0100010101010101010000011 0100110001001001010001000.

8.3.3. Image Display and Post-processing

Before the computer processing output, or the digital image, can be shown to an observer on a monitor, it needs to be converted into an analog signal. This type of conversion is determined by the digital-to-analog conversion function (DAC). In order to improve diagnosis, the image that was initially shown can be processed using a collection of steps and methods known as postprocessing techniques. These steps and methods convert the original image into an output image that is suitable for the observer (radiologist) and meets their needs. These operations can be used, for instance, to stitch together multiple images to create a single image, improve sharpness and contrast, or decrease noise in images. Figure 8.6 illustrates the impact of a widely used digital image processing technique called grayscale mapping.

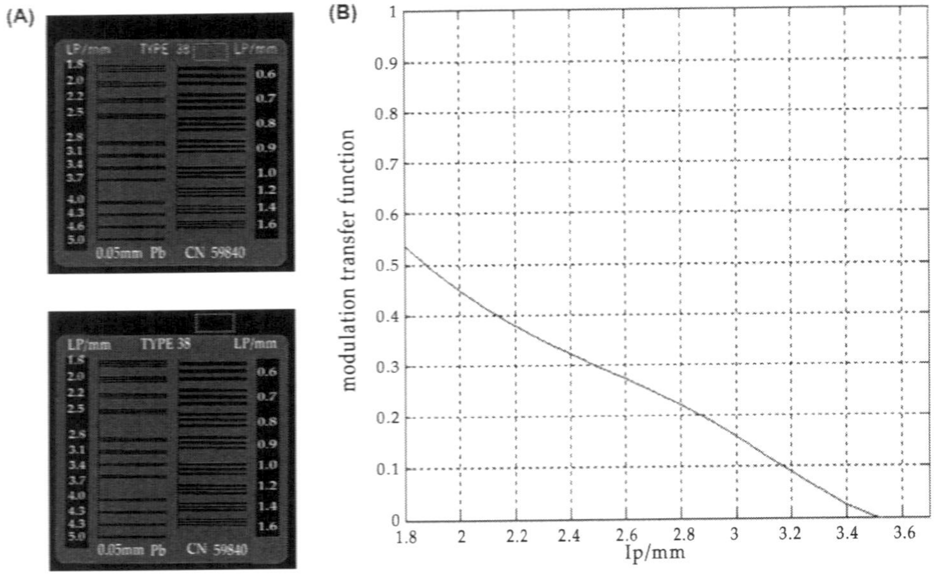

Figure 8.6. *Bar phantom image obtained from the PDR to calculate the signal-to-noise ratio (SNR), contrast-to-noise ratio (CNR) and spatial resolution (A). Line-squares on the phantom images indicated the regions of interest for SNR and CNR measurements. A modulation transfer function (MTF, 10%) curve was used for resolution evaluation (B). The 10% MTF value is 3.17 lp/mm (157μm) on the image obtained from the PDR.*

Source: *Kim, T-H., Heo, D-W., Jeong, C-W., Ryu, J-H., Jun, H. Y., Han, S-J., Ha, T., & Yoon, K-H. Development of portable digital radiography system with a device for monitoring x-ray source-detector angle and its application in chest imaging. Sensors. 2017; 17(3), 531. https://doi.org/10.3390/s17030531.*

8.3.4. Image Storage

The enormous volume of images produced for the various digital radiology exams needs to be kept for medicolegal as well as retrospective analysis. These days, a variety of storage systems and devices, including magnetic tapes, disks, and laser optical disks for long-term storage, are employed for this purpose. A RAID (redundant array of independent disks) storage system, for instance, is frequently used in a PACS environment. It is significant to remember that photos kept in a system for short-term archiving are removed by the institution after a predetermined amount of time.

8.3.5. Image and Data Communications

The use of computer communication networks to transfer images from the acquisition phase to the display/viewing and storage phase is known as image and data communications. Local area networks (LANs) are used if the image transmission occurs within the hospital (through the Intranet). However, networks like wide area networks (WANs) must be used if the images need to be sent to distant locations outside of the hospital via the Internet.

The digital radiology department uses Picture Archiving and Communication Systems (PACS) for image archiving, communication, and storage. Additionally, in order to manage patient data effectively, information systems like HL-7 (Health Level-7) and DICOM (Digital Imaging and Communications in Medicine) are being used to integrate hospital information systems (HIS) and radiology information systems (RIS) with PACS via computer networks.

Image compression is a crucial component of data and image communications. Image compression is used to shorten image transmission times and save storage space, which in turn lowers costs. In digital radiology, lossless or reversible compression and lossy or irreversible compression are two commonly used compression techniques. When an image is decompressed in the former case, no information is lost; in the latter case, some information is lost (Figure 8.7).

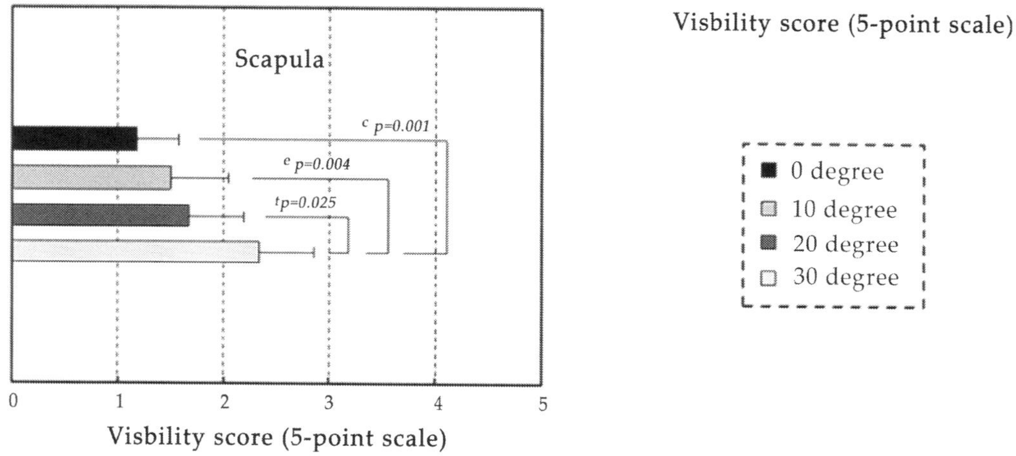

Figure 8.7. *Mean anatomic landmark visibility scores according to different angle degrees. The significant difference between different angle degrees was analyzed with repeated-measures ANOVA and Tukey's post hoc test: [a] 0 vs. 10; [b] 0 vs. 20; [c] 0 vs. 30; [d] 10 vs. 20; [e] 10 vs. 30; and [f] 20 vs. 30. Note that the scores including the border of the heart, the fifth rib and the scapula were significantly different from angle degrees ($p < 0.05$). Five-point scale: 1, definitely seen; 2, probably seen; 3, equivocal; 4, probably not seen; and 5, definitely not seen.*

Source: *Kim, T-H., Heo, D-W., Jeong, C-W., Ryu, J-H., Jun, H. Y., Han, S-J., Ha, T., & Yoon, K-H. Development of portable digital radiography system with a device for monitoring x-ray source-detector angle and its application in chest imaging. Sensors. 2017; 17(3), 531. https://doi.org/10.3390/s17030531.*

8.3.6. Image and Information Management

Using databases and file management software, image and information management refers to the use of PACS and information systems like RIS and HIS to manage the enormous amount of images and text data generated in a digital radiology department. As for the hospital's business operations, the PACS deals with images produced by the various digital imaging modalities, while the RIS and HIS primarily handle textual information (Seeram, 2011; Bushberg et al, 2012; Seeram, 2016; Bushong, 2018).

8.4. Integrating the Healthcare Enterprise

Integrating the Healthcare Enterprise (IHE) is a crucial component of PACS-RIS-HIS integration and digital image acquisition. IHE is a model for making sure that communication standards like HL-7 and DICOM function well to support integration. In 1998, the Radiological Society of North America (RSNA) and the Healthcare Information and Management Systems Society (HIMSS), two significant organizations, created what they refer to as a technical framework based on three fundamental components: an actor, an integration profile, and a data model. This is how the idea of IHE was born (Seeram, 2011; Bushberg et al, 2012; Seeram, 2016; Bushong, 2018).

8.5. Digital Radiography Modalities

Based on the aforementioned technologies, digital radiography consists of a number of imaging modalities connected to the PACS-RIS-HIS image and information systems. Computed radiography (CR), flat-panel digital radiography (FPDR), digital mammography (DM), and digital fluoroscopy (DF) are among the imaging modalities. Complete integration between imaging modalities and PACS-RISHIS systems is necessary for overall successful and productive operations.

8.5.1. Computed Radiography

Utilizing storage or photostimulable phosphors, computed radiography (CR) generates digital images with the help of pre-existing X-ray imaging technology. To create digital images of the patient, radiographic data is processed using a digital computer. A CR imaging system for use in clinical practice was introduced by Fuji Medical Systems in 1983. Other businesses that now produce CR imaging systems include Agfa, Kodak, Konica, and Cannon, to name a few. In CR, the imaging plate (IP), which is housed in a cassette that resembles a film-screen cassette, is coated with a photostimulable phosphor, like barium fluorohalide, to protect it from damage and exposure to foreign materials. In CR, the IP is regarded as the digital detector at that point.

The basic steps in the production of a CR image are shown in Figure 8.8 and include the following:

1. The IP is exposed to X-rays, which causes electrons in the phosphor to move to another energy level, where they remain trapped to create a latent image.
2. The plate is then taken to the CR reader/processor (digital image processor) where it is scanned by a laser beam which causes the trapped electrons return to their original orbit, and in the process, light is emitted.
3. This light is collected by a light guide and sent to a photomultiplier tube (PMT). The output electrical signal from the PMT is subsequently converted into digital data.
4. A digital processor processes the digital data to produce a CR image.
5. The CR image is subsequently displayed for viewing.
6. The IP is exposed to a bright light to erase it (remove residual latent image).
7. The IP can now be used again.

One of the main distinctions between film-screen radiography and CR is that the latter's exposure latitude is approximately 10^4 times narrower than CR's. The inability of CR systems to image detail (spatial resolution) is a significant disadvantage. While a CR's spatial resolution is roughly 3–5 line pairs/mm, film-screen radiography imaging systems have a spatial resolution of roughly 10–15 line pairs/mm. Conversely, for CR systems, the contrast resolution is better and adjustable, but for filmscreen systems, it is fixed.

The detective quantum efficiency is a significant objective measure of the quality of digital images (DQE). The DQE is a metric that quantifies the effectiveness of a digital detector in producing a usable image from the X-rays obtained from the patient. Compared to film-screen systems, the DQE for CR is substantially better. This indicates that, in comparison to film-screen detectors, CR can convert X-rays from the patient into meaningful data over a larger exposure range.

8.5.2. Flat-Panel Digital Radiography

To address the drawbacks of CR systems, flat-panel digital radiography (FPDR) systems were created. The digital detector, as its name suggests, is a flat-panel design that differs greatly from the CR detector (IP) in both structure and functionality. Based on the kind of detector being utilized, there are currently two types of flat-panel digital radiography imaging systems, which are commonly known as:

1. Indirect conversion digital radiography systems.
2. Direct conversion digital radiography systems.

X-rays are first transformed into light by means of a phosphor like cesium iodide. A matrix array of electronic components is exposed to the phosphor's emitted light, which causes electrical charges to be created and stored in direct proportion to the X-ray exposure. The charges result in electrical signals, which a digital computer then digitizes and processes to create an image. X-rays are directly converted to electronic signals by detectors in direct conversion digital radiography systems. X-rays strike the photoconductor (e.g., selenium) that generates electrical signals when connected to a matrix array of electronic components. An image is created by digitally processing and digitizing these signals.

Unlike the first type, which is represented by an array of electronic elements, the indirect type makes use of an array of charge-coupled devices (CCDs) (Figure 8.9a). As seen, the CCDs are connected to a cesium iodide scintillator phosphor. When X-rays strike a phosphor, they produce light. This light then strikes a CCD array, which transforms it into electrical signals. A digital computer then digitizes and processes the signals to create an image.

It's crucial to remember that the flat-panel digital detector can be cleaned and put back to use once all electrical charges have been read out. Furthermore, flat-panel detectors have a number of benefits, such as a high DQE and spatial resolution that is on par with CR systems. Additionally, the characteristic curve of the digital detectors used in CR and flat-panel digital radiography differs significantly from the film characteristic curve. The output signal of the digital detector is linear in the radiation exposure input. In contrast to the film characteristic curve, which has limited exposure latitudes (defined by their slopes), this linear response results in wider exposure latitudes. This represents one of the digital detector's main advantages. The digital detector's wide exposure latitude allows for acceptable image quality even with low or high input exposures. In contrast, film-screen radiography results in either overexposed dark images or underexposed light images, requiring retakes to achieve optimal film density and potentially exposing the patient to increased radiation (Table 8.1).

Table 8.1. The Application of Radiography in Imaging – SNR, CNR, Distortion and Visibility Values on Chest AP Images According to Different Angles

SNR, CNR, Distortion and Visibility Values on Chest AP Images According to Different Angles					
Angle Degree / Value	**0°**	**10°**	**20°**	**30°**	***p*-Value ***
SNR	408.7 ± 160.0	408.8 ± 157.8	428.0 ± 176.3	463.4 ± 155.9	0.082
CNR	82.3 ± 23.0	100.0 ± 30.9	102.8 ± 33.1	98.2 ± 28.8	0.114
Distortion †					
CTD (size, mm)	101.9 ± 0.3	104.4 ± 0.3	106.6 ± 0.4	107.5 ± 0.3	<0.001 [abcdef]
(deformity, %)	(100.0%)	(102.5%)	(104.6%)	(105.5%)	
TTD (mm)	278.0 ± 0.3	278.5 ± 0.1	278.7 ± 0.1	279.4 ± 0.3	<0.001 [abcdef]
(%)	(100.0%)	(100.2%)	(100.3%)	(100.5%)	
TLD (mm)	250.2 ± 1.0	260.7 ± 1.3	266.3 ± 1.3	273.7 ± 1.4	<0.001 [abcdef]
(%)	(100.0%)	(104.2%)	(106.4%)	(109.4%)	
Visibility ‡					
Border of Heart	1.67 ± 0.52	2.17 ± 0.75	2.50 ± 0.55	3.00 ± 0.00	0.044 [bce]
Clavicle	1.00 ± 0.00	1.33 ± 0.52	1.50 ± 0.55	1.83 ± 0.41	0.110
1st Rib (Rt-side)	1.00 ± 0.00	1.33 ± 0.52	1.50 ± 0.55	1.67 ± 0.52	0.292
5th Rib (Rt-side)	1.33 ± 0.52	1.67 ± 0.52	2.33 ± 0.52	3.00 ± 0.00	<0.001 [bcdef]
Scapula	1.17 ± 0.41	1.50 ± 0.55	1.67 ± 0.52	2.33 ± 0.52	0.032 [cef]

Source: *Kim, T-H., Heo, D-W., Jeong, C-W., Ryu, J-H., Jun, H. Y., Han, S-J., Ha, T., & Yoon, K-H. Development of Portable Digital Radiography System with a Device for Monitoring X-ray Source-Detector Angle and Its Application in Chest Imaging. Sensors. 2017; 17(3), 531. https://doi.org/10.3390/s17030531.*

Abbreviation: CNR, contrast-to-noise ratio; CTD, cardiac transverse diameter; SNR, signal-to-noise ratio; TTD, thoracic transverse diameter; TLD thoracic longitudinal diameter. Data are presented as mean ± SD after six measurements at each point. * The significant difference between different angle degrees was analyzed with repeated-measures ANOVA with Tukey's post hoc test: [a] 0 vs. 10; [b] 0 vs. 20; [c] 0 vs. 30; [d] 10 vs. 20; [e] 10 vs. 30; and [f] 20 vs. 30. † The image distortion according to the changes of angulation was calculated the deformity as the percentage changes in the sizes of the diameter. The statistical analysis was used with repeated-measures ANOVA and Tukey's post hoc test as follows: [a] 0 vs. 10; [b] 0 vs. 20; [c] 0 vs. 30; [d] 10 vs. 20; [e] 10 vs. 30; and [f] 20 vs. 30. [‡] The value of each anatomical landmark on the chest image was analyzed according to the radiological diagnosis on a five-point scale: 1, definitely seen; 2, probably seen; 3, equivocal; 4, probably not seen; and 5, definitely not seen.

8.5.3. Digital Fluoroscopy

Digital fluoroscopy is the term used to describe fluoroscopy that uses digital image processing. Using digital image processing software, one of the main objectives of digital fluoroscopy is to increase the perceived contrast resolution when compared to conventional fluoroscopy. To name a few benefits of digital fluoroscopy, there are also edge enhancement, grayscale processing, and temporal frame averaging.

Radiography captures still images, while fluoroscopy captures live, real-time images that show the movement of organs and hollow internal structures like the gastrointestinal tract and blood circulatory system. A typical fluoroscopy imaging system includes a fluoroscopic X-ray tube, an image intensifier tube (the radiation detector), related optics, a television (TV) or CCD camera tube, and a television monitor for viewing and displaying images.

On the other hand, in a digital fluoroscopy system, the ADC digitizes the electrical output signal from the TV/CCD video system and sends it to a digital computer for image processing in digital fluoroscopy. Since the image intensifier tube records the radiation entering the patient, it serves as both the detector and the detector in digital fluoroscopy. Recently, some digital fluoroscopy systems have also been using flat-panel digital detectors.

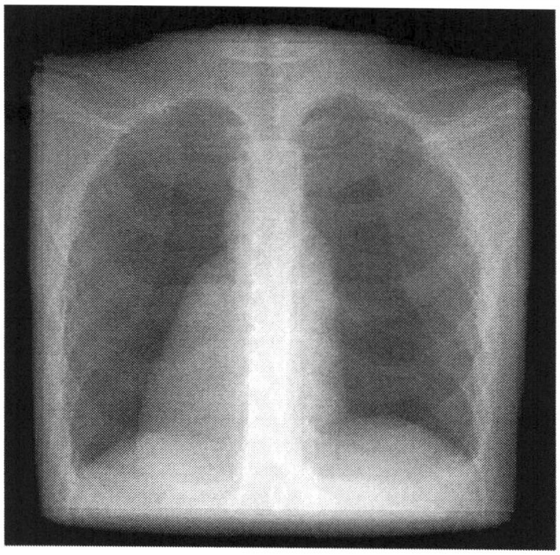

Figure 8.8. *An example result for fluoroscopy imaging.*

Source: *Yan Z, Li L, Qiu R, Chen Z. Research on X-ray Fluorescence Enhanced Fluoroscopy Imaging Technology. Photonics. 2021; 8(10):441. https://doi.org/10.3390/photonics8100441.*

A digital subtraction angiography (DSA) is a type of angiography in which pre- and post-contrast images are digitally subtracted in real time using digital fluoroscopy. By reducing or eliminating the tissues that obstruct the view of vascular structures, these procedures aim to enhance the observer's impression of low-contrast vessels. These subtraction techniques include temporal subtraction, which subtracts images based on time, and energy subtraction, which subtracts images based on various kilovoltages (Seeram, 2011; Bushberg et al, 2012; Seeram, 2016; Bushong, 2018).

8.5.4. Digital Mammography

Mammography, also known as soft tissue imaging, is simply radiography of the breast. To detect breast cancer using film-screen mammography, many specific technical considerations must be made. All of the previously mentioned shortcomings of film-screen radiography also affect film-screen mammography. Digital mammography offers numerous advantages in addition to overcoming these drawbacks. The ability to use digital image processing tools to improve the image's diagnostic interpretation is one of the major advantages of digital mammography.

To image the breast, digital mammography systems currently use CCD arrays, CR detectors, and flat-panel digital detectors, including direct and indirect conversion detectors. Furthermore, digital mammography offers the "second-reader" approach and employs computer-aided diagnosis (CAD) software to assist radiologists in improving their detection of malignant lesions and microcalcifications (Mahesh, 2004).

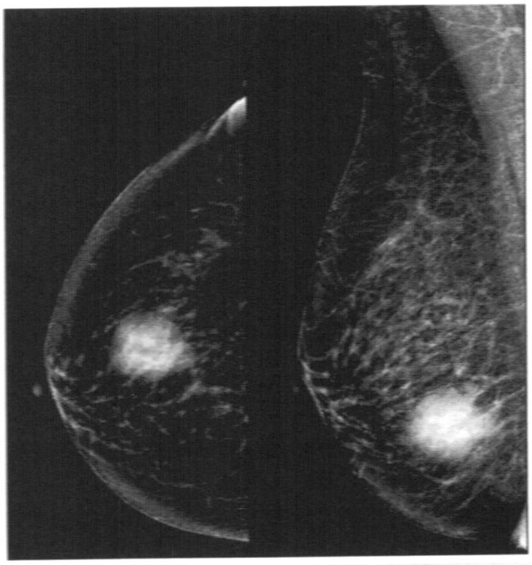

Figure 8.9. *Digital mammography-an example tumor detection.*

Source: *Püsküllüoğlu M, Świderska K, Konieczna A, Rudnicki W, Pacholczak-Madej R, Kunkiel M, Grela-Wojewoda A, Mucha-Małecka A, Mituś JW, Stobiecka E, et al. Discrepancy between tumor size assessed by full-field digital mammography or ultrasonography (cT) and pathology (pT) in a multicenter series of breast metaplastic carcinoma patients. Cancers. 2024; 16(1):188. https://doi.org/10.3390/cancers16010188.*

8.6. Picture Archiving and Communication Systems

The digital images produced by the aforementioned digital radiography modalities must be displayed for interpretation, saved and archived for medicolegal reasons and retrospective analysis, and transmitted to remote locations to meet the needs of other users, including emergency physicians and surgeons in the operating room, both inside and outside of an institution. Using a Picture Archiving and Communication System (PACS) is necessary to complete this task quickly and effectively. PACS are therefore now typical in departments of digital radiology.

A Picture Archiving and Communication System (PACS), a computer system for managing the enormous volume of digital images produced by the various digital image acquisition modalities, is the foundation of a digital imaging department. The various tasks carried out by this technology have also been referred to as image management and communication systems (IMACS); however, PACS is currently a more widely used and common term.

8.6.1. Definition of PACS

Picture archiving and communication system (PACS) is a medical imaging technology used primarily in healthcare organizations to securely store and digitally transmit electronic images and clinically-relevant reports. Technologies such as PACS are becoming increasingly important as the volume of digital medical images grows throughout the healthcare industry and sophisticated data analytics of images becomes more prevalent. This is not only because PACS can handle many types of images from many different imaging devices, but also because it enables easy access to the images for diagnostic and medical decision-making purposes.

8.6.2. Major System Components

The main parts of PACS are depicted below and consist of display workstations, interface devices, PACS computers, and image acquisition devices. These parts are connected to the HIS and RIS via digital communication networks (Figure 8.10).

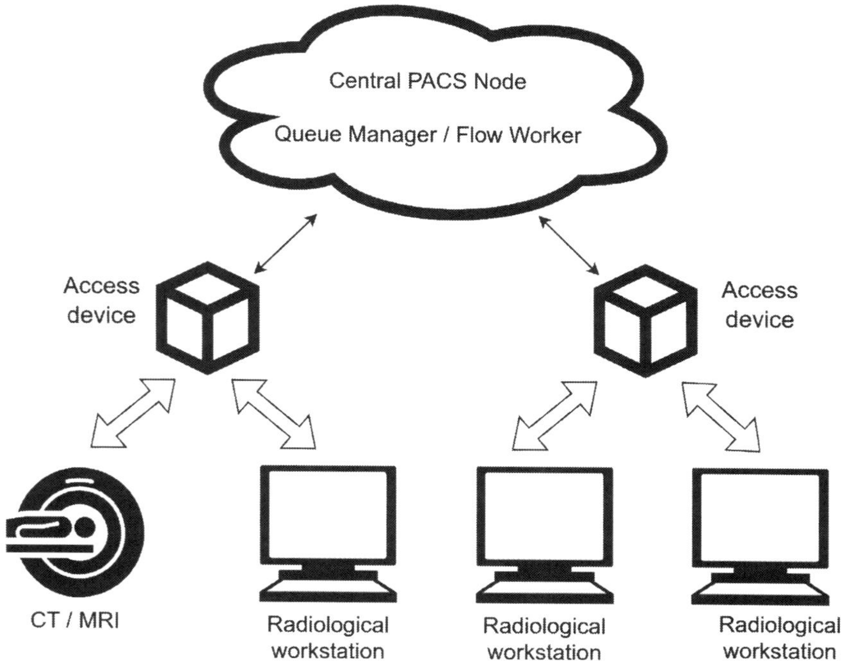

Figure 8.10. *A scheme of a PACS system*

Source: *Kawa J, Pyciński B, Smoliński M, Bożek P, Kwasecki M, Pietrzyk B, Szymański D. Design and implementation of a Cloud PACS architecture. Sensors. 2022; 22(21):8569. https://doi.org/10.3390/s22218569.*

The PACS computer, a "high-end" computer or server, is the brains of the entire system. Photos and medical records (e.g., demographics) are subsequently transferred to the PACS computer, which has both a database server and an archive system, from the digital image acquisition modalities, the HIS, and the RIS. A redundant array of independent disks (RAID), magnetic tapes, and laser optical disks are common archiving methods used in PACS environments.

Soft-copy workstations, also known as display workstations, are used to display images on a monitor for the purpose of image interpretation. Furthermore, the types of these workstations vary based on how much the observer uses them. Technologists frequently use review workstations for a general evaluation of image quality prior to the images being sent to the PACS, even though radiologists are required to have high-resolution diagnostic workstations in order to interpret images and diagnose the patient's medical condition.

One of the main functions of workstations is that they enable users to enhance diagnosis through digital post-processing of images. For instance, compressing images can shorten image transmission times and save storage space.

Other conditions must be satisfied for the PACS to function effectively and efficiently. Using industry healthcare standards for data and image communications is one such mandate. HL-7 (Health Level-7) and DICOM (Digital Imaging and Communication in Medicine) are two standards that are currently utilized in a PACS environment. HL-7 is primarily concerned with textual information from the HIS and RIS, whereas DICOM is primarily concerned with images from the digital image acquisition modalities.

Data security is crucial in both a digital hospital and a PACS setting since the PACS hold private patient data and information.

The interfaces allow users to easily communicate with the PACS computer and the HIS/RIS through image acquisition modalities. They also enable users to access the PACS computer via the World Wide Web (Samei et al, 2004).

8.7. Quality Assurance in Digital Radiography

Quality assurance (QA) and quality control (QC) procedures are valuable techniques to promote ongoing quality enhancement in a product. In the field of radiology, policies, procedures, and activities related to QA/QC all serve the purpose of:

1. Ensure that patients are exposed to minimum radiation using the ALARA (as low as reasonably achievable) philosophy.
2. Produce optimum image quality for diagnosis.
3. Reduce the costs of radiology operations.

QA and QC for digital radiography systems are still developing, and specialized instruments are now available to test the functionality of PACS components as well as digital imaging equipment. For instance, technologists are already regularly conducting quality control (QC) tests for CR systems, dark noise, exposure index calibration, and other related topics. These tests are becoming routine.

8.8. Medical Imaging Informatics

The term "informatics" has been derived from the term "information." For computer applications in general, information refers to useful, meaningful, and organized data. In other words, computers convert data into information, to be used by humans for solving problems in the real world.

Imaging informatics (II) has replaced the term medical imaging informatics (MI) and is now commonplace in the imaging community. The Society of Imaging Informatics in Medicine (SIIM) states that the "science of imaging informatics is the study and application of processes of information and communications technology for the acquisition, manipulation, analysis, and distribution of image data."

8.8.1. Informatics

Informatics is the process of converting data into information, and as such, the process heavily relies on computers and communication technologies.

- **Informatics Subspecialties:** Healthcare informatics, biomedical informatics, nursing informatics, imaging informatics (radiology informatics), cardiology informatics, clinical informatics, and other subspecialties have all emerged as a result of the application of informatics to various disciplines.

- **Healthcare Informatics/Medical Informatics:** Healthcare informatics and medical informatics are the terms used to describe the use of information technology in healthcare and medicine, respectively. There are several definitions in the literature and on various medical informatics websites; however, Healthcare Information and Management Systems Society (HIMSS) has defined both terms as "the interdisciplinary study of the design, development, adoption, and application of IT-based innovations in healthcare services delivery, management, and planning."
- **Scope of Health Informatics:** Health informatics encompasses a broad spectrum of subjects. For example, a number of health informatics textbooks offer guidance in this area. The common themes that emerge are generally focused on major components: information science and technology, computer science, healthcare information systems, the electronic health record, health data analytics, security concerns, data mining and machine learning, artificial intelligence, decision support, Internet technologies, and so on. Core concepts are the fundamental ideas of informatics related to models, data, information, and system theory.

  The study of clinical information systems, which include nursing, laboratory, cardiology, and radiology information systems, as well as administrative systems that handle tasks like patient scheduling and registration, falls under the broad topic of health information systems. In addition, information systems-related topics include disaster recovery, electronic health records, system integration, security and confidentiality concerns, training, and regulatory issues, to name a few.

  Lastly, the use of computers in research and education will be covered under the topic of specialized applications in a healthcare informatics curriculum. Furthermore, healthcare informatics courses must cover decision support systems and telehealth concepts and issues.

8.8.2. Imaging Informatics

These days, the digital hospital and digital imaging departments function within the information technology (IT) space. Information Technology concepts are used in digital image acquisition technologies, digital image processing, digital image display, storage, and archiving, and digital image communications. The field of information technology is expanding and gaining popularity across society. It involves applying communications and computer technology to address societal issues, such as those pertaining to healthcare and medical imaging.

Imaging informatics is defined by the Society for Imaging Informatics in Medicine (SIIM) as "the study and application of processes of information and communications technology for the acquisition, manipulation, analysis, and distribution of image data."

Because images can be used for diagnosis, assessment, planning (to determine the extent of a tumor and assist in preparing a management strategy), guidance during procedures, communication, education, training, and research, medical imaging is important to the healthcare industry. Information technology is needed to perform these tasks (IT). IT is the application of communications technology and computer technology to address societal issues, such as healthcare and medical imaging. These days, IT plays a significant role in digital medical imaging.

Information systems, standards for exchanging text and image data, computer communication networks, web technology, handling text and images, concerns about privacy, security, and confidentiality, and digital image processing are just a few of the subjects covered by IT. Picture Archiving and Communication Systems (PACS) have been widely implemented in radiology departments in more recent times.

8.8.3. Health Information Systems

An information system is a computer-based system designed to gather and analyze data in order to give its users the knowledge they need to solve problems and make decisions. Hospital information systems (HIS) and healthcare information systems (HIS) are systems used in hospitals and other healthcare facilities to support and improve patient care and management.

Clinical information systems (CISs) and administrative information systems (AISs) are the two main component systems of the HIS. Order entry, monitoring, nursing, laboratory, and radiology information systems (RIS) are just a few of the information systems that are included in CISs. Information systems for registration, scheduling, payroll and finance, human resources, quality control, and contract management are all included in AISs.

A few characteristic and essential features of an RIS are as follows:

- Order entry: requested radiology examinations ordered by physicians are entered into the system. This is also known as registration of patients.
- Scheduling of various imaging procedures.
- Report generation: radiologists enter image interpretation reports. These reports are obviously linked to the appropriate patient and examination.
- Billing preparation: costs associated with various procedures done on patients are generated and sent to a billing system.
- Other related functions: these include functions such as quality assurance, inventory monitoring, and statistical analysis as well as communications that are important to the daily operations of the imaging department.

It is clear that the information contained in the RIS can be shared with the HIS, so that physicians in the hospital, for example, can access related information on their patients from their offices if required.

8.8.4. The Electronic Health Record

The adoption of HIS, RIS, and PACS is paving the way for the transition from paper-based medical records to electronic health records (EHR) to address the constraints of traditional records. A key drawback of paper-based records is their inability to incorporate images from systems like PACS. Additionally, paper-based records lack the functionality to effectively utilize decision support and other related systems.

8.8.4.1. Definition and Components

HIMSS states that the EHR "is a longitudinal electronic record of patient health information generated by one or more encounters in any care delivery setting. Included in this information are patient demographics, progress notes, problems, medications, vital signs, past medical history, immunizations, laboratory data and radiology reports. The EHR automates and streamlines the clinician's workflow. The EHR has the ability to generate a complete record of a clinical patient encounter—as well as supporting other care related activities directly or indirectly via interface—including evidence-based decision support, quality management, and outcomes reporting." There is a ton of medical data in the EHR, including patient information (e.g., demographic data), as well as other pertinent health data (like pictures from diagnostic tests, for example). Data and information from order entry, clinical documentation, data repositories, and decision support, results reporting, clinical messaging, and e-mail are all contained in the EHR. In addition to offering numerous advantages to medical professionals, such as doctors, the EHR also benefits the healthcare organization as a whole. Improved data integrity and care quality, for instance, as well as higher provider productivity and satisfaction, are some of these advantages.

8.8.5. System Integration

Integration is a key idea in imaging informatics because it addresses the idea that information systems, PACS, and imaging modalities (data acquisition devices) must be able to exchange data and communicate with one another seamlessly for them to be effective and efficient.

8.8.5.1. Requirements for System Integration

System integration requires a number of things in order to be successful and efficient. These consist of the master patient index (MIP), uniform language, data dictionary, interface, and communication (data exchange) standards.

Systems are connected through an interface so that data can be shared between them. Because the early interfaces allowed two systems to communicate with one another, they were point-to-point interfaces. These days, more advanced interfaces known as interface engines—computer programs, or software—make it easier for data to move between multiple systems. A clinical data repository and the mapping technique are used to enable this kind of communication. When terms from one system must match similar terms from another, this is referred to as "mapping." Although a data dictionary defines terms used in a specific enterprise (e.g., healthcare organization), the MIP is a database that includes all data (e.g., demographics) about the patient and is crucial in identifying and locating the patient's records that are being studied.

Radiologists, technologists, and other related staff members working in the imaging department must understand the concept of using standards for data exchange in imaging informatics (e.g., physicists and biomedical engineers and IT personnel). DICOM (Digital Imaging and Communications in Medicine) and HL-7 (Health Level-7) are the two standards that are used in the imaging department to transmit textual data and images, respectively. Although DICOM was designed primarily to handle image communication between image acquisition devices and PACS, as well as between PACS and other enterprise systems, HL-7 was created to manage text data interchange between different information systems, including HIS and RIS.

Lastly, it's critical to remember that one of the major imaging informatics topics is the Integrating the Healthcare Enterprise (IHE) initiative. The Radiological Society of North America (RSNA) and the Healthcare Information and Management Systems Society (HIMSS) collaborated to launch this project in

1998. Ensuring seamless communication (data exchange) between image acquisition devices, PACS, and information systems from various vendors is the overarching goal of the IHE initiative.

8.8.6. The Next Era in Imaging Informatics

At least six key areas in medical imaging informatics that have drawn more attention in the literature are part of the field's upcoming era. These include enterprise imaging, Big Data, cloud computing, machine learning and deep learning, and artificial intelligence.

- **Enterprise Imaging:** Although traditional vendor-neutral archives (VNAs) and PACS are still used in medical imaging and hospitals, there has been a growing focus on the transition to enterprise imaging systems in an attempt to centralize workload and data into a single system. In addition to saving operating expenses for healthcare facilities, this approach will help to increase the effectiveness of patient management.

  These efforts have led to the introduction and development of enterprise imaging, a term defined by the Healthcare Information and Management Systems Society (HIMSS) and the Society for Imaging Informatics in Medicine (SIIM) as "a set of strategies, initiatives and workflows implemented across a healthcare enterprise to consistently and optimally capture, index, manage, store, distribute, view, exchange, and analyze all clinical imaging and multimedia content to enhance the electronic health record."
- **Cloud Computing:** Cloud computing is another idea that has surfaced in the field of imaging informatics. This term refers to "the access of computing resources through the Internet for purposes of data storage, aggregation, synthesis, and retrieval, together with the capacity to act on the data with computational algorithms and software packages." Infrastructure as a Service (IaaS), Platform as a Service (PaaS), and Software as a Service (SaaS) are the three cloud computing models that are currently available.
- **BigData:** Big Data is the most recent "emerging science" in medical imaging informatics. "The four Vs—Volume, which describes the sheer number of data elements within these extraordinarily large data sets; Variety, which describes the aggregation of data from multiple sources; Velocity, which describes the high speed at which data is generated; and Veracity, which describes the inherent uncertainty in some data elements—define big data, which are extremely complex data sets. Personalized image interpretation, the identification of novel imaging markers, value quantification, and workflow characterization are just a few of the ways that Big Data will impact medical practice. Imaging departments will be able to "venture confidently into the next era of informatics and data science" thanks to potential applications.
- **Machine Learning and Deep Learning:** The study of computer

algorithms that can recognize intricate patterns or relationships from empirical data and arrive at reliable conclusions is known as machine learning. This multidisciplinary field is closely related to statistical physics, artificial intelligence, data mining, statistics, probability theory, optimization, and theoretical computer science. Medical image segmentation and registration, computer-aided detection and diagnosis systems for computed tomography (CT), and magnetic resonance imaging (MRI) are among the applications of machine learning in medical imaging.

Conversely, deep learning is another field that will see increasing use in medical imaging. "The advantage of deep learning is that features are identified as part of the learning process; it does not require image feature identification and calculation as a first step," according to the description of the machine algorithm.

- **Artificial Intelligence:** Artificial intelligence (AI) is a component of computer science that "aims to mimic human cognitive functions... and can be applied to various types of healthcare data (structured and unstructured) and popular AI techniques include machine learning methods for structured data, such as the classical support vector machine and neural network, and the modern deep learning, as well as natural language processing for unstructured data." Major disease areas that use AI tools include cancer, neurology, and cardiology.

8.8.7. The Technologist as an Informaticist

IT-related extra skills will be necessary for technologists working in the entire digital medical imaging department. These departments already have someone known as a PACS Administrator, who works exclusively to maintain the integrity of the PACS. In some departments, this person is an IT specialist, and in others, a technologist. Technologists need to keep up their education in the digital realm of radiology, which includes digital image processing, in order to be productive and successful in this position. The technologist will thus take on a new role as an informaticist.

8.8.8. The Benefits of Imaging Informatics

With the widespread adoption of digital image acquisition, processing, display, storage, and communications technologies, imaging informatics developed. As a result of the EHR's development and the data that radiologists refer to as the entire patient entity (EPE), imaging informatics now offers substantial advantages to the healthcare industry as a whole as well as the imaging department.

The more educated those who assist patients in regaining their health are, the more effectively, efficiently, and dependably they can contribute to patient care. Such assistance is provided by those with training in imaging informatics, a subspecialty of radiology, and ultimately the patient gains from their knowledge.

8.8.9. Certification in Imaging Informatics

The Certified Imaging Informatics Professional (CIIP) was developed as a result of the PACS administrator certification and the idea of going above and beyond. The American Board of Imaging Informatics (ABII), the American Registry of Radiologic Technologist Technologists (ARRT), and the Society for Imaging Informatics in Medicine (SIIM) collaborated to create the CIIP certification. The SIIM website has information about the examination development process, content, eligibility requirements, goals, and mission. The SIIM and the ASRT founded the ABII in 2007. The mission of ABII is "to enhance patient care, professionalism, and competence in imaging informatics. ABII has created and manages the Imaging Informatics Professional (IIP) certification program and awards the Certified Imaging Informatics Professional (CIIP) designation to qualified candidates."

8.10. Advances in Digital Radiography

When German scientist Wilhelm Conrad Röntgen first observed X-rays in 1895, it laid the groundwork for contemporary diagnostic imaging and radiography, more than a century ago. He was the first person to receive the Nobel Prize in Physics in 1901 in recognition of his discovery. These days, radiography is changing due to digitization, just like all other industries.

Digital mobile radiography, AI-assisted X-ray interpretation, dual-energy imaging, tomosynthesis, computer-aided diagnosis, automatic image stitching, and many other developments have been made in the field of digital radiography in recent years. Improvements in image quality have contributed to better patient outcomes and improved patient care. Furthermore, using digital radiography minimizes the need for repeats, which offers the advantage of less radiation exposure.

The advantages are below:

- Shorter exposure times
- Improved detail detectability
- Extremely high image quality
- Faster processing and diagnosis
- Images that are easier to store and share with doctors
- Capability for remote viewing from connected digital devices

8.10.1. Differences Between X-rays and Digital Radiology

Image detection, image capture, and image data storage are common features of both digital radiography and traditional X-rays. A person's body is exposed to an X-ray beam during a radiography procedure. A portion of the X-rays are taken up by the internal organ systems. The remaining X-rays are sent to a detector—a film or digital detector, for example—where they form a pattern that is recorded for later analysis.

The primary differences between traditional X-rays and digital radiography are as follows:

- Traditional X-rays use film to capture images of internal structures in the body.
- In digital radiography, digital detectors instantly produce a digital radiographic image and store the images separately on a digital medium such as a computer.

Through electronic health records (EHRs) or other devices that store patient data, radiographers, physicians, and other medical professionals can easily access images electronically thanks to digital radiography.

It can be categorized into two types:

- Computed radiography (CR) works through an indirect process. It replaces traditional film used in traditional radiography with an imaging plate (IP). The information is then transferred over to a computing device for analysis.

- Digital detector array radiography (DDA) is also known simply as digital radiography, which uses a digital detector array or flat panel detector to convert X-rays directly into a digital image.

Digital radiography is centered on digital technology. Over the past ten years, the field of medical imaging has seen a rise in the use of this sophisticated type of X-ray inspection. New developments in radiology keep changing the field. For example, applications such as:

- Virtual reality and augmented reality to create immersive training for future radiology professionals
- Deep mind to reduce false results for cancer screening
- Cardiac MRI segmentation to deliver real-time diagnosis
- Augment intelligence to automate mundane manual tasks

8.10.2. AI-Aided X-ray Interpretation

The field of radiology has made significant progress in the analysis and interpretation of imaging data thanks to developments in computer vision, machine learning (ML), artificial intelligence (AI), and deep learning algorithms. Radiology professionals can enhance patient care by using AI-assisted X-ray interpretation to diagnose and treat injuries and illnesses more quickly and accurately.

AI-aided X-ray interpretation works as follows:

- Using algorithms, it analyzes data and images at high speed from public and proprietary medical databases.
- It then compares images with previous findings to identify patterns and anomalies.

Benefits of AI-aided X-ray interpretation in diagnostic imaging include the following:

- Faster tracking of crucial information for diagnosis
- The ability to prioritize critical cases better
- Reduction of errors in reading electronic health records (EHRs)

8.10.2.1. Use Cases for AI-Aided X-ray Interpretation

Over the past few years, artificial intelligence (AI) has made significant progress in the interpretation of X-rays, particularly in the area of chest radiography—the most frequently performed diagnostic imaging test in emergency rooms. It keeps progressing in a lot of areas. Below are a few examples:

- AI-aided X-ray interpretation was used to help diagnose COVID-19. According to a *European Radiology* study, AI-assisted chest X-ray assessments helped radiologists differentiate COVID-19-positive from COVID-19-negative patients and improved the precision of diagnoses from 65.9% to 81.9%.
- A study published in *JAMA* found that AI algorithms performed as well as radiology residents when making preliminary interpretations of chest radiographs. The findings of the study suggest that AI can therefore improve radiology workflows, strengthen overall accuracy for more precise diagnoses, help address issues with resource scarcity, and lower healthcare costs.

8.10.3. Dual-Energy Imaging

Dual-energy imaging is a type of digital radiography, specifically computed tomography (CT). CT, also known as computed axial tomography (CAT), works this way:

- It uses a standard X-ray tube that produces X-ray beams that pass through the body at multiple angles and are captured by digital detectors.
- A computer then assembles the captured data to make cross-sectional images of the body that resemble "slices."

Similar principles apply to a dual-energy CT scanner, which additionally employs a second, lower-voltage X-ray tube in addition to the conventional X-ray tube. Compared to standard CT, the technique of using two distinct X-ray energy sources of varying powers has advantages because it generates faster and clearer images for the detection of lesions and abnormalities.

Radiology experts occasionally employ materials referred to as contrast agents to facilitate imaging. For instance, a frequently used tool that makes it possible to examine blood vessels is iodine-based contrast. Compared to a standard CT scanner, a dual-energy CT scanner can detect iodine more clearly, resulting in more detailed images that can aid in diagnosis.

8.10.3.1. Use Cases for Dual-Energy Imaging

Dual-energy imaging is not a novel idea. Studies conducted as early as the 1970s and 1980s showed how dual-energy technology could be used to improve tissue characterization. Dual-energy imaging's utility for diagnostic imaging was, however, limited by the lengthy data acquisition process.

Today's faster processors in new technology enable faster data acquisition and analysis, which boosts dual-energy imaging's acceptance in the medical field.

Dual-energy imaging may be used for the following use cases:

- To produce better images of blood vessels
- To reduce the number of examinations a patient has to undergo
- To detect abnormalities in the body, for example detecting what type of kidney stone is present in a patient
- To improve image quality if a patient has metal inserts in their body structure
- To produce images that are well-designed for advanced 3D reconstruction and visualization of structures

8.10.4. Tomosynthesis

Tomosynthesis is a sophisticated form of digital mammography that was approved by the FDA in 2011. It is also referred to as digital breast tomosynthesis (DBT), 3-D mammography, and breast tomosynthesis.

Sometimes radiologists find it challenging to identify cancer due to the flat images generated by traditional 2D mammography, even to the point where abnormal areas appear in the images. Patients are frequently called back for follow-up testing as a result of this.

Tomosynthesis uses an alternative imaging technique to help prevent this. It uses 2D and 3D-like images to create multiple images of the breast, which are then sent to a computer that assembles the images using algorithms to provide a more comprehensive view of the patient's breasts.

8.10.4.1. Use Cases for Tomosynthesis

One kind of digital radiography that has several advantages is tomosynthesis. The following figures demonstrate the benefit of tomosynthesis:

- Johns Hopkins Medicine reports that tomosynthesis can detect 41% more invasive cancers.
- According to Stanford Health Care, tomosynthesis reduces false positives by approximately 15%.
- A study published in *European Radiology* reveals that radiologists can improve cancer detection and reduce the time to read images with an AI reading support system.

Overall accuracy can be raised by tomosynthesis, particularly when combined with traditional mammography.

Additional benefits for radiology professionals and patients include:

- Detection of breast cancer in the early stages or in patients not showing any symptoms
- Greater accuracy for breast cancer screening for people with dense breasts
- Identification of tumors that traditional mammograms can miss
- Reduction of callbacks and false-positive results

8.10.5. Computer-Aided Diagnosis

Computer science and medicine converge in computer-aided diagnosis, or CAD. This type of digital radiography technology is intended to help medical professionals make more accurate diagnoses.

For radiologists to analyze and assess, diagnostic imaging methods such as MRI, CT, X-ray, and ultrasound diagnostics provide vital information. Radiologists typically have to read images in a condensed amount of time due to the urgency of learning the results.

Computer-aided diagnosis (CADx) and computer-aided detection (CADe) are two types of CAD.

- **Computer-Aided Detection (CADe):** Marks areas of images that appear abnormal to reduce the chances of missing pathologies and to spotlight anomalies.
- **Computer-Aided Diagnosis (CADx):** Provides support for assessing and classifying pathologies, such as tumors and lesions, presented in medical images.

8.10.5.1. Use Cases for Computer-Aided Diagnosis

For a long time, CAD has been a standard in the medical field. Early CAD iterations relied on user domain knowledge and manual engineering.

Using AI and machine learning is one of the more recent methods for increasing knowledge in CAD. Large amounts of intricate clinical data are also processed by these intelligent systems to generate new knowledge and enhance diagnostic performance.

To aid radiologists in the interpretation of medical images and the production of more precise diagnoses, CAD software finds extensive use in the medical field. The most popular medical uses are for the detection of breast cancer and the identification of pulmonary nodules that may be indicative of lung cancer. It is used in detecting the following:

- Colon cancer
- Prostate cancer

- Bone metastases
- Coronary artery disease
- Alzheimer's disease
- Diabetic retinopathy

8.10.6. Automatic Image Stitching

Several fields use image stitching in digital radiography, which is the process of joining smaller images to create a larger one. For instance, a satellite has a limited range but can capture images of the Earth's surface. It is capable of capturing an image of the topography of a specific area within the United States, but not the entire nation. Using clever technology, image stitching joins the disparate images of different regions to produce a sizable topographic map of the United States.

Similar to this, a digital radiology scanning system in a medical setting can scan specific body parts, but not the entire body at once. Radiology experts can "stitch" together images of various body parts using image stitching technologies to see a picture of a patient's entire bone structure in order to search for anomalies that may be indicative of possible medical problems.

Image registration and image mosaicking are other terms that are used in the context of image stitching. Medical image stitching is essential to medical robotics and intelligent systems, ranging from real-time guidance and post-procedural assessment to diagnostics and surgical planning. It does this by combining two or more sets of imaging data into a single coordinate system.

The technique of piecing together multiple images automatically, without the need for human intervention, is known as automatic image stitching. In situations where a single scan does not provide a complete view of the area being investigated, automatic image stitching uses AI and ML algorithms to overlap regions of the same area to create a panoramic image that helps doctors diagnose a disease.

8.10.6.1. Use Cases for Automatic Image Stitching

There are several ways that automatic image stitching can be used in medicine. For instance, preoperative planning for procedures like leg alignment operations can be accomplished by surgeons through the stitching of images. In order to diagnose scoliosis, medical professionals can also view the full image of a patient's spine.

Recent studies offering insight into use cases for automatic image stitching include:

- A recent article in the *Sensors* journal published on MDPI points out how a panoramic stitching algorithm used in cone beam computed tomography reduced the need for patients to reposition themselves when images are being taken.
- An article in *Scientific Reports* notes that image stitching can be used to bring together different images of a single area for comparison purposes. For example, scans taken at different times can help to determine the growth of a tumor or determine the effects of surgery.

8.10.7. Digital Mobile Radiography

With wheels, digital mobile radiography equipment is portable and easy to move to a patient's bedside in medical environments like hospitals. For instance, a mobile X-ray unit can image patients who have limited mobility after surgery in order to assist the surgeon in assessing the surgical result. Disinfection is made easier by the mobility of digital mobile radiography equipment.

Before referring patients for more sophisticated imaging procedures, doctors in digital radiography use mobile digital radiography equipment to evaluate and diagnose patients. For instance, hospitals saw a significant influx of patients in need of diagnostic imaging during the COVID-19 pandemic. Digital mobile radiography units have been a vital triaging and screening instrument for evaluating patients' lung conditions.

8.10.7.1. Use Cases for Digital Mobile Radiography

A few examples are given below:

- Digital mobile radiography equipment allows patients who cannot be moved to a radiology department to get chest radiography.
- Because of its unique size, digital mobile radiography equipment can be positioned within tight spaces and between beds and other equipment, such as in surgical or endoscopic suites.
- According to a study published in *BMC Health Services Research*, digital mobile radiography equipment can be used outside of the hospital, including in nursing homes for the elderly, group dwellings for people with intellectual disabilities, and shelters (Seeram, 2011; Bushberg et al, 2012; Seeram, 2016; Bushong, 2018)

A Closer Look

Applications in Healthcare and Medical Imaging

Pannu has identified and described the general areas of AI. These areas include language understanding, learning, and adaptive systems; problem-solving; perception; modeling; robotics; and games such as chess. AI has specific applications in healthcare and medical imaging.

In healthcare, Jiang et al. surveyed the literature on the current status of AI, its future direction. They reviewed four areas of concern: the motivation for applying AI techniques to healthcare, the types of data subject to AI techniques, the AI techniques used, and the types of disease currently being examined in which AI techniques can be applied to generate useful and valid results. The data types include both structured and unstructured data in medical imaging, genetics, electrodiagnosis, monitoring, physiologic, disability evaluation, mass screening, and so forth. Popular AI techniques used are machine learning for structured data and natural language processing for unstructured data. Additionally, they identified major areas using AI tools such as cancer, neurology, and cardiology and reviewed ten disease types examined in the literature.

The applications of machine learning in everyday human activity include its use in banking, finance, marketing, and the Internet. In medical imaging, a number of applications have been identified and discussed in the literature. For example, machine learning and deep learning applications in medical imaging range from image segmentation, image registration, automatic labeling and captioning, computer-aided detection and diagnosis to reading assistant and automatic dictation and integration with Healthcare Big Data: Towards Precision Imaging. The integration with healthcare Big Data is linked to what has been referred to as precision medicine which "involves the prevention and treatment strategies that consider individual variability by assessing large sets of data, including patient information, medical imaging, and genomic sequences. The success of precision medicine is largely dependent on robust quantitative biomarkers. In general, deep learning can be used to explore and create quantitative biomarkers from medical big data obtained through internet of things, genetics and genomics, medical imaging, and mobile monitoring sources (Figure 8.11). In particular, imaging is non-invasively and routinely performed for clinical practice, and can be used to compute quantitative imaging biomarkers. Many radiomic studies have correlated imaging biomarkers with the genomic expression or clinical outcome. Deep learning techniques can be used to generate more reliable imaging biomarkers for precision medicine."

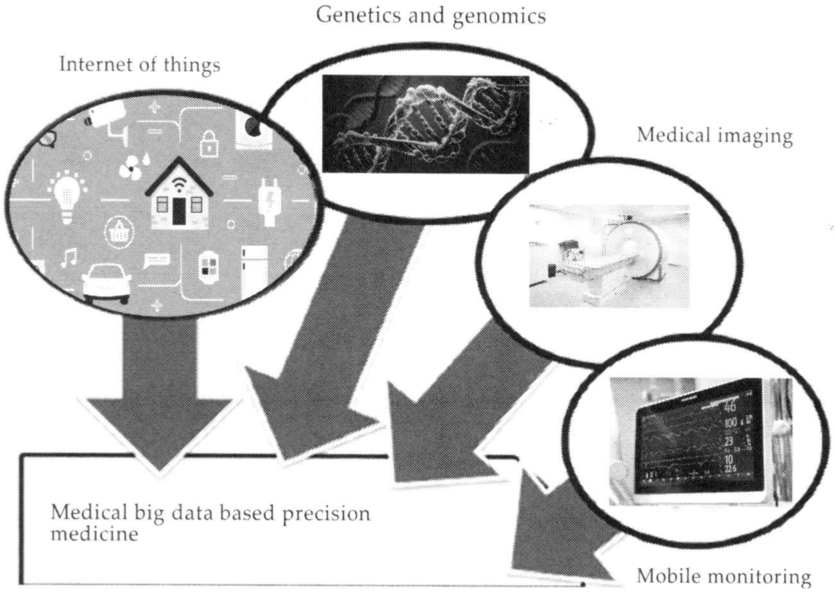

Figure 8.11. *The use of deep learning to explore and create quantitative biomarkers from medical Big Data obtained through Internet of things, genetics and genomics, medicinal imaging, and mobile monitoring sources.*

Source: *E. Seeram. Digital Radiography. Springer. https://doi.org/10.1007/978-981-13-3244-9_1.*

It is important to note that AI, machine learning, and deep learning are at the introductory stages of their development and applications in medical imaging. Furthermore, several experts have stated categorically that as these emerging topics in imaging informatics evolve, they will gain acceptance and become useful tools in medical imaging technologies. Imaging technology students and practicing technologists should make every effort to understand AI, machine learning, and deep learning and their applications in imaging informatics, in order to communicate effectively with radiologists and medical physicists and, later through more formal coursework on these topics, be able to assume leadership in imaging informatics. These tools can only help in restoring the health of patients.

Summary

- Digital radiography is filmless, and allows immediate acquisition, deletion, editing and transfer of films to a computer system which generates the image almost at once.
- Digital detection is based on the conversion of absorbed X-ray energy into electrical charge, which must then be represented digitally in grayscale images to show the quantified X-ray energy that was absorbed at each point in the digital image.
- Film-based imaging consists of X-ray interaction with electrons in the film emulsion, production of a latent image, and chemical processing that transforms the latent image into a visible one.
- Data acquisition refers to the collection of X-rays transmitted through the patient. It is the first step in the production of the image. For digital radiography, special electronic detectors (digital detectors) are used and replace the X-ray film cassette used in film-based radiography. These detectors are of several types that utilize technologies to convert X-rays to electrical signals (analog signals).
- Picture Archiving and Communication Systems (PACS) are being used for storing/ archiving and communicating images in the digital radiology department. In addition, information systems, such as the radiology information systems (RIS) and the hospital information systems (HIS), are now being integrated with the PACS via computer networks, using communications standards such as DICOM (Digital Imaging and Communications in Medicine) and HL-7 (Health Level-7), for effective management of patient information.
- Image and information management refers to the use of PACS and information systems such as RIS and HIS to manage the vast number of images and text data produced in a digital radiology department, using databases and file management software.
- Computed radiography (CR) makes use of photostimulable or storage phosphors to produce digital images using existing X-ray imaging equipment. A digital computer is used to process data collected by radiographic means to produce digital images of the patient.
- Mammography is radiography of the breast and is often referred to as soft tissue imaging. Film-screen mammography requires a great deal of special technical considerations to detect breast cancer.
- Informatics refers to the process of changing data to information, and therefore computers and communication technologies are central elements to the process.
- An information system is a computer-based system used to collect and process data to provide its users with information needed for problem-solving and decision-making. A healthcare information system and hospital information system (HIS) are systems used within a hospital or enterprise that support and enhance the care and management of patients.

References

1. Bushberg, J. T., Seibert, J. A., Leidholdt Jr., E. M., & Boone, J. M. (2012). *The Essential Physics of Medical Imaging* (3rd ed.). Philadelphia, PA: Lippincott Williams & Wilkins, Philadelphia, PA, USA, 2012. 1048 pp.
2. Bushong, S. (2018). *Radiologic Science for Technologists* (11th ed.). St Louis, MO: Elsevier. ISBN: 9780323429443
3. Erickson, B. J., Korfiatis, P., Akkus, Z., & Kline, T. L. (2017). Machine learning. *Radiographics, 37*, 505–515.
4. Jiang, F., Jiang, Y., Zhi, H., Dong, Y., Li, H., Ma, S., et al. (2017). Artificial intelligence in healthcare: past, present and future. *Stroke and Vascular Neurology, 2*(4), 230–243.
5. Kansagra, A. P., Yu, J. -P. J., Chatterjee, A. R., Lenchik, L., Chow, D. S., Prater, A. B., et al. (2016). Big data and the future of radiology informatics. *Academic Radiology, 23*, 30–42.
6. Mahesh, M. (2004). Digital mammography: an overview. *Radiographics, 24*, 1747–1760.
7. Mendelson, D. S., & Rubin, D. L. (2013). Imaging informatics: essential tools for the delivery of imaging services. *Academic Radiology, 20*, 1195–1212.
8. Pisano, E. D., & Yaffe, M. J. (2005). Digital mammography. *Radiology, 234*, 353–362.
9. Roth, C., Lannum, L., & Persons, K. (2016). A foundation for enterprise imaging: HIMSS-SIIM collaborative white paper. *Journal of Digital Imaging, 29*, 530–538.
10. Samei, E., Seibert, J. A., Andriole, K., Badano, A., Crawford, J., Reiner, B., Flynn, M. J., & Chang, P. (2004). General guidelines for purchasing and acceptance testing of PACS equipment. *Radiographics, 24*, 313–334.
11. Seeram, E. (2011). *Digital Radiography: An Introduction*. Clifton Park, NY: Delmar Cengage Learning. ISBN : 9781401889999.
12. Seeram, E. (2016). *Computed Tomography: Physical Principles, Clinical Applications, and Quality Control* (4th ed.). St Louis, MO: Elsevier.
13. Seeram, E., & Brennan, P. (2017). *Radiation Protection in Diagnostic Imaging*. Burlington, MA: Jones and Bartlett Learning.

Chapter

RAMAN SPECTROSCOPY IN MEDICINE

9

Contents

Introduction

The Raman Effect, or the inelastic scattering of photons, was discovered by CV Raman in 1928 and is the foundation of Raman spectroscopy. Photons entering a sample are either scattered or absorbed by the light source. Elastic scattering is the process of scattering a photon while preserving its energy; if it is absorbed, the photon's energy is transferred to the molecules. A tiny percentage of scattered photons, or one in every 10 billion, can, nevertheless, be scattered inelastically, meaning that their energy will slightly alter. The Raman Effect is caused by this tiny energy difference between the incident and scattered photons. For biomedical applications, Raman spectroscopy offers various benefits such as nondestructiveness, speed of acquisition, and molecular information. Water also exhibits weak Raman scattering, which indicates that its presence in the sample has no effect on the spectrum under study. The very weak Raman signal and the existence of undesired noise sources, such as the strong fluorescence background found in biological materials, are the primary drawbacks of Raman spectroscopy.

Raman spectroscopy is a widely recognized and effective tool for the study of biological tissues and the diagnosis of various diseases. It provides spectral information related to the specific molecular structures of substances.

Orientation and Directional Terms

Term	Definition	Illustration
Raman scattering	Raman scattering, commonly referred to as the Raman effect, is an optical phenomenon in which the interaction of incoming excitation light with a sample generates scattered light. The energy of the scattered light is reduced by the vibrational modes of the chemical bonds present in the specimen.	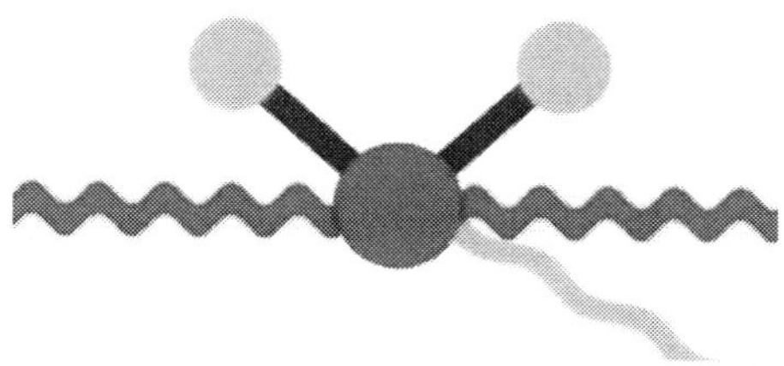
Resonance Raman spectroscopy (RRS)	Resonance Raman spectroscopy (RRS) is an advanced technique used to study vibrational bands in the group frequency region and the information obtained is similar to that obtained by Fourier transform infrared (FTIR) and Raman studies.	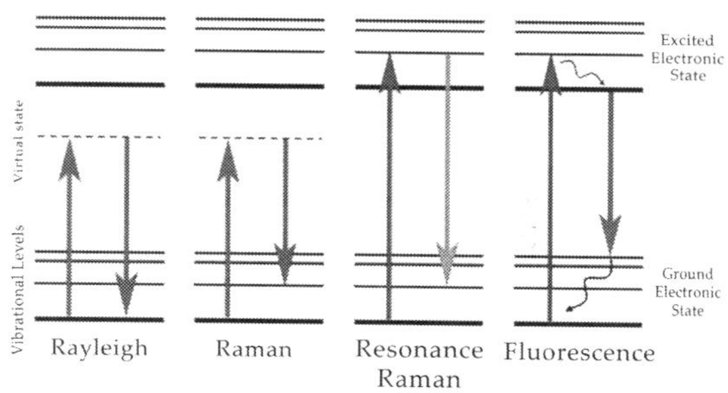
Spatially offset Raman spectroscopy (SORS)	Spatially offset Raman spectroscopy (SORS) is a spectroscopic technique that allows for the non-invasive chemical characterization of diffusely scattering materials, ranging from opaque plastics to biological tissues. SORS has been explored for a range of applications, including disease diagnosis, the detection of explosives through unopened containers and the in-depth, non-destructive analysis of pharmaceutical products and objects of art.	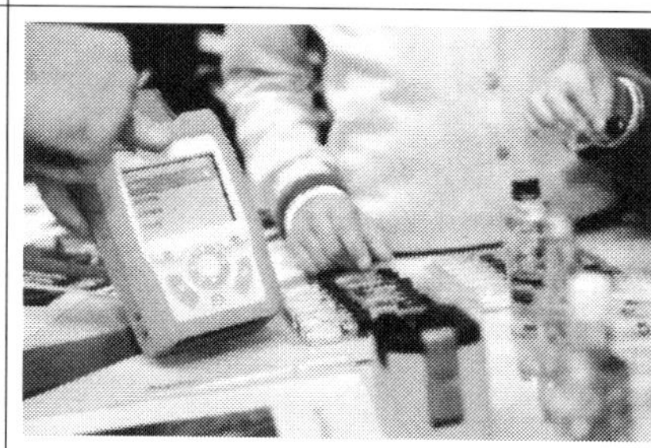
Lyotropic liquid crystals	Lyotropic liquid crystals result when amphiphiles, which are both hydrophobic and hydrophilic, dissolve into a solution that behaves both like a liquid and a solid crystal. This liquid crystalline mesophase includes everyday mixtures like soap and water.	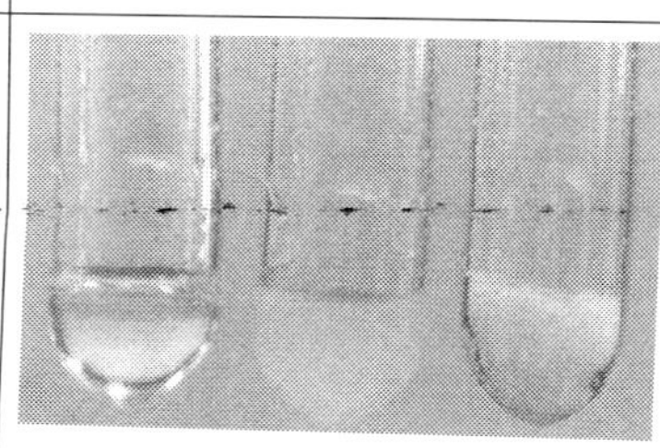

9.1. Raman Spectroscopy

A non-destructive method of chemical analysis, Raman Spectroscopy yields precise data on molecular interactions, phase and polymorphy, crystallinity, and chemical structure. It is predicated on how light interacts with a material's chemical bonds.

9.1.1. Principles of Raman Spectroscopy

Materials based on the Raman Effect, which is the inelastic scattering of incoming light of a material and its frequency changes owing to the power of excited molecular vibrations, were studied using Raman spectroscopy. When starting from the vibrational ground state, Stokes scattering can cause a frequency redshift; however, when starting from an excited vibrational state, the incident photon may gain energy when scattered (anti-Stokes scattering). Since every fingerprint is different from the other, the resulting Raman spectrum shows a high degree of individualization and scientific distinctiveness and is closely related to the molecular structure and vibrational characteristics of various materials. In general, rotational or other low-frequency modes can be detected using Raman spectroscopy; however, these are unrelated to the clinical uses covered in this article. "Low-frequency modes" in the context of Raman spectroscopy generally refer to molecular vibrational modes involving large-scale or collective motions, such as translational movements of entire molecular segments and molecular rotations. Compared to high-frequency vibrational modes, which involve localized atomic vibrations within the molecule, these modes have lower frequencies.

The molecules that make up the relevant cells and tissues vibrate in ways that cause the energy of scattered sunlight to vary noticeably. Since this approach uses light to examine disease-specific molecular changes, it can be applied noninvasively, particularly in scenarios where fiber-optic access is practical. It is possible to differentiate between various cell and tissue types as well as between diseased and healthy tissues using the molecular information that has been collected. Devices based on Raman spectroscopy can offer clinical tools that are accurate, minimally invasive, and possess unique qualities that match or surpass gold standard techniques. The type and structure of the molecules can be determined by utilizing the distinct spectral signals produced by various chemical bonds and functional groups. These vibrational alterations in molecules can be found using Raman spectroscopy, which also sheds light on the molecular makeup and organization of the molecules within cells. Through a comparative analysis of the Raman spectra of both normal and epigenetically altered cells, scientists can pinpoint the molecular alterations linked to various illnesses. These alterations could involve modifications to the composition or structure of proteins, lipids, nucleic acids (NAs), or other biological molecules, providing important new information for the study of molecular diseases (Baker et al, 2018).

9.1.2. Different Types of Raman Spectroscopy

The results can be evaluated in a non-destructive and high-throughput manner using Raman spectroscopy. Additionally, it is reasonably priced and needs little prior training, showing great promise for clinical applications. The Raman scattering signal, however, has a low anti-interference capacity and is weak in intensity. As a result, spectral images cannot be quickly captured for clinical applications, and a lengthy time period is needed to obtain an acceptable signal-to-noise ratio (SNR) for practical applications. The majority of biological samples examined in clinical settings also have high background fluorescence, which lowers the Raman spectrum's signal-to-noise ratio even more.

Table 9.1. Summary of Some of the Raman Techniques Used for Monitoring the Effects of Anticancer Drugs on Cancer Tissues

Monitoring Approach	Nanoparticles	Anticancer Drug	Raman Instrumentation	Target
Cancer response to anticancer drugs	Targeted Cet-PLGA- b-PEG and Non-targeted PLGA- b-PEG	Microtubule targeted vascular disrupting agents (MTVDA)	Confocal Spontaneous Raman Microscopy (λ = 532 nm; laser power on sample = 10 mW; integration time = 5 s; number of spectra acquired for each sample = 10)	Ex-vivo hepatocellular carcinomas
Monitoring of concentration of anticancer drug in cancer cell nucleus/cytoplasm	Squalene	Doxorubicin	Confocal Spontaneous Raman Microscopy (λ = 785 nm; laser power on sample = 60 mW; integration time = 20 s; number of spectra acquired for each sample = 30)	Murine lung carcinomas and Human breast cancer
Assessing profiles of the release of anticancer drugs	Diatomic NP decorated with Au NPs and enclosed in gelatin shell	Galunisertib	SERS (λ = 638 nm; He-Ne laser power = 50 mW; laser power on sample = 1 mW; acquisition time = 1 s; SERS spectra collected from 30 cells) Raman imaging (λ = 638 nm; He-Ne laser power = 50 mW; laser power on sample = 20 mW; Raman images acquired by raster scanning with step size of 0.5 µm; number of spectra acquired per cell = 1500/2000)	Colorectal cancer

Source: *Canetta E. Current and Future Advancements of Raman Spectroscopy Techniques in Cancer Nanomedicine. International Journal of Molecular Sciences. 2021; 22(23):13141. https://doi.org/10.3390/ijms222313141*

Several techniques for enhancing Raman signals have been investigated to address this issue; the most widely applied is SERS. Table 9.1 enumerates the uses various Raman spectroscopy techniques in cancer nanomedicine.

9.1.3. Recent Experimental Studies of Different Raman Spectroscopy

An ideal signal-to-noise ratio (SNR) can be obtained from the zero-offset diffuse beam used to identify lesions at the surface-to-epidermal-to-dermal junction sampling volume. This SNR will form the foundation for upcoming Raman spectroscopy in the identification of skin cancer. Spatially offset Raman spectroscopy (SORS) can gather Raman signals from deep layers of skin tissue, help identify lesions, and yield more precise diagnostic data when it comes to the detection of skin cancer. In a similar vein, SORS can be utilized in bone tissue regeneration monitoring to gauge variations in the concentration of collagen protein in deep bone tissue, allowing an evaluation of the state of skeletal health. Dooley and associates examined whether it would be possible to track the concentrations of collagen (0–0.84 g cm^{-3}) during the regeneration of bone tissue using SORS.

Li et al. used a coherent anti-Stokes Raman microscope to image cells. The relationship between two-photon fluorescence, second-harmonic generation, and coherent anti-Stokes Raman scattering (CARS) has enabled the analysis of various biological phenomena involving lipid metabolism, cancer formation, cardiovascular disease, and skin biology.

In order to obtain deeper signals in vivo than traditional Raman instruments, surface-enhanced spatial offset Raman spectroscopy (SESORS) combines the signal enhancement provided by SERS with the diffusion scattering provided by SORS. Berry along with others initially proved that SESORS signals could be found in nanotags at a 48 mm depth. Many studies have been done using CARS imaging to image molecules in cells and tissues. In order to produce a distinct signal that can be used to create detailed chemical images of samples without the need for exogenous labels, CARS uses the coherent interactions between laser beams and molecular vibrations. They have found important uses in material analysis and biological systems research. Mizuguchi along with others. made a noteworthy discovery about the potential applications of CARS imaging, allowing for the visualization of the whole intracellular lipid structure.

Furthermore, this exceptional ability can be used to track live cells with intracellular lipid structures in real time. Expanding upon this basis, Fueser and associates carried out thorough studies using CARS microscopy on *Caenorhabditis elegans*, demonstrating its applicability for single-organism imaging. These investigations demonstrate the great promise of CARS microscopy for medical diagnostics. Additionally, Kaneta et al. utilized ultra-multiplex CARS microscopy, a cutting-edge method, to thoroughly investigate the distribution of water concentration in human skin in vitro. This novel method makes it possible to identify possible pathological changes brought on by an imbalance in the water distribution of the human skin. Taken as a whole, these studies highlight the clinical applicability and adaptability of CARS microscopy in various scientific fields.

SRS microscopy and second-harmonic generation (SHG) microscopy have been used to visualize tissue sections from cancer patients and healthy individuals' gastrointestinal tracts. Rapid developments in artificial intelligence and machine learning have resulted in impressive progress in image-based medical diagnostics in recent years. A number of research teams have effectively created SRS histology techniques combined with deep learning algorithms to facilitate the quick diagnosis of a variety of human tumors, such as laryngeal cancers and brain tumors. Consider Zhang et al. used a coherent nonlinear optical microscopy method to perform label-free histology on human pancreatic tissue by combining SRS and SHG. They also looked into how important histological features could be automatically identified and analyzed using machine and deep learning. These studies are important for reasons other than just technology in the field of medical image diagnostics. Additionally, they give medical professionals quicker and more accurate diagnostic instruments, which are especially important for the early diagnosis and treatment of diseases like cancer. To confirm the viability of these approaches and broaden their use in clinical practice, more research is needed (Amal et al, 2012; Allegrini et al, 2013; Acquarelli et al, 2017; Atkins et al, 2017).

9.1.4. Raman Spectrometers

The three primary components of a Raman instrument are the excitation laser, detector, and spectrometer. The central component of the Raman apparatus, the spectrometer, is in charge of separating and measuring the various wavelength components that are present in the light that the sample scatters. To obtain spectral resolution and measurement precision, optical elements like gratings or interferometers are utilized to accomplish this task. On the other hand, segregated spectral signal capture is greatly dependent on the detector. It successfully transforms these signals into their electrical equivalents, which are then thoroughly examined and processed. A key element in the creation of an excitation light source is an excitation laser. These lasers can be gas, solid-state, or laser diodes, among other varieties. Different excitation light source variations have different wavelength and power characteristics, which allow for customized selection according to the particular needs of the sample in question. An excitation light source is passed through an optical fiber to the sample, stimulating its molecules to undergo Raman scattering.

Additionally, optical alignment and calibration, sample light delivery and collection, sterility and durability, and detection system sensitivity are needed for a clinical Raman system. Furthermore, the gadget needs to be compact and lightweight. These characteristics are comparable to those of typical medical equipment. The components that make up a clinical Raman system can be broadly grouped using the excitation and detection branches. When light from a specific laser source is transmitted to a target tissue spot via an articulated light delivery arm or fiber-optic probe, excitation takes place. A standard delivery method is then used to send the collected Raman-scattered light to a spectrograph and detector. There are many intricate challenges involved in the design and deployment of clinical Raman systems. To ensure consistent and accurate measurements, it is essential to precisely align and calibrate the optical pathway. Secondly, when developing optical delivery and sample collection mechanisms, the complexities of real-world operations in a clinical setting must be taken into account. Furthermore, since clinical situations frequently call for extended instrument use, the device needs to be sturdy and sterile to ensure dependability and security. The non-invasive nature of clinical Raman systems is one of their distinguishing features. By using light-guided arms or fiber-optic conduits, light can be smoothly directed into target tissues without the need for sampling or incisions. This reduces discomfort and risk for the patient and makes real-time monitoring easier. Additionally, Raman spectroscopy offers insights that are inherently linked to the chemical composition, which promotes a variety of applications in advanced biological research as well as drug surveillance and disease diagnostics. As technology for in vivo clinical assessments has advanced, so too has the range of individual components that have been studied and cleared for use in these systems (Baker et al, 2018).

9.1.5. Raman Spectroscopy for Signal Enhancement

After going through a revolutionary evolution to become one of the most adaptable modalities for the sensitive detection and complex visualization of chemical and biological analytes, SERS was first employed for the identification of single molecules. Chemical and physical enhancement mechanisms are the main components of SERS. Metal nanostructures like Ag and Au are the main source of physical enhancement. These structures are very easy to prepare, highly repeatable, and relatively stable. They have the ability to cause free electrons on the surface to oscillate collectively, greatly increasing the intensity of Raman signals. The latter requires the materials under examination to be directly adhered to or glued to a rough metal substrate in order to enhance the Raman signal via a charge-transfer mechanism. To improve the Raman signal, these materials can transfer charges to the metal surface. Furthermore, by measuring the Raman strength, SERS can be used to analyze a molecule and determine its location and concentration. Additionally, this method can be used to determine the analytes' spatial distribution. SERS is now a crucial tool in molecular analyzes thanks to technological advancements. An advanced platform for the qualitative and quantitative evaluation of different analytes is presented by the special combination of nanostructures, charge transfer, and accurate Raman measurements, which makes a significant contribution to analytical chemistry, biomedicine, and materials science.

In the field of plasma antennas, metal nanostructures have become essential components that enhance Raman signals for SERS-based molecular detection. It appears that certain nanoenvironments, such as nanopores, ion bond gaps, or nanotips, can greatly enhance the Raman signal. Zhang and associates. explored the use of dual-template technology to create porous metamaterials in an intricate 3D fabrication process. This method gives you more precise control over the structural characteristics of the plasma used in SERS. A firm template made of porous poly (methyl methacrylate) (PMMA) was used in their study's dual-templating methodology to create hierarchically ordered porous metamaterials in a three-dimensional arrangement. Precursors for this dual-templating approach were lyotropic liquid crystals (LLCs) made from octaethylene glycol monohexadecyl ether (C16EO8).

Research on porous metamaterials, nanostructured plasma antennas, and various substrate architectures contributes to our knowledge of enhanced Raman signal generation in the context of SERS. This emphasizes how material engineering, plasma interactions, and nanostructures interact intricately to improve the sensitivity and accuracy of molecular detection applications.

Song el.al. examined a top-down approach to high-performance SERS substrate preparation. Using a top-down method, scalable nanolaminated SERS substrates were created. Song and associates. Initially, polymer nanopillar arrays were created on polyester (PET) films and replicas were made using a UV-curable device with a UV-curable polyurethane (PU) polymer resist and a nanostructured polydimethylsiloxane (PDMS) stamp. Au and SiO_2 film layers were deposited alternately after multilayered MIM nanostructures with numerous vertically oriented plasmonic nanogaps on individual nanopillars were constructed. Lastly, they exposed the embedded nanogap hotspots using a buffered oxide etchant (10:1) (BOE) and a wet chemical etching technique to improve the performance of SERS. By carefully adjusting the plasmonic elements and nanogaps, SERS efficiency is increased, making the substrate more sensitive and useful for detecting target analytes. This all-inclusive method demonstrates the methodical creation of nanolaminated SERS substrates characterized by finely tuned plasmonic nanogaps and complex nanopillar arrays. The joint endeavors to create, manufacture, and refine these configurations highlight how crucial it is to fully utilize SERS substrates to improve analytical capabilities.

Furthermore, Dong et al. engineered a "slow light effect" on a macroporous TiO_2 inverse opal (MIO) structure that was modeled after beehives and demonstrated remarkable SERS performance. The MIO structure extracts exosomes from the plasma of cancer patients and analyzes them without the need for labeling techniques. A schematic of this procedure is shown in Table 9.2, and the outcomes show increased efficacy and precision in the identification of several malignancies. In this study, exosomes from the plasma's 1087 cm^{-1} SERS peak were utilized to provide a label-free, flexible, affordable, and fast way to obtain accurate tumor liquid biopsy. This technique offers a great deal of clinical promise for quick in vitro cancer screening. Dong's thought process is intriguing and offers insights into future developments.

Table 9.2. Summary of Current Cancer Raman Bioimaging Techniques in Cancer

Raman Imaging	Application	Nanoparticles	Raman Instrument	Target
Spontaneous Raman microscopy	Cancer screening and grading	No	Raman microscope (λ = 785 nm; power on sample = 5–10 mW; integration time = 1 s; 10 scans per spectrum)	Osteosarcoma
Spontaneous Raman microscopy	Cancer progression and grading	No	Raman microscope (λ = 532 nm; power on sample = 5–10 mW; integration time = 1 s; 10 scans per spectrum)	Enchodroma and Chondrosarcoma
Topically Applied Surface Enhanced Resonance Raman Ratiometric Spectroscopy (TAS3RS)	Visualization of microscopic residual of ovarian cancer tissues	Targeted functionalized NPs with IR780 Raman reporter and Non-targeted NPs with IR140 Raman reporter	Raman microscope (λ = 785 nm; diode laser power = 300 mW; power on sample = 100 mW; acquisition time < 100 ms)	Murine animal model of ovarian adenocarcinoma
Raman multiplexing	Visualization of true extension of brain cancer	Targeted-RGD-SEERS and Non-targeted RAD-SEERS	SERS (λ = 785 nm; diode laser power = 300 mW; power on sample = 10–100 mW; acquisition time = 1.5 s)	Glioblastoma multiforme (GBM) Cancer

SESORRS	In-vivo visualization of cancer tissues	Integrin-targeting SERRS active nanostars	SORS (λ = 785 nm; laser power = 400 mW; power on sample for conventional Raman imaging = 20 mW; power on sample for SORS measurements = 130 mW)	Deep-seated GBM tumor through intact skull
Multicolor/ multitarget SERS imaging	Characterization of expression of different cancer protein biomarkers on the same cancer cell	SERS Au/Au core satellite NPs with 6 distinct Raman reporters on the core	6-color/ 1-target iSERS microscope (λ = 785 nm; He-Ne laser power on sample = 1.2 mW; integration time = 100 ms)	Breast cancer

Source: *Canetta E. Current and Future Advancements of Raman Spectroscopy Techniques in Cancer Nanomedicine. International Journal of Molecular Sciences. 2021; 22(23):13141. https://doi.org/10.3390/ijms222313141.*

Using Raman spectroscopy, SERS retains a wealth of chemical fingerprint information while improving the plasmon's sensitive excitation and scattering properties. Specifically, the measurements are easily conducted in both ambient and aqueous environments, and the majority of Raman peaks have narrow widths that make them appropriate for multiplex analyzes. SERS is widely acknowledged as a dependable analytical technique for determining the molecular signatures of analytes that may be of clinical interest. The synthesis of highly sensitive SERS substrates has advanced significantly in a number of biomedical applications, most notably in the diagnosis of disease. However, their direct clinical application in biological fluids has been severely hindered by the effect of fouling on substrates with SERS activity. In order to achieve the clinical conversion of SERS in the future, this is another challenge that needs to be addressed (Amal et al, 2012; Allegrini et al, 2013; Acquarelli et al, 2017; Atkins et al, 2017).

9.2. Instrumentation

For in vivo measurements, a Raman spectrometer should be an integrated system capable of real-time spectrum acquisition and analysis. A light source, sample light delivery and collection, spectrograph with detector, and computer interface are the components of an in vivo Raman system. Because they can supply the sample with enough power to detect Raman spectra in an acceptable integration time, lasers are the excitation source used in Raman spectroscopy. To optimize the Raman system for in vivo biomedical applications, however, vital factors like laser wavelength, power, and integration time must be taken into account. For instance, taking into account the maximum allowable exposure and temperature increase is necessary to prevent tissue damage. Thus, getting a good signal to noise ratio and minimizing tissue damage are necessary for choosing the right laser power. Many strategies, such as excitation in the near infrared (NIR), have been proposed to prevent fluorescence background. In biological tissue, fluorophores can produce signals that obscure or overwhelm the weak Raman signal. In contrast to visible or UV excitation, the majority of biological fluorophores are known to have lower fluorescence backgrounds because they do not exhibit peak emission in this spectrum. Owing to these benefits, the majority of Raman spectroscopy systems used for skin diagnosis employ a 785-nm diode laser as the excitation source because it is an affordable light source with low fluorescence and a deep tissue penetration range. Optical fibers are the most widely used method for sample light delivery and collection in clinical applications.

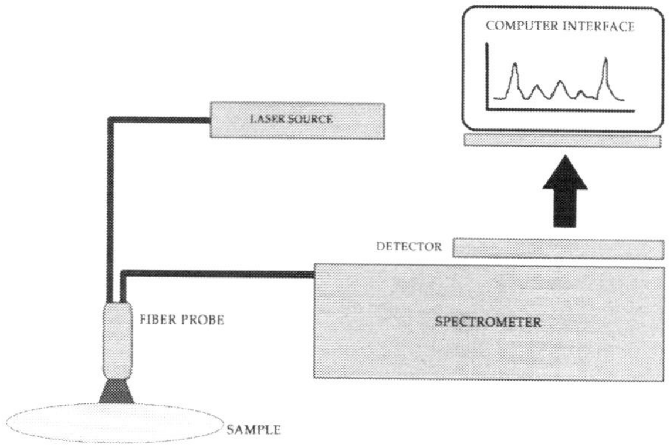

Figure 9.1. *Schematic of a typical Raman system for in vivo biomedical applications.*

Source: Ramírez-Elías, M. G., & González, F. J. (2018). Raman Spectroscopy for In Vivo Medical Diagnosis. InTech. doi: 10.5772/intechopen.72933.

The clinical application determines the design of the Raman fiber probe. The probe used in skin Raman spectroscopy is made up of multiple collection fibers encircling a single central delivery fiber. An essential part of Raman spectroscopy is choosing an appropriate detection system. In biomedical applications, a spectrograph connected to a cooled charge coupled device (CCD) is the standard Raman detection system. To minimize thermal noise, the majority of CCDs employ a thermoelectric (TE) system to cool the detector to -70°C. A spectrograph connected to both the CCD and the Raman probe is also necessary for the detection system. For the spectrograph to give comprehensive information on biological Raman bands, a spectral resolution of 8–10 cm^{-1} is advised. The diffraction grating, the CCD pixel size, and the spectrograph optical parameters all affect the spectral resolution. Figure 9.2 depicts a schematic of how these components are usually arranged.

9.3. Raman Effect

The inelastic scattering of photons by matter, also known as the Raman Effect or Raman scattering, involves both an energy exchange and a change in the direction of light. This effect usually involves the gain of vibrational energy by a molecule due to the shifting of incident photons from a visible laser to a lower energy. We refer to this as typical Stokes-Raman scattering.

There is a chance that a substance will scatter light. The majority of scattered photons are elastically scattered, or Rayleigh scattered; that is, they have different directions but the same energy (frequency, wavelength, and color) as the incident photons. In general, the intensity of Rayleigh scattering is between 0.1 and 0.01% of the radiation source's intensity. Raman scattered photons are an even smaller subset of scattered photons (roughly 1 in a million) that can be scattered inelastically, meaning that their scattered photon energy differs from the incident photon energy (usually lower). The material either gains or loses energy during the process due to energy conservation.

Chemists and physicists use different types of Raman spectroscopy to take advantage of this effect and learn more about materials for a range of uses. In addition to these and other options, a variety of other variations of Raman spectroscopy enable the examination of electronic energy levels and rotational energy (if gas samples are employed). There are more sophisticated methods that use multiple laser beams, pulsed lasers, and other elements.

9.3.1. Theory

The theory of normal (non-resonant, spontaneous, vibrational) Raman scattering of light by discrete molecules is the main topic of this article. While the concepts of X-ray Raman spectroscopy are similar, electronic energy levels are excited instead of vibrational ones.

9.3.1.1. Molecular Vibrations

In general, Raman scattering provides information about a molecule's vibrations. It is also possible to learn about rotational energy in the case of gases. Phonon modes can also be seen in solids. Raman scattering is similar to infrared absorption in terms of molecular vibrations, but the selection criteria are different.

- **Degrees of Freedom:** There are a total of 3N degrees of freedom for any given molecule, where N is the number of atoms. The fact that each atom in a molecule can move in three dimensions accounts for this number. It is more typical to think about a molecule's movement as a whole when working with molecules. As a result, the three dimensions of freedom—molecular translation, rotation, and vibration—are divided into three groups. A molecule's overall translational motion (along each of the three spatial dimensions) is reflected in three of the degrees of freedom. Similarly, rotations of the molecule about the x, y, and z axes correspond to three degrees of freedom. Because rotations along the bond axis do not alter the atoms' positions within the molecule, linear molecules only have two rotations. The vibrational modes of molecules correspond to the remaining degrees of freedom. These modes involve the molecule's chemical bonds bending and stretching. The number of vibrational modes in a linear molecule is 3N-5, while the number in a non-linear molecule is 3N-6.
- **Vibrational Energy:** Since molecular vibrational energy is known to be quantized, it can be represented by a Dunham expansion when anharmonicity is significant, or by the quantum harmonic oscillator (QHO) approximation. The vibrational energy levels according to the QHO are:

$$E_n = h\left(n+\frac{1}{2}\right)\nu = h\left(n+\frac{1}{2}\right)\frac{1}{2\pi}\sqrt{\frac{k}{m}}$$

where n is a quantum number. Since the selection rules for Raman and infrared absorption generally dictate that only fundamental vibrations are observed, infrared excitation or Stokes Raman excitation results in an energy change of

$$E = h\nu = \frac{h}{2\pi}\sqrt{\frac{k}{m}}$$

The vibrating medium has an energy range of roughly 5 to 3500 cm^{-1}. A Boltzmann distribution describes the percentage of molecules that occupy a specific vibrational mode at a given temperature. A photon of the right energy, which is in the terahertz or infrared range, can directly absorb a molecule to excite it to a higher vibrational mode. This is where infrared spectroscopy starts. Alternatively, an inelastic scattering process can generate the same vibrational excitation. Similar to the Stokes shift in fluorescence that George Stokes discovered in 1852, this phenomenon is known as Stokes Raman scattering because it emits light at a longer wavelength than the incident light that is absorbed, which is now known to correspond to lower energy. Rather than light, neutrons or electrons can theoretically produce effects that are conceptually similar. Anti-Stokes scattering is the name given to an increase in photon energy that lowers the vibrational energy state of the molecule.

9.3.1.2. Raman Scattering

The energy of the stimulating laser photons is thought to be involved in the virtual electronic energy level that is involved in Raman scattering. Raman or Rayleigh scattering results from the molecule being excited to an imaginary state through photon absorption and subsequent re-emission. While the final state in each of the three scenarios has the same electronic energy as the initial state, it has a different vibrational energy in the case of Stokes Raman scattering (higher), anti-Stokes Raman scattering (lower), or Rayleigh scattering (the same).

Normally this is thought of in terms of wavenumbers, where $\tilde{\nu}_0$ is the wavenumber of the laser and $\tilde{\nu}_M$ is the wavenumber of the vibrational transition. Thus Stokes scattering gives a wavenumber of $\tilde{\nu}_0 - \tilde{\nu}_M$ while

$\tilde{\nu}_0 + \tilde{\nu}_M$ is given for anti-Stokes. When the exciting laser energy corresponds to an actual electronic excitation of the molecule then the resonance Raman Effect occurs. Raman scattering can be explained by a model based on classical physics, which also predicts an increase in intensity that increases with the fourth power of the light frequency. An induced electric dipole oscillates in response to a molecule scattering light. An induced dipole that follows the alternating electric field that is modulated by molecular vibrations may be caused in a molecule by the oscillating electric field component of electromagnetic radiation. Thus, beat frequencies arising from the external field and vibrations of the normal mode are observed together with oscillations at the frequency of the external field.

The Raman spectrum is the name given to the spectrum of the scattered photons. Known more popularly as a Raman shift, it plots the scattered light's intensity as a function of its frequency difference Δν to the incident photons. Around the Rayleigh Δν=0 line, the locations of corresponding Stokes and anti-Stokes peaks form a symmetric pattern. Due to the fact that the frequency shifts reflect the energy differential between the same upper and lower resonant states, they are symmetric. However, the pairs of features' intensities will usually vary. They are dependent upon the populations of the material's initial states, which are dependent upon temperature. The lower state will have a higher population than the upper state when thermodynamic equilibrium is reached. As a result, the rate of Stokes transitions—transitions from the lower, more populated state to the upper state—will be higher than the rate of anti-Stokes transitions, which occur in the opposite direction. Following this, anti-Stokes scattering peaks are weaker than Stokes scattering peaks. Their ratio can be used to measure temperature since it is dependent on it:

$$\frac{I_{\text{Stokes}}}{I_{\text{anti-Stokes}}} = \frac{(\tilde{\nu}_0 - \tilde{\nu}_M)^4}{(\tilde{\nu}_0 + \tilde{\nu}_M)^4} \exp\left(\frac{hc\tilde{\nu}_M}{k_B T}\right)$$

9.3.1.3. Selection Rules

Raman scattering necessitates a change in polarizability, in contrast to IR spectroscopy, which requires a change in dipole moment for vibrational excitation to occur. A Raman transition between two states can only occur if there is a difference in the molecular polarizability of those states.

For a vibration, this means that the derivative of the polarizability with respect to the normal coordinate associated to the vibration is non-zero: $\frac{\partial \alpha}{\partial Q} \neq 0$. In general, a normal mode is Raman active if it transforms with the same symmetry of the quadratic forms $(x^2, y^2, z^2, xy, xz, yz)$ which can be verified from the character table of the molecule's point group. As with IR spectroscopy, only fundamental excitations $\Delta v = \pm 1$ are allowed according to the QHO. There are however many cases where overtones are observed. The rule of mutual exclusion, which states that vibrational modes cannot be both IR and Raman active, applies to certain molecules.

The specific selection rules state that the allowed rotational transitions are $\Delta J = \pm 2$where J is the rotational state. This generally is only relevant to molecules in the gas phase where the Raman linewidths are small enough for rotational transitions to be resolved.

Only phonons with zero phase angle can be detected by IR and Raman, with the exception of situations in which phonon confinement is evident, according to a selection rule that only applies to ordered solid materials.

9.3.1.4. Symmetry and Polarization

Understanding the relationships between molecular symmetry and Raman activity through the monitoring of the scattered photons' polarization can help identify peaks in Raman spectra. Certain Raman-active modes are only accessible when light is polarized in a single direction; other modes can be accessed by rotating the polarization. Based on its symmetry, each mode is divided.

The symmetry of a vibrational mode is deduced from the depolarization ratio ρ, which is the ratio of the Raman scattering with polarization orthogonal to the incident laser and the Raman scattering with the same polarization as the incident laser: $\rho = \frac{I_r}{I_u}$. Here I_r is the intensity of Raman scattering when the analyzer is rotated 90 degrees with respect to the incident light's polarization axis, and I_u the intensity of Raman scattering when the analyzer is aligned with the polarization of the incident laser. When polarized light interacts with a molecule, it distorts the molecule which induces an equal and opposite effect in the plane-wave, causing it to be rotated by the difference between the orientation of the molecule and the angle of polarization of the light wave.

9.3.1.5. Stimulated Raman scattering and Raman Amplification

The above-described spontaneous Raman-scattering process occurs when one of the numerous incoming photons is scattered by the material at random intervals of time. Therefore, this phenomenon is known as spontaneous Raman scattering.

Conversely, stimulated Raman scattering can occur when one or more Stokes photons are purposefully injected along with the pump light, or when some Stokes photons have already been generated spontaneously by Raman scattering and are somehow forced to remain in the material. In that scenario, pump photons are transformed into additional Stokes photons more quickly than in the case of spontaneous Raman scattering, increasing the total Raman-scattering rate. More Stokes photons are added more quickly the more that are already there. This is used in Raman amplifiers and Raman lasers to effectively enhance the Stokes light when the pump light is present.

- **Requirement for Space-coherence**: Suppose that the distance between two points A and B of an exciting beam is *x*. Generally, as the exciting frequency is not equal to the scattered Raman frequency, the corresponding relative wavelengths λ and λ' are not equal. Thus, a phase-shift $\Theta = 2\pi x(1/\lambda - 1/\lambda')$ appears. For $\Theta = \pi$, the scattered amplitudes are opposite, so that the Raman scattered beam remains weak.
- A crossing of the beams may limit the path x.

Several tricks may be used to get a larger amplitude:

- A light beam may propagate in two ways in an optically anisotropic crystal, each with a distinct polarization and index of refraction. If a quadrupolar (Raman) resonance can transfer energy between these modes and the phases stay coherent throughout, there could be a significant energy transfer. This generation is optical parametric.
- It is possible to pulse light to prevent beats from showing. The pulse lengths in Impulsive Stimulated Raman Scattering (ISRS) have to be less than all pertinent time constants. Under ideal circumstances, the interference between incident and Raman light is too brief to permit beats, resulting in a frequency shift that is approximately inversely proportional to the cube of the pulse length.

Femtosecond laser pulses are required in laboratories because longer pulses cause the ISRS to become significantly weaker. Therefore, nanosecond pulses that produce regular time-incoherent light cannot be used to observe ISRS.

9.3.2. Inverse Raman Effect

The form of Raman scattering known as the inverse Raman Effect was first observed by Boris P. Stoicheff and W. J. Jones. When anti-Stokes scattering is greater than Stokes scattering, there will be an absorption line (intensity dip) at $\nu L+\nu M$ on the continuum as it exits the material. The application of this phenomenon is known as inverse Raman spectroscopy, the phenomenon itself is known as the inverse Raman Effect, and a record of the continuum is known as an inverse Raman spectrum.

Both absorption from a continuum of lower frequencies and absorption from a continuum of higher frequencies are covered by the authors of the first description of the inverse Raman Effect. They point out that if the material is in thermal equilibrium and its Raman frequency originates from vibrations, absorption from a continuum of lower frequencies won't be seen.

- **Supercontinuum Generation:** A wide bandwidth supercontinuum for high-intensity continuous wave (CW) lasers can be achieved through stimulated Raman scattering. The two incident photons' frequencies are equal in this process, and the emitted spectra are found in two bands that are separated from the incident light by the phonon energies. This can also be thought of as a special case of four-wave mixing. Spontaneous emission builds up the first Raman spectrum, which is then amplified. The Raman spectrum can be used as a new starting point to create a chain of new spectra with decreasing amplitude at high pumping levels in long fibers, resulting in higher-order Raman spectra. A spectrum can be seeded at the start to mitigate the intrinsic noise caused by the initial spontaneous process. Alternatively, a feedback loop, like that found in a resonator, can be used to stabilize the process. Raman amplification and spectrum generation may find widespread application in the near future due to the technology's easy integration into the rapidly developing fiber laser field and the need for transversal coherent high-intensity light sources (i.e., broadband telecommunication, imaging applications).

9.4. Data Preprocessing

Unwanted background components from various sources, such as intrinsic fluorescence, noise from external sources, and noise from the equipment being used, are a major problem in biological Raman spectroscopy.

9.4.1. Smoothing and Denoising

The shot noise, flicker noise, dark current, thermal noise, and fluorescence background are the primary sources of noise found in Raman spectra obtained from biological samples. An alternative is to use a Raman system with high-end, thermoelectric-cooled spectrometers to reduce the thermal noise and dark signal. The shot noise is typically the most prominent noise in Raman spectra, and it is related to the particle nature of light. The shot noise that is roughly related to the measurement of n counts is $n^{1/2}$. By increasing the number of counts n, it is possible to improve the signal to noise ratio (S/N). Put another way, because the signal increases proportionately with time, S/N can be enhanced by lengthening the averaging period. There are numerous methods for removing multitude noise from Raman spectra. Because noise manifests as high-frequency fluctuations while signals are thought to be low frequency, smoothing is frequently used to remove high-frequency components from Raman spectra. Fourier filtering is one method of smoothing. By using this method, it is possible to reconstruct Raman spectra noise-free by eliminating the higher frequency fluctuations, which are merely noise. This method's disadvantage is that removing the higher frequency noise can frequently cause distortion and artifacts in the Raman spectra. The Savitzky-Golay (SG) filtering method is a frequently employed smoothing technique. The SG filter is a local polynomial fitting technique based on moving windows. Some of the Raman bands may vanish as the moving window size increases. To prevent losing Raman data, it is crucial to select the right parameters, such as the moving window size and polynomial order. Other smoothing techniques include wavelet filtering, which uses the discrete wavelet transform to break down the spectrum and isolate the noise by localizing it in frequency and space, and locally weighted scatter plot smoothing (LOWESS). After it has been isolated, the data can be rebuilt using the inverse wavelet transform and it can be set to zero. All of the aforementioned techniques require careful parameter selection to prevent the removal of significant Raman bands during smoothing.

9.4.2. Background Removal

The background fluorescence in biological Raman spectra is one source of noise. Since biological tissues' Raman scattering intensity is several orders of magnitude lower than that of the intrinsic fluorescence emission, fluorescence appears as a strong band that obstructs Raman signals and needs to be eliminated in order to analyze the Raman spectra. Two methods have been used to eliminate background: computational and experimental. Shifted excitation, photo bleaching, and time gating are some of the experimental techniques that are connected to modifications in the equipment. These methods' relatively complicated instrumentation, lengthy acquisition times, and sample modifications are some of their drawbacks, which may make the analysis of biological samples challenging. On the other hand, employing computational methods for background removal offers benefits like speed, affordability, and ease of implementation. These techniques include the following: morphology operators, linear programming, polynomial fitting, Fourier transform, wavelet transform, first- and second-order differentiation, multiplicative signal correction, geometric approach, asymmetric least squares, and methods based on iterative reweighted quantile regression. However, because of its ease of use, polynomial fitting is the most popular approach. This method removes background effects by fitting a polynomial and then subtracting it from the Raman spectrum. A higher order polynomial fitting may take into account Raman bands as background and may be impacted by high frequency noise, so choosing the right polynomial order is crucial. Several modified polynomial fitting techniques were put forth to address this problem.

9.4.3. Normalization

If Raman spectra from the same sample were obtained under different experimental conditions, such as shifting laser power levels, or at different times, they might have different intensities. By ensuring that the intensity of a particular Raman band of the same material is the same or as close to it as possible in all the spectra recorded under the same experimental parameters, the normalization process addresses these variations in intensity levels. Normalization to area is one strategy. Using this method, the intensity is divided by the square root of the sum of squares of all intensities at each frequency in the spectrum. It is preferable to normalize the spectra such that the total area under the spectrum is 1.0. This normalization is helpful when the spectra do not share a common band. One benefit of this approach is that it is not reliant on any particular band; however, a drawback is that background noise may affect the normalization process. Peak normalization is an additional method that uses the intensity corresponding to the reference (internal or external) central frequency of a specific Raman band. The amide I at 1660 cm^{-1} and the C–H vibrations at 1450 cm^{-1} band are frequently utilized as benchmarks because of their consistent intensities that remain unaffected by other modifications in the specimen. This method is not appropriate when the nature of the samples could cause a shift in the band position because it assumes that the reference does not change from one spectrum to another.

9.5. Chemometrics

Chemometrics extracts chemical and physical information from chemical data, or in this case, spectroscopic data, using statistical and mathematical techniques. One way to identify components in a sample is to use individual bands; however, this is not the best approach because multiple molecules can have the same band in the same localization, making one band non-specific for a given molecule. To achieve a more accurate identification, utilize the entire spectrum or multiple bands. This method views every point in a spectrum as a variable, and spectroscopic data can be shown as a matrix with rows denoting observations (Raman spectra) and columns representing variables (Raman shift or wavenumber). Multivariate data analysis is used to analyze data that contains multiple variables. The proper application of any one of the numerous multivariate data analysis techniques depends on the analysis's goal. Data description, exploratory analysis, discrimination, classification, clustering, regression, and prediction are some examples of possible objectives. Additionally, there are two categories of data analysis techniques: supervised and unsupervised. When a priori knowledge is not available, supervised methods are employed. They are highly helpful in uncovering hidden structures within unlabeled data and are occasionally utilized as a precursor to supervised methods. Unsupervised techniques include principal component analysis (PCA) and hierarchical cluster analysis (HCA). Conversely, supervised approaches require predetermined information, like class labels, and their analysis uses a training data set to identify patterns in the data, which is then used to validate the model on a test set. Partial least squares is one instance of a supervised technique (PLS).

9.5.1. Principal Component Analysis (PCA)

An unsupervised technique called principal component analysis (PCA) is frequently used to minimize the number of variables in exploratory data analysis. The foundation of PCA is the eigenvector decomposition of the spectra matrix's covariance matrix into eigenvalues and eigenvectors. The principal components, also known as eigenvectors, are arranged in decreasing order by each associated eigenvalue and are orthogonal along n-dimensional axes. This indicates that, in contrast to the original components, which might have been correlated, the principal components are uncorrelated and independent of one another. Additionally, because of their decreasing order, the first principal component accounts for the greatest amount of the original data's variance, followed by the second, which accounts for a greater amount than the third, and so forth. One way to conceptualize the original data would be as an M×N matrix of M spectra sampled at N wavenumbers. Three results are obtained from applying PCA to this matrix: N principal components, N eigenvalues that indicate the significance of the corresponding principal components, and an N×N matrix with the coefficients for the transformation between the original data and the principal components. A new set of N "synthetic" spectra known as principal components is created from the original N experimental spectra. In conclusion, one benefit of principal component analysis (PCA) is that it can be used to find a smaller set of variables that account for the most variance, thereby reducing the original dataset's dimension. This is achieved by assessing the relative importance of the successive principal components. Furthermore, random noise and significant spectral changes will be separated into separate principal components due to the uncorrelated nature of changes in the Raman signal. As a result, noise can be eliminated from the Raman signal without compromising its usefulness by discarding numerous principal components.

9.5.2. Partial Least Squares (PLS)

In addition to vibrational spectroscopy, PLS is one of the most popular multivariate data analysis methods for estimating and quantifying sample constituents. Since it's a supervised method, the calibration samples' constituent concentrations are all known. Similar to PCA, the noise seen in the spectra is divided into distinct latent variables (LVs) that are excluded from the calibration process, increasing the accuracy of predictions. Multiple LVs can also be included in a PLS model to account for nonlinear relationships between the properties of interest and intensity.

9.5.3. Classification and Clustering Models

Finding differences between the spectra is the main goal of a number of data analysis techniques, which enable the identification and classification of groups of spectra. In biomedical Raman spectroscopy, k-nearest neighbors (KNN), support vector machines (SVM), discriminant analysis (DA), hierarchical cluster analysis

(HCA), and artificial neural networks (ANNs) are the most often utilized techniques. Using metrics of similarity between spectra, such as the Euclidean distance, the KNN method compares every spectrum in the dataset. This technique has been applied to the diagnosis of colon cancer in conjunction with Raman spectroscopy and PCA. HCA is one of the techniques used in Raman and infrared imaging, and it employs a number of multivariate distance computations, including Euclidean and Mahalanobis metrics, to identify similar spectra. In a similar vein, cluster identification and pattern recognition in complex data can be achieved with artificial neural networks. ANNs are computer models that are based on the structure and functions of the central nervous system. These networks are made up of interconnected nodes, or neurons, that perform various tasks like data input, output, storage, and forwarding. ANN is made up of multiple layers, each with a certain number of neurons. One can distinguish between patients suffering from Alzheimer's disease, other forms of dementia, and healthy individuals by using ANNs in the data analysis of blood serum Raman spectra. As a supervised method of data analysis, DA necessitates prior knowledge of each sample group's membership. Using linear combinations of variables, DA calculates a set of discriminant functions that, in accordance with Fisher's criterion, maximize variance between groups and minimize variance within groups. Combining PCA and LDA techniques can be very helpful at times. This is known as the PC-LDA model, which increases classification efficiency by automatically identifying the most diagnostically significant features. SVMs are kernel-based algorithms that take input data and convert it into a high-dimensional space. They then build a hyperplane that maximizes the distance between any given input class's closest data point. SVM and Raman spectroscopy have both been employed as cancer screening techniques.

9.6. Clinical Applications of Raman Spectroscopy

Clinical trials currently frequently employ immunohistochemistry, imaging methods, and cytological evaluations. These techniques lack automation and are costly and time-consuming. Although it has a number of drawbacks, histopathological testing is widely used in the diagnosis of cancer and is regarded as the standard test procedure. In most cases, pathologists' assessment of microscopic sample staining is the primary method used to detect cancer. However, because it uses dyes that are not specific to cancer cells, this method is invasive, time-consuming, and has limited sensitivity. Secondly, there aren't many pathologists qualified to perform expert evaluations. Furthermore, this approach lacks objectivity and is unduly reliant on the subjective assessment of pathologists. Misdiagnosis therefore frequently occurs during tissue evaluations. To overcome these constraints and satisfy the clinical requirements, more advanced clinical diagnostic techniques are needed.

In a range of medical samples, Raman spectroscopy is sensitive to the biochemical indicators of disease. Because of the versatility of these vibrational approaches, tailored analyzes—which might involve signature-based strategies—can be created in response to clinical requirements in an effort to comprehend the complexities of disease profiles for the purpose of diagnosis or to pinpoint a specific, highly sensitive target molecule. The majority of vibrational spectroscopy methods are easy to use, dependable, and reliant on basic sample preparation techniques. Furthermore, the equipment can be customized for particular uses (such as handheld, imaging, and probe-based). Due to their ability to distinguish between diseased and non-diseased states with extreme sensitivity and specificity, as well as the ability to determine the severity of a disease in specific circumstances, these advantages make them medically useful and suitable for clinical settings. Recent years have seen a rapid advancement in the application of Raman spectroscopy to clinical problems, demonstrating the spectroscopy's ability to provide objective data to support clinical decision-making and broaden our basic understanding of the interactions between light and matter.

9.6.1. Cancer Diagnosis

Due to the ability to measure biological samples minimally invasively, in vivo, and without labeling, cancer is one of the most frequently studied clinical targets with Raman spectroscopy. One significant development that makes it possible to perform in vivo measurements of cancer in hollow organs is the creation of fiber-optic Raman probes that can be used in endoscopy procedures.

- **Lung Cancer:** Short et al. created a Raman probe for autofluorescence bronchoscopy, which they used to detect lung cancer in vivo. By lowering the number of false positives from autofluorescence bronchoscopy, they showed the potential of Raman for lung cancer in vivo diagnosis.
- **Gastrointestinal Cancer:** Bergholt et al. conducted an in vivo diagnostic trial in 2014 to categorize Barrett's esophageal dysplasia (BE). Real-time Raman spectroscopy can be used prospectively to screen patients with suspicious BE in vivo, as evidenced by their reported diagnostic sensitivity of 87.0% and specificity of 84.7%. Taketani et al. studied colon cancer-stricken mice. discovered changes in the molecular makeup of collagen type I and lipids, as well as its progression. With 86.8% accuracy, the tumor lesion could be distinguished from the control mouse's normal tissues. The diagnostic of stomach cancer has also been a use for biomedical Raman spectroscopy. Bergholt and associates have also published a statistically sound study in which 450 patients had Raman endoscopy to detect precancerous lesions in the stomach using PLS-DA. The same group evaluated unique biomolecular variations of various anatomical locations in the colorectum for cancer diagnosis and used in vivo Raman spectroscopy to characterize the properties of normal colorectal tissues. They draw the conclusion that, in comparison to cancer tissue, the interanatomical Raman spectral variability of normal colorectal tissue is less pronounced. For the diagnosis of colorectal cancer, their PLS-DA model yielded 88.8% diagnostic accuracy, 93.9% sensitivity, and 88.3% specificity.
- **Oral Cancer:** PCA-LDA was used to classify Raman spectra of oral diseases from 18 patients into a benign or malignant category. The method yielded a 77% sensitivity with 100% specificity. We discussed how Raman spectroscopy can be used to detect early alterations in the oral mucosa and the effectiveness of this method in treating oral cancer. When noncancer locations were compared in a population with and without smokers, prediction accuracy ranged from 75% to 98%. A different

group reported 82–89% accuracy in differentiating between different lesion categories and normal oral tissue. Lately, Lin and colleagues... revealed how useful fiber-optic-based Raman spectroscopy is for nasopharyngeal carcinoma (NPC) in vivo real-time diagnosis during endoscopy. A total of 95 subjects' in vivo Raman spectra totaling 3731 were obtained in real time. The Raman spectra of cancerous and healthy nasopharyngeal tissues differ markedly from one another. Their approach yielded a 93.1% diagnostic accuracy (sensitivity of 93.6%; specificity of 92.6%) for the identification of nasopharyngeal cancer using PCA-LDA. Oral squamous cell carcinoma (OSCC), oral submucosa fibrosis (OSMF), and oral leukoplakia (OLK) are all visible in the Raman spectra of the diseased tissue. For the three diseased groups and the normal group, the study's diagnostic accuracy was good (89, 85, 82, and 85%, respectively).

- **Skin Cancer:** A 2012 study by Lui et al. examined various forms of skin cancer through a clinical investigation involving 453,537 patients. The authors' equipment provided an acquisition time of roughly one second, and the software preprocessed the spectra right away, enabling real-time analysis of skin lesions. Using multivariate analysis tools with sensitivity ranging from 95 to 99%, benign and malignant skin lesions such as melanomas, basal cell carcinomas, squamous cell carcinomas, actinic keratoses, atypical nevi, melanocytic nevi, blue nevi, and seborrheic keratosis were examined and distinguished. Lim along with others. assessed the diagnostic potential of a multimodal spectrum diagnosis for noninvasive in vivo disease diagnosis of skin cancers other than melanoma. Using optical fiber-based systems, they obtained reflectance, fluorescence, and Raman spectra from 137 lesions in 76 patients. Using a multimodal approach, they were able to obtain the best classification for skin cancers other than melanoma. However, the best way to classify melanoma was to use Raman spectroscopy in isolation. Jermyn et al. developed a Raman probe to detect invasive brain cancer in situ in real time in patients. They showed that during human brain cancer surgery, Raman spectroscopy can reliably identify grade 2–4 gliomas in vivo and distinguish between the normal brain and the brain invaded by cancer cells with a sensitivity and specificity greater than 90%. This method is also able to classify in real time, which makes it a very useful tool for decision-making and surgical procedures.

9.6.2. Skin Diseases

- **Atopic Dermatitis:** The molecular makeup of skin has been analyzed using Raman spectroscopy in many published studies, and the results have been correlated with atopic dermatitis (AD) history and mutations in the FLG gene; Kezic et al. examined 137 Irish children with a history of moderate to severe AD and measured NMFs noninvasively on their skin. Gonzalez along with others used PCA and Raman spectroscopy to identify the presence of the protein filaggrin in newborn skin as a method of early detection for AD linked to filaggrin. The coefficients of the principal components for each skin spectra of newborns were determined in order to look for the presence of filaggrin in the Raman spectra. 93.86% of the variance in the original data that could be explained was accounted for by the first and second principal components.

This finding suggests that this strategy can be used to identify individuals who are more likely to develop AD, opening the door to the possibility of using this technique as an early detection method for AD. Gonzalez along with others confirmed the efficacy of Raman spectroscopy as a non-invasive method for identifying mutations in the filaggrin gene. The pure filaggrin Raman spectrum and the skin spectra of Mexican AD patients were correlated in this study to estimate the amount of filaggrin present. The genetic analysis revealed that 8 out of the 19 patients (42%) had an FLG mutation. Out of the eight patients, two (10%) were homozygous and six (31%) heterozygous for the 2282del4 FLG mutation, while one (5%) developed a compound heterozygote for both the 2282del4 and R501X mutations. A lower correlation value between the spectra and the filaggrin spectrum suggests a lower concentration of filaggrin. These genetic results were compared to the estimated amount of filaggrin.

- **Skin Aging:** Tfayli noted a small amount of variation in skin lipids as people aged. As the volunteer ages increased, the Raman spectral features of skin lipids changed in lateral packing. Gonzalez et al. distinguished between photoinduced skin damage and chronological aging using PCA of in vivo Raman spectra from the skin that was exposed to and shielded from the sun.
- **Nickel Allergy:** Alda et al. found biochemical variations in the skin's structure between individuals with nickel allergy and healthy individuals. PCA was used to classify the group differences in Raman spectra.
- **Melasma:** Moncada and associates employed Raman spectroscopy on patients with melasma receiving treatment with a triple combination cream (Tretinoin, Fluocinolona, and Hydroquinone) and discovered variations in the melanin-related peaks at 1352 and 1580 cm^{-1}. Patients who did not respond to treatment had poorly defined peaks in their Raman skin spectrum, which is consistent with protein breakdown and molecule degradation.

9.6.3. Other in Vivo Applications: UV/Vis Raman, Raman Imaging, and SERS

Generally, near-infrared (NIR) excitation sources are preferred in in vivo Raman applications.

When compared to visible or UV excitation, NIR wavelengths between 780 and 1100 nm reduce the fluorescence background in the tissue and make it easier to analyze the Raman bands. Numerous biomedical Raman applications have made use of the visible excitation sources. However, there are several drawbacks to using visible wavelengths for in vivo biomedical Raman applications, including heat generation, autofluorescence, and a decrease in penetration depth. Because UV radiation is mutagenic, it is not used for in vivo measurements. A laser spot scans the sample region and records Raman spectra at predetermined intervals in Raman imaging. An image is constructed from cells and tissues based on the intensity of a particular Raman band or bands. Additionally, chemometric analysis can be used to distinguish between the Raman spectra, producing what is known as a Raman chemical image—a picture of the sample that includes chemical information. Coherent anti-Stokes Raman spectroscopy (CARS) and stimulated Raman scattering are two more techniques for Raman imaging. The study of biochemical interactions in cells and tissues has made use of these techniques. Nevertheless, only animal models have been used for in vivo applications. The drawback of Raman imaging is that it requires lengthy integration times, which makes it unsuitable for in vivo human measurement. In vivo biomedical applications have employed surface-enhanced Raman spectroscopy (SERS) to identify biomarkers in animal models. However, this technique is not practical for in vivo Raman measurements of human tissue due to toxicity concerns with the nanoparticles used in SERS.

For in vivo biomedical applications, combining Raman spectroscopy with other optical techniques is another option. For instance, diffuse reflectance, fluorescence spectroscopy, confocal reflectance microscopy, and optical coherence tomography have all been used in conjunction with Raman spectroscopy. The multimodal approach's drawbacks include the more expensive and complicated system required to carry out the measurements. When compared to Raman spectroscopy alone, however, the multimodal approach has an advantage because it offers additional, in-depth information about the illness and a more precise diagnosis in terms of both sensitivity and specificity (Atkins et al, 2017; Baker et al, 2018).

9.7. Raman Spectroscopy: A Novel Technology for Gastric Cancer Diagnosis

Because stomach cancer is typically advanced when it is diagnosed, it ranks fifth in the world for cancer diagnoses and third for cancer-related deaths. The pathogenesis of gastric cancer involves multiple stages, such as intestinal metaplasia, dysplasia, invasive carcinoma, multifocal atrophic gastritis, and chronic non-atrophic gastritis. The course of the disease has a direct impact on the prognosis of gastric cancer; in early cases, over 90% of patients survive for five years following effective treatment. The best chance of improving the prognosis and survival of gastric cancer is early detection. Thus, improving early detection rates requires the use of sensitive and effective examination techniques.

Clinical gastric cancer diagnosis frequently makes use of endoscopic diagnosis, pathological diagnosis, and medical imaging. These diagnostic methods have significant drawbacks, including lengthy diagnosis times, severe trauma, a high rate of error, and a reliance on the subjective experience of doctors. Thus, there is an urgent need for a new, quick, non-invasive, extremely accurate, and sensitive method of diagnosing stomach cancer. By obtaining fingerprints from molecules, Raman spectroscopy, a molecular vibrational spectroscopy technique, can identify the structures and properties of different substances. Many different types of tumors can currently be diagnosed using Raman spectroscopy.

9.7.1. Raman Spectroscopy and Tumor Diagnosis

When it comes to Raman scattering, the type of scattering that involves part of the photon's energy being transferred to the molecule is known as Stokes Raman scattering, and the type of scattering that involves the photon receiving energy from the molecule's rotation and vibration is known as anti-Stokes Raman scattering. The difference between the frequency of the scattered light and the frequency of the incident light (Rayleigh scattering) during Raman scattering is known as the Raman shift, which is the transverse coordinate of the Raman spectrum that we see. Regardless of the excitation wavelength, the vibrational energy level of the molecule is what determines the Raman shift and varies depending on the chemical group. The vertical coordinate of the Raman spectrum is the intensity of the Raman peak, which is determined by the excitation light wavelength, power, concentration, and molecular polarization rate of the material being tested in addition to the collection efficiency of the instrument system. Every molecule has a unique Raman spectrum, including gas, solid, and liquid molecules. Thus, without sample labeling, Raman spectroscopy can ascertain the characteristics and composition of diverse substances.

A Raman spectrometer's components include the excitation light source, focusing system, filter, dispersion system, detector, and recording system. The term used to identify different types of Raman scattering is spontaneous Raman spectroscopy. Due to their low intensity and poor resistance to interference, Raman signals are inconvenient for spectral acquisition and quick imaging because they require a lengthy integration time in real-world applications to produce a spectrum with a respectable signal-to-noise ratio. Furthermore, in biological samples, the fluorescence background can have an impact on the Raman signal. Numerous methods for improving Raman signals have been developed to overcome the problems of low signal-to-noise ratio and sluggish acquisition speed. The most widely used Raman signal enhancement methods are stimulated Raman spectroscopy (SRS), surface-enhanced Raman spectroscopy (SERS), tip-enhanced Raman spectroscopy (TERS), and resonance Raman spectroscopy (RRS). These methods show promise in the fields of biology and medicine because they are all highly selective and sensitive to biochemical changes without requiring the labeling of the sample. Some overlapping peaks are unavoidable during the signal acquisition process because of the intricate nature of the surroundings and the properties of the Raman spectroscopy signal. It has been shown that combining symmetric zero-area conversion with L-M fitting allows for the identification of overlapped spectral peaks. With excellent specificity and accuracy in a wide range of applications, the developing spectral pre-processing and classification algorithms substantially offset the impact of the spectrometer and surrounding environment on the quality of the spectra. When it comes to the diagnosis of various tumors, researchers use data processing techniques like statistics, machine learning, and deep learning to analyze Raman spectroscopy data from samples of tumor tissues, cancer cells, bodily fluids, or tumor markers. These days, malignant tumors in the bladder, breast, brain, cervix, colorectum, esophagus, gastrointestinal tract, liver, lung, and oral cavity can all be diagnosed with Raman spectroscopy. It can also be used to diagnose ovarian, nasopharyngeal, and laryngeal carcinomas (Bergholt et al, 2011a; Bergholt et al, 2011b; Bergholt et al, 2011c; Bergholt et al, 2014).

9.7.2. Raman Spectroscopy for the Diagnosis of Gastric Cancer

Currently used to detect gastric cancer are endoscopic diagnosis, histopathology, clinical imaging, tumor markers, and other clinical methods. Endoscopic and histopathological diagnosis, which is carried out at the tissue and cellular levels, is considered the "gold standard" in clinical tumor diagnosis. After staining the tissues, the tissue types of normal gastric mucosa, precancerous lesions, and gastric cancer can be identified by looking under a microscope at the size, density, and nucleoplasmic ratio of the cells as well as the structure, number, and arrangement of the glands. It takes roughly three days to detect. However, this calls for biopsy sampling to diagnose tissue, which may cause bleeding or perforation in the gastrointestinal tract. In addition, test procedures take time, and results may not be available right away. Pathologists' subjective factors also have an impact on the accuracy of pathological diagnosis.

As clinical diagnostic tools, X-ray contrast radiography examinations, computed tomography examinations, magnetic resonance imaging (MRI), and other imaging diagnostic techniques are frequently employed; however, they are limited in their ability to identify the form and composition of pathological tissues. These techniques have a poor detection rate for microscopic tumors and early-stage gastric cancer because they can only make an approximate assessment of the shape and nature of pathological tissues and have a low spatial resolution. Clinical markers like CEA, CA19–9, CA125, and CA72–4 are frequently utilized. Tumor markers have limited specificity and sensitivity, making them unsuitable for use in the diagnosis of gastric cancer. They can also be affected by individual differences and benign diseases. It requires several days to be detected. It requires several days to be detected. What's more, tumor markers are incredibly hard to find. This demonstrates how important Raman spectroscopy is for the early identification of stomach cancer.

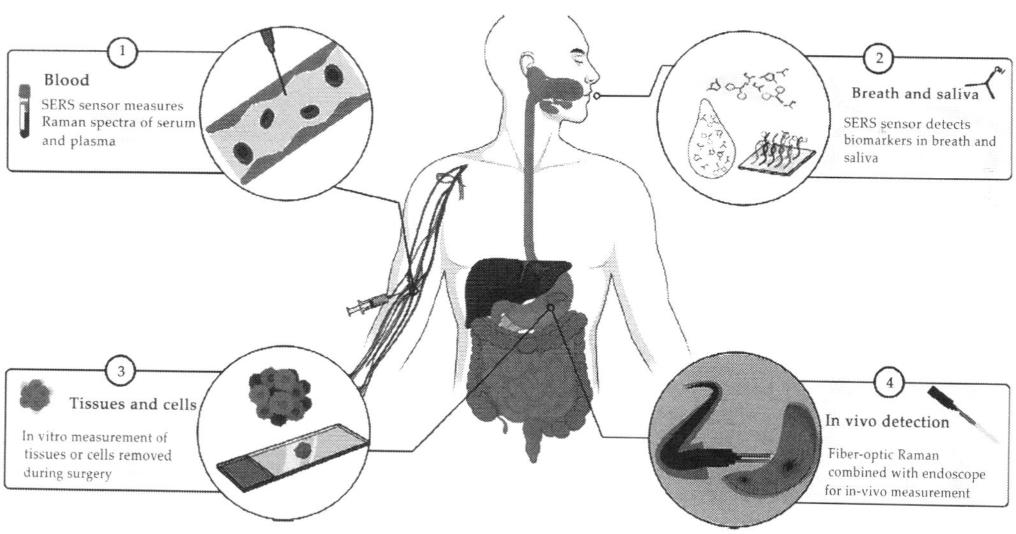

Figure 9.2. *Sample types for Raman spectroscopy in the diagnosis of gastric cancer.*

Source: Liu K, Zhao Q, Li B and Zhao X (2022) Raman Spectroscopy: A Novel Technology for Gastric Cancer Diagnosis. Front. Bioeng. Biotechnol. 10:856591. doi: 10.3389/fbioe.2022.856591.

The Raman spectra's corresponding characteristic peaks and intensity can be used to directly reflect the changes in the chemical composition and content of stomach tissues or cells that occur during the cancerous process. Using histopathology as the reference standard, the comprehensive sensitivity and specificity of Raman spectroscopy for the diagnosis of gastric cancer are 0.89 and 0.92, respectively. Because of this, Raman spectroscopy is an easy-to-use, non-invasive optical diagnostic method that is sensitive and objective for identifying gastric cancer. It also permits real-time diagnosis.

9.7.3. In Vitro Diagnosis of Gastric Cancer by Raman Spectroscopy

Ex vivo samples were obtained and subjected to Raman spectroscopy to distinguish and categorize chemical variations between samples.

9.7.3.1. Raman Spectroscopy of Gastric Tissue and Cell Samples In Vitro

The most common and direct use of Raman spectroscopy in diagnosing the type of gastric tumor is data collection and classification of gastric tissues or cells. The Raman spectroscopy-based approach for diagnosing gastric cancer can gather data straight from fresh tissues, whereas traditional intraoperative histological diagnosis necessitates workflows like tissue transport, sample processing, and section preparation.

In Raman studies of isolated gastric tissues and cells, the most frequently used samples are frozen, fresh tissue, and formalin-fixed paraffin-embedded (FFPE) samples. FFPE samples can be studied once the diagnostic results are known, but the tissue's biochemical makeup may change as a result of the fixation process, changing the Raman peaks. The signal-to-noise ratio and reproducibility of frozen tissues' Raman spectra are better than those of fresh tissues. However, compared to fresh tissues, the freezing and thawing process seems to alter the intensity of some Raman peaks, decreasing the accuracy of detection. For Raman spectroscopy of isolated tissues, a desktop Raman spectroscopy system is usually utilized. Due to the relatively low absorption coefficient of NIR light by molecules in biological tissues that primarily absorb light (e.g., melanin, water, and lipids), NIR light sources, in particular 785 nm lasers located in the high transmittance "optical window" of biological tissues, are frequently used in medical Raman measurement systems. Although NIR light with wavelengths of 785 nm and 1,064 nm is more effective at reducing tissue autofluorescence and has been used more frequently in diagnostic studies of gastric cancer, visible light with a wavelength of 532 nm has a higher scattering intensity than NIR light.

The sample is exposed to light through the transmission system, and the detector and spectrometer gather and process the Raman signal produced by the tissue sample. The wavenumber region in which Raman spectra are usually obtained is 400–3,500 cm^{-1}. This region can be further classified into three areas: the high wavenumber region (HW, 2,800–3,200 cm^{-1}), the intermediate region (FP, 400–1800 cm^{-1}), and the Raman fingerprint region (FP, 400–1800 cm^{-1}). The intermediate region is usually devoid of Raman characteristic peaks. The majority of studies only obtain spectral data in the FP region or both the FP and HW regions because the acquisition range of the spectra influences the acquisition time and redundancy of subsequent data processing. Analyzing the FP region alone is preferable to analyzing the HW region alone, and analyzing the FP and HW regions concurrently is preferable to analyzing the FP and HW regions independently, per related research. Additionally, research indicates that while increasing the integration time can greatly increase prediction accuracy, increasing the laser power has little effect overall. The desired experimental conditions should be selected based on the characteristics of the sample under investigation, as the selection of various spectral ranges and spectral acquisition conditions can impact the diagnostic outcomes.

Raman spectroscopy has advanced significantly as a quick and non-invasive way to identify stomach tissues. Other studies have demonstrated that the use of Raman detection on isolated gastric tissues can be used to diagnose gastric dysplasia, distinguish between precancerous and cancerous tissues, identify malignant gastric mucosal tissues, and diagnose gastric cancer (Bergholt et al, 2011a; Bergholt et al, 2011b; Bergholt et al, 2011c; Bergholt et al, 2014).

9.7.3.2. Raman Spectroscopy for Body Fluid Samples In Vitro

Plasma, red blood cells, white blood cells, and platelets are vital bodily fluids that are used to track a variety of disease states. For over 40 years, blood components and whole blood have been detected using Raman spectroscopy. The SERS technique is more sensitive than other methods and is primarily used in research to detect the small changes that the constituent parts of cancerous blood undergo.

The creation of enhanced substrates or nanoenhanced materials is essential to SERS because molecules that are adsorbed on metal surfaces at a specific nanometer size exhibit abnormally large Raman scattering cross-sections. Studies on SERS have demonstrated that 3D nanostructured gold nanoparticle/silicon nanowire array (Au/SiNWA) SERS substrates are also an effective means of differentiating between gastric and normal serum SERS-active substrates. Gold and silver nanomaterials are frequently employed in SERS investigations.

Ancient Greek physicians associated particular diseases with particular breath odors. Studies conducted since 1971 have revealed that breath is made up of a complex mixture of almost 3,000 volatile organic compounds (VOCs). Particular VOCs are produced by cancer cells or tissues when they are under oxidative or metabolic stress. They can therefore be employed as VOC biomarkers for cancer without having an impact on clinical symptoms. Furthermore, saliva has clear advantages for use in the diagnosis of gastric cancer and can reflect a person's health status directly. Research has indicated that early and advanced gastric cancer can be distinguished by employing gas chromatography–mass spectrometry in conjunction with solid phase microextraction (SPME) and surface enzymatic respiration (SERS) to detect organic compound biomarkers in saliva or breath. This non-invasive, quick, and accurate analysis technique, which is based on the SERS sensor, provides a novel approach to identifying gastric cancer patients in the general population.

9.7.4. In Vivo Diagnosis of Gastric Cancer by Raman Spectroscopy

Fiber optic Raman technology enables in situ testing as well as biomedical in vivo testing in the field, and many researchers aim to bring Raman spectroscopy technology from the lab to in situ testing in the field. Any portion of a sample can be detected by the fiber optic Raman probe, which consists of an optical fiber and a tiny lens. This allows it to gather Raman spectral information for the sample detection site. In addition to obtaining real-time images of the tumor, the combination of fiber optic Raman and endoscopy in the diagnosis of gastric cancer enables the simultaneous acquisition of Raman spectral data for flexible and non-destructive detection of the digestive tract. It is essential to look for adhesions or fluids through the gastroscope on the gastric mucosa and the gastric lumen before utilizing fiber-optic Raman to obtain Raman spectra in vivo. Endoscopy can be used to locate the target Raman acquisition site after the adherent has been rinsed and aspirated away to rule out interference from other tissues and blood vessels.

Raman spectroscopy is currently used to detect biological tissues. Quartz-based optical fibers offer unparalleled advantages in terms of light transmission, in vivo compatibility, and bending flexibility. The application dictates the fiber optic probe's structural design; for in vivo stomach detection, for instance, the probe needs to be more flexible and smaller. Moreover, an earlier investigation discovered that the Raman spectrum was not significantly affected by alterations in the probe's angle or tissue pressure (Bergholt et al, 2011a; Bergholt et al, 2011b; Bergholt et al, 2011c; Bergholt et al, 2014).

9.7.5. Data Processing and Analysis of Raman Spectroscopy

A typical Raman spectroscopy spectral analysis workflow includes feature selection, data preprocessing, and multivariate modeling.

The spectral signal undergoes preprocessing to get rid of anomalies and undesired changes. Common preprocessing methods include scaling, baseline correction, noise reduction, and scattering correction. Moreover, spectrum normalization (e.g., maximum value, average intensity normalization, spectral area, etc., can lessen the impact of variations in the excitation intensity, making it easier to compare spectral shapes and relative peak intensities between various tissues. The most widely used filtering technique in research utilizing Raman spectroscopy to examine gastric cancer is Savitzky-Golay (SG) filtering. The most important feature of the SG filter, a filtering technique based on local polynomial least square fitting in the time domain, is its ability to remove noise while maintaining the signal's width and shape.

Spectral data contain a large amount of invalid information, which is why feature selection is used. Directly analyzing the entire spectrum may have an impact on the diagnostic effect and increase computational costs. In addition to manually truncating the spectrum or choosing specific peaks based on prior knowledge, algorithms are commonly used to perform feature selection and spectral extraction of the raw spectra. In Raman studies on gastric cancer, principal component analysis (PCA) is the most often utilized feature extraction technique. One well-liked unsupervised technique for making spectral data analysis easier before feeding it into multivariate models is the PCA algorithm. Reducing variables, however, might cause the original pattern of the spectral data to change and result in the loss of important information.

An equation linking the spectrum and the label must be established to derive the class information of the sample to be measured from the Raman spectral data. As a result, multivariate modeling is utilized to enable sample identification and diagnosis. Although Raman peak intensity comparison is the simplest method of classification, its accuracy is not very high. Diagnostic accuracy can be increased by using the ant colony optimization algorithm (ACO) to identify the best Raman features and the analysis method to distinguish peak feature intensities based on the Mahalanobis distance. However, it is typical to use a range of multivariate analysis tools to examine various spectral data when working with large amounts of data. When using Raman spectroscopy to diagnose gastric cancer, partial least squares (PLS) and linear discriminant analysis (LDA) are more frequently employed. After projecting the data into a low-dimensional space, the LDA algorithm aims to make the data as compact as possible for the same class and as dispersed as possible for different classes. The PLS algorithm transforms the combined information of the dependent and independent variables linearly to extract the features from the sample data. Additional algorithms that have been employed are the artificial neural network (ANN), quadratic discriminant analysis (QDA), characteristic ratio method (CRM), multinomial logistic regression (MNLR), and classification and regression tree (CART).

To increase the stability of the diagnostic model, adequate supporting data and both internal and external validation are needed. Using a subset of the dataset as a test set, internal validation is the process of repeatedly training a model, usually with cross-validation (e.g., leave-one-out cross-validation). External validation is the process of testing the developed model using a freshly measured dataset. Without external validation, the results could be unduly optimistic (Amal et al, 2012; Allegrini et al, 2013; Acquarelli et al, 2017; Atkins et al, 2017).

A Closer Look

In Vivo Raman Spectroscopy of Skin

With a surface area of about 1.6 m^2, the skin is the largest organ in the human body and makes up 16% of our body weight. Terrestrial life would not be possible without skin. Skin functions as a semi-permeable barrier to help stop excessive water loss, which could otherwise cause death and desiccation. Additionally, it thwarts undesired outside dangers like chemical insult, microbial invasion, mechanical harm, and UV light damage to the body. This is the skin function according to the so-called "outside in-inside out" paradigm. The stratum corneum (SC), or outer 20 μm or so of the skin, has long been recognized as the primary barrier component of the skin. It is a heterogeneous structure that is commonly compared to bricks and mortar, where the mortar is made of lipid and the bricks are flattened coenocyte cells. It is an extremely powerful barrier. It was formerly believed to be a dead layer, but over time, it was discovered to have significant metabolic activity and function as a responsive, intelligent material. It is a dynamic membrane with a complex structure.

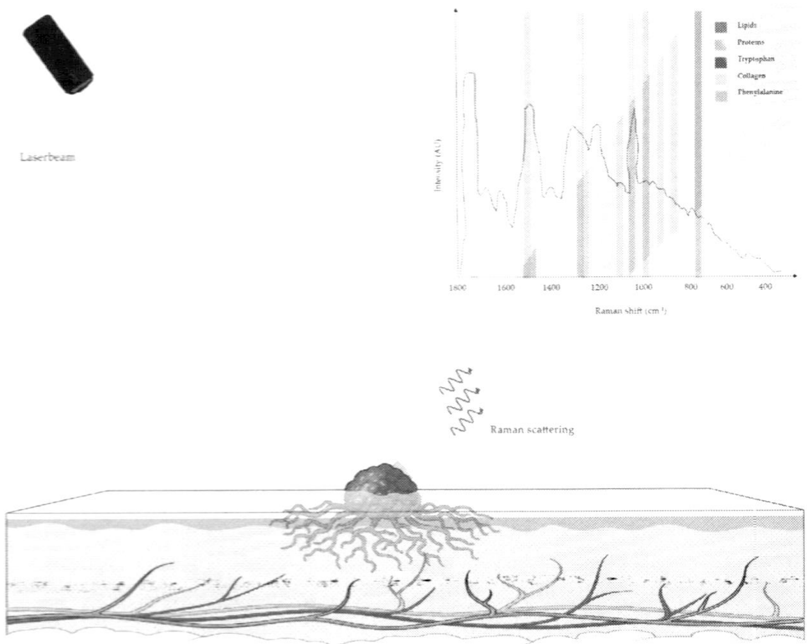

Source: Delrue C, Speeckaert R, Oyaert M, De Bruyne S, Speeckaert MM. From Vibrations to Visions: Raman Spectroscopy's Impact on Skin Cancer Diagnostics. Journal of Clinical Medicine. 2023; 12(23):7428. https://doi.org/10.3390/jcm12237428.

Thus, there are ramifications for numerous aspects of industry and health from comprehending the structure and function of the SC. It can malfunction and lead to a variety of diseases, some of which are extremely common. For instance, in the UK alone, eight million people suffer from a skin condition. Some are tolerable, while others are deadly serious. These include various cancers in addition to other conditions like acne, psoriasis, and eczema (especially atopic dermatitis). To avoid the digestive system, the pharmaceutical industry, for example, is interested in delivering medications through the skin. By moisturizing and focusing on skin actives and evaluating their impact, the cosmetics industry is interested in enhancing the health and appearance of SCs. As a result, techniques for characterizing the structure and its modifications are desperately needed.

While there are many spectroscopic techniques that can advance knowledge, Raman spectroscopy has been hailed as being at the forefront of skin research. It should be noted that Edwards et al. did not publish the first complete Raman spectrum of skin until 1992. its development has been astounding. Like with other biological systems, it was discovered that Raman spectroscopy has several built-in benefits. Its molecular sensitivity can reveal a great deal about the state or order of the molecules as well as identify which ones are present in many situations. Its relative insensitivity to water also makes it possible to see other molecules in the spectrum, but it can also be used to gauge the skin's level of hydration. Additionally, since the method relies on scattering, non-invasive depth profiling is possible due to the application of the confocal principle. As a result, it not only satisfies all criteria for examining skin, but it may also do so in vivo and non-invasively.

- **Composition of the Skin and Its Changes:** This was originally worked on by Gerwin Puppels et al. late in the decade of the 1990s. The complex Raman spectrum originating from the SC is a result of its numerous constituent parts. Nonetheless, these constituents are widely recognized and consist primarily of water, lipids (ceramides being the primary class), natural moisturizing factors (NMF), molecules from sweat, and keratin, the principal structural protein. The primary component of NMFs, which are derived from the breakdown of the significant skin protein filaggrin (FLG), is a variety of hydroscopic amino acids. They play a crucial role in controlling the SC's elasticity, pH, and water content. The method of analysis used is to model the spectra obtained from the SC using the spectra of the primary constituents present; this approach is effective in the majority of situations. Consequently, each spectrum can be modeled to provide a depth profile of the primary components of the SC when Raman spectra are obtained as a depth profile confocally through the SC. The ones that are typically extracted from the fingerprint region include trans-urocanic acid, keratin, NMF, ceramide 3, cholesterol, urea, and lactic acid (pH4). Moreover, a profile of the water content can be obtained by utilizing the high wavenumber region. The ratio of the Raman intensities of the protein's CH3 stretch at 2935 cm^{-1} and the water's OH stretch vibration at 3390 cm–1 is used to calculate this. Thus, Raman spectroscopy can measure in vivo all of the essential components that comprise the SC in great detail. Considering that this has been demonstrated to be possible, numerous applications are possible.
- **Atopic dermatitis (AD):** Atopic dermatitis, sometimes referred to as atopic eczema, is a recurrent, inflammatory, itchy, and non-contagious type of dermatitis that is becoming more and more common. It has been demonstrated that in 50% of cases, single mutations

in the filaggrin gene are a risk factor for AD. As was previously mentioned, filaggrin is a crucial protein in the development of the SC and the source of the hydroscopic amino acids known as NMFs, which aid in the regulation of SC hydration. In a large study, NMF levels were measured using in vivo Raman spectroscopy after 3149 participants were tested for polymorphisms in the filaggrin gene.

- **Different Skin Types: Axilla and Scalp (With and Without Dandruff):** Even though skin covers the majority of the body, it is known to be uneven; this is probably so it can adapt to the various stresses placed on anatomically distinct areas. The number of cell layers and, consequently, the thickness of the SC, are among the observed variations. For example, palmo-plantar skin is particularly thick and has several well-known variations. Additional body regions exhibiting discernible variations are the axilla and the scalp. A new, smaller pen-shaped probe has been developed because these areas are hard to access with the in vivo Raman instrument in its standard configuration. It makes it possible to position the window against the subject in more recessed and curved parts of their body and makes them more comfortable while the measurements are being taken. This probe can be used to study the scalp and axilla. The "normal" SC of the volar forearm differs significantly from the scalp and axilla SC. For example, in the same subjects, the scalp is found to have lower levels of NMFs than the volar forearm. Although the cause is obviously different, this is at a similar lower level as was seen with the subjects' mutations in the filaggrin gene as previously described. Furthermore, the lipids in the scalp and axilla differ from one another and from the lipids in the volar forearm in terms of order. 4 These Raman spectroscopy findings undoubtedly advance our current understanding of the composition and capabilities of the body's various skin regions. A thorough investigation of dandruff and the effectiveness of anti-dandruff shampoo containing zinc pyrithione (ZnPTO) has been finished, utilizing the same Raman probe. This revealed several alterations in the SC of the dandruff scalp, such as an additional decrease in the NMF levels to 0.16 au as opposed to 0.39 au in the healthy scalp; normal forearm levels are greater than one. When the anti-dandruff shampoo is used, the levels return to what is seen in a healthy scalp.
- **Skin Hydration:** The water content of the skin is known to reflect the health of the skin and is associated with changes in surface morphology, elasticity, flexibility, and sensory perception. It is acknowledged that the water content throughout the SC determined by in vivo Raman spectroscopy is a dependable, standard technique. Since the water content is low outside and plateaus inside the viable epidermis, this depth profile is also used to calculate the SC thickness. The method for obtaining the SC thickness from the water profile is more debatable. Numerous analysis techniques have been proposed, but the performance of the various models varies greatly because the profile shape varies with varying skin thickness and hydration levels. In a recent study, Tom Hancewicz and colleagues demonstrated the need for a consensus-building approach to the problem, which involved averaging several different approaches, in order to accurately model and quantify the wide range of water profile types encountered in typical in vivo Raman spectroscopy water measurements. After that, these findings were confirmed by measurements made using reflectance confocal microscopy. Because of its ability to provide non-invasive, spatially

resolved depth profiling of skin hydration, in vivo confocal Raman spectroscopy is now the most effective way to investigate a wide range of medical, cosmetic, and pharmaceutical issues where skin hydration is a key component.

- **Pene**tration of Actives Into Skin: How molecules enter the skin is of interest to the cosmetic and pharmaceutical industries. The primary goal of the pharmaceutical industry is to prevent any potential gastrointestinal tract side effects from drugs. If the skin is the target for both industries, figuring out how and where an active molecule enters the skin is essential to comprehending any potential benefits. Thus, in vivo Raman spectroscopy has a very useful application in this case. A thorough investigation of the skin active retinol, both with and without penetration enhancers, and from a variety of delivery methods, provides a clear picture of what can be accomplished. It displays the quantitative amount and timing of retinol's penetration through the SC and into the target tissue, the viable epidermis. Additionally, the significant impact of penetration enhancers such as triton 100 and oleic acid was described. Raman spectroscopy measures all constituents, not just the active molecule. It also indicates the penetration depth of the vehicle, which was always observed to be ahead of the active molecule.

The bulk of studies on skin penetration are conducted in vitro and are thought to be representative of the in vivo environment. A recent study compared in vivo penetration with in vitro. Correlations between in vivo data and these kinds of in vitro studies are extremely rare. The best way to accomplish this is with Raman spectroscopy. Niacinamide, the model active in this study, was administered in a variety of vehicles. The amount of niacinamide that penetrated the skin in vitro and the strength of the niacinamide signal found in the stratum corneum in vivo were found to be well correlated. Similar to the retinol study, the amount of active that was delivered also depended on how well the vehicle penetrated. It also made clear how much more research of this kind is required to help validate the in vitro results and gain a deeper understanding of the skin penetration process' mechanistic details. As a result, in vivo Raman spectroscopy is set to contribute even more significantly to this crucial field of skin research.

Summary

- Raman spectroscopy provides spectral information related to the specific molecular structures of substances and has been well established as a powerful tool for studying biological tissues and diagnosing diseases.
- Raman Spectroscopy is a non-destructive chemical analysis technique which provides detailed information about chemical structure, phase and polymorphy, crystallinity and molecular interactions.
- Raman spectroscopy was used to study materials based on the Raman Effect, which is the inelastic scattering of incoming light of a material and its frequency changes due to the power of excited molecular vibrations.
- The spectrometer, detector, and excitation laser are the three main parts of a Raman instrument. The spectrometer serves as the central element within the Raman instrument and is responsible for the separation and measurement of distinct wavelength components inherent in the light scattered by the sample.
- Metal nanostructures have emerged as crucial elements in the field of plasma antennas, contributing to the augmentation of Raman signals in SERS-based molecular detection.
- A Raman spectrometer useful for in vivo measurements should be an integrated system that can provide real-time spectral acquisition and analysis.
- Raman effect or Raman scattering the inelastic scattering of photons by matter, meaning that there is both an exchange of energy and a change in the light's direction.
- Raman scattering is conceptualized as involving a virtual electronic energy level which corresponds to the energy of the exciting laser photons.
- Monitoring the polarization of the scattered photons is useful for understanding the connections between molecular symmetry and Raman activity which may assist in assigning peaks in Raman spectra.
- The main sources of noise present in Raman spectra from biological samples are the shot noise, fluorescence background, flicker noise, dark current, and thermal noise.
- Chemometrics uses mathematical and statistical methods to provide chemical/physical information from chemical data or for the subject under consideration, spectroscopic data.
- Principal component analysis (PCA) is an unsupervised method often used to reduce the number of variables and exploratory analysis of data.
- In most of the in vivo Raman applications, near infrared (NIR) excitation sources are preferred. NIR wavelengths in the range of 780–1100 nm result in lower fluorescence background in the tissue and simplify the analysis of the Raman bands in comparison to visible or UV excitation.
- In Raman scattering, the scattering in which a portion of the energy of the photon is transferred to the molecule is called Stokes Raman scattering, while the scattering in which the energy of the vibration and rotation of the molecule is transferred to the photon is anti-Stokes Raman scattering.

References

1. Acquarelli, J., van Laarhoven, T., Gerretzen, J., Tran, T. N., Buydens, L. M. C., & Marchiori, E. (2017). Convolutional Neural Networks for Vibrational Spectroscopic Data Analysis. *Analytica Chimica Acta, 954*, 22–31.
2. Allegrini, F., & Olivieri, A. C. (2013). An Integrated Approach to the Simultaneous Selection of Variables, Mathematical Pre-processing and Calibration Samples in Partial Least-Squares Multivariate Calibration. *Talanta, 115*(17), 755–760.
3. Amal, L., Ding, L., Liu, B. B., Tisch, U., Xu, Z. Q., Shi, D. Y., et al. (2012). The Scent Fingerprint of Hepatocarcinoma: In-Vitro Metastasis Prediction with Volatile Organic Compounds (VOCs). *International Journal of Nanomedicine, 7*, 4135–4146. https://doi.org/10.2147/IJN.S32680.
4. Atkins, C. G., Buckley, K., Blades, M. W., & Turner, R. F. B. (2017). Raman Spectroscopy of Blood and Blood Components. *Applied Spectroscopy, 71*(5), 767–793.
5. Auner, G. W., Koya, S. K., Huang, C., Broadbent, B., Trexler, M., Auner, Z., et al. (2018). Applications of Raman Spectroscopy in Cancer Diagnosis. *Cancer Metastasis Reviews, 37*(4), 691–717.
6. Avram, L., Iancu, S. D., Stefancu, A., Moisoiu, V., Colnita, A., Marconi, D., et al. (2020). SERS-Based Liquid Biopsy of Gastrointestinal Tumors Using a Portable Raman Device Operating in a Clinical Environment. *Journal of Clinical Medicine, 9*(1), 212.
7. Baker, M. J., Byrne, H. J., Chalmers, J., Gardner, P., Goodacre, R., Henderson, A., et al. (2018). Clinical Applications of Infrared and Raman Spectroscopy: State of Play and Future Challenges. *Analyst., 143*(8), 1735–1757.
8. Bergholt, M. S., Zheng, W., Ho, K. Y., Teh, M., Yeoh, K. G., & Yan So, J. B. (2014). Fiberoptic Confocal Raman Spectroscopy for Real-Time In Vivo Diagnosis of Dysplasia in Barrett's Esophagus. *Gastroenterology, 146*(1), 27–32.
9. Bergholt, M. S., Zheng, W., Lin, K., Ho, K. Y., Teh, M., Yeoh, K. G., et al. (2011a). Characterizing Variability in In Vivo Raman Spectra of Different Anatomical Locations in the Upper Gastrointestinal Tract toward Cancer Detection. *Journal of Biomedical Optics, 16*(3), 037003.
10. Bergholt, M. S., Zheng, W., Lin, K., Ho, K. Y., Teh, M., Yeoh, K. G., et al. (2011b). Combining Near-Infrared-Excited Autofluorescence and Raman Spectroscopy Improves In Vivo Diagnosis of Gastric Cancer. *Biosensors and Bioelectronics, 26*(10), 4104–4110.
11. Bergholt, M. S., Zheng, W., Lin, K., Ho, K. Y., Teh, M., Yeoh, K. G., et al. (2011c). In Vivo Diagnosis of Gastric Cancer Using Raman Endoscopy and Ant Colony Optimization Techniques. *International Journal of Cancer, 128*(11), 2673–2680.
12. Bovenkamp, D., Sentosa, R., Rank, E., Erkkilä, M., Placzek, F., & Püls, J., et al. (2018). Combination of High-Resolution Optical Coherence Tomography and Raman Spectroscopy for Improved Staging and Grading in Bladder Cancer. *Applied Sciences, 8*(12), 2371.

Chapter

ANGIOGRAPHY

10

Contents

Introduction

Angiography, also known as arteriography, is a type of medical imaging that shows images of the body's internal organs and blood vessels, specifically the heart chambers, veins, and arteries. Using X-ray-based methods like fluoroscopy, modern angiography is carried out by injecting a radio-opaque contrast agent into the blood vessel and imaging.

An angiograph, more commonly known as an angiogram, is a film or image of blood vessels. While the term can refer to both arteriograms and venograms, in everyday language angiogram and arteriogram are often used interchangeably, while venogram is used more specifically. The term angiography includes radionuclide angiography and newer vascular imaging techniques like CO_2 angiography, CT angiography, and MR angiography. Isotope angiography has also been used, but is more accurately called isotope perfusion scanning.

Orientation and Directional Terms

Term	Definition	Illustration
Cerebral angiography	Cerebral angiography also known as cerebral arteriography or neuroangiography, this technique focuses on imaging blood vessels within the brain and is used to diagnose conditions such as aneurysms, Arteriovenous Malformations (AVMs), and stenosis.	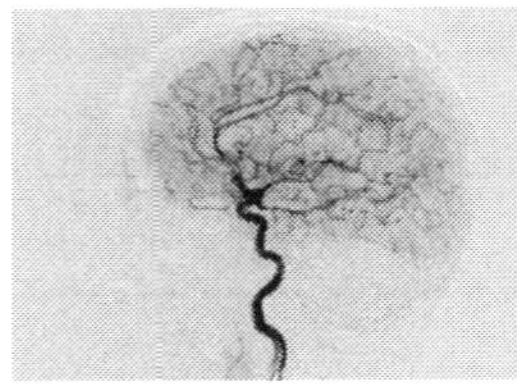
Coronary angiography	Coronary angiography involves imaging the blood vessels supplying the heart (coronary arteries) and is a critical tool for diagnosing coronary artery disease and planning coronary interventions like angioplasty and stent placement.	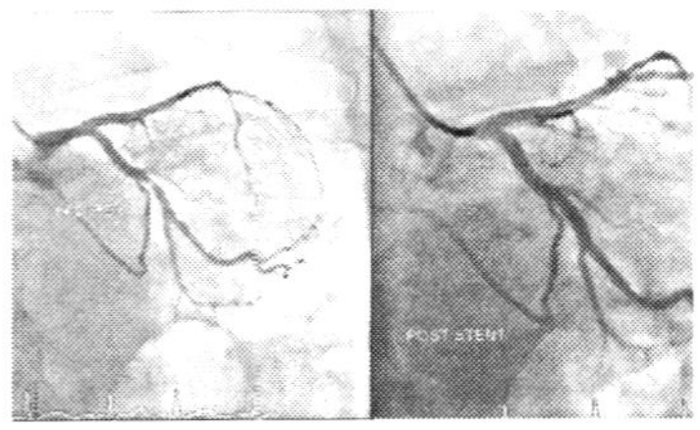
Renal angiography	Renal angiography is employed to evaluate the blood vessels within the kidneys and is useful in diagnosing renal artery stenosis and other kidney-related vascular conditions.	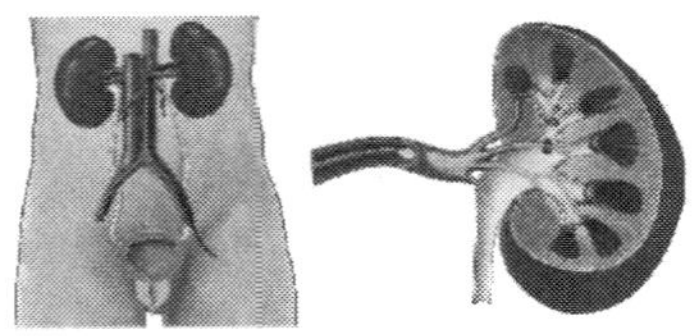
Pulmonary angiography	Pulmonary angiography visualizes the blood vessels in the lungs and is mainly utilized to diagnose pulmonary embolism, a potentially life-threatening condition caused by blood clots in the lung arteries.	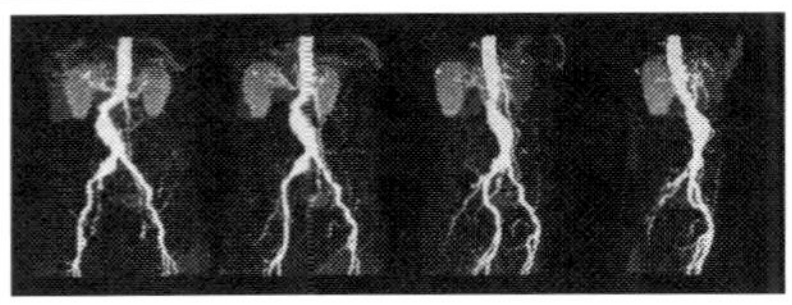
Peripheral angiography	Peripheral angiography is used to assess blood flow and detect vascular abnormalities in the arms, legs, and other peripheral regions of the body. It is particularly useful in diagnosing Peripheral Artery Disease (PAD) and identifying blockages or narrowed vessels.	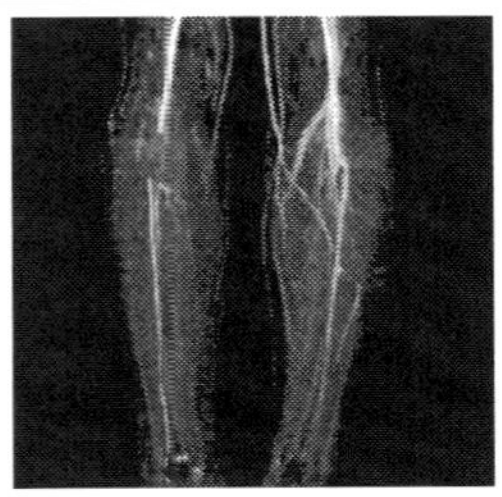

10.1. Historical Perspective

The general term for the radiographic analysis of the blood vessels is angiography. Using contrast agents injected into particular vascular system segments, these studies image pathologic and physiologic changes in visceral, cerebral, peripheral, and cardiac anatomy.

The right and left ventricles of a horse's heart were catheterized by Claude Bernard in 1844. Through this initial phase, researchers were able to create novel methods that were eventually applied to human subjects. In order to outline the anatomy of deceased bodies, investigators injected radiopaque materials into their vessels in the late 1800s, giving rise to the field of angiography. Because they were so toxic, these early contrast agents were not suitable for use on living people.

A method for imaging the ventricular system of a living person's brain was created by Walter Dandy, a neurosurgeon at The Johns Hopkins University, between 1918 and 1919. Pneumoencephalography was the name of the technique. The discovery of additional materials that might be utilized to image anatomic structures that are difficult to see with traditional radiography sparked interest as a result of this advancement.

The radiopaque chemical sodium iodide was found to be safe to use in living subjects at the beginning of 1920. Moniz, Egas, and J. P. Caldas started doing brain angiograms. They imaged the brain's vascular system using the radiocarousel and sodium iodide as the contrast agent. Caldas invented the radiocarousel, which could image at a rate of one image per second for up to six simultaneous dots. Brooks was looking into femoral artery imaging using sodium iodide. The age of angiography officially began with this.

The first human cardiac catheterization is credited to Werner Forssmann, who looked for a way to deliver medication directly to the site of need. He inserted a 65-cm catheter into his right atrium from his left antecubital vein when he was 25 years old in 1929. He showed off this accomplishment with a chest X-ray that showed where the catheter was positioned. Numerous researchers employed his work as a basis for their investigations into cardiovascular physiology.

Throughout the early 1970s and these initial attempts at angiography, many modifications were made to contrast agents, tools, and techniques. In addition to image intensifiers, generators, and X-ray tubes, rapid sequence cassette changers were being developed further during the 1940s. The bolus of contrast agent was administered to the intended location in the 1950s and 60s using automatic injection devices. The Schonander cut film changer was unveiled along with enhanced rapid sequence imaging devices.

The use of catheters to deliver contrast agents directly to a target site was being researched. A human cardiac catheterization was reported to have gone well by Zimmerman. Direct approach was the preferred technique for inserting the catheter during the early days of angiography. This required cutting a hole, exposing the target vessel, and inserting the catheter all the way into the lumen of the vessel.

In 1953, S. I. Seldinger provided a technique for inserting the catheter by means of a percutaneous needle replacement. This method streamlined the process and increased the safety of angiographic studies. 1959 saw J. Ross Jr. and C. Cope gave an explanation of the transseptal catheterization process. Cope experimented with different catheter shapes in order to perfect a technique for selective coronary arteriography. During this time, serial magnification methods and subtraction were introduced, and research into the use of computer systems in conjunction with radiography equipment was starting.

Improvements in digital techniques throughout the 1980s led to the advancement of fundamental subtraction principles and the introduction of digital subtraction angiography as the modality most frequently utilized for cardiac catheterization. The usage of angiography as the main diagnostic tool was further diminished with the introduction of computed tomography and magnetic resonance imaging. During this time, nonsurgical interventions were refined, and angiography evolved from a solely diagnostic modality to an adjunct in numerous disease processes. Vascular and cardiac therapy now primarily focuses on interventional radiography. Although the discussion of these principles may pertain to diagnostic procedures, a transfer to interventional radiography is only a short step away. The fundamental concepts underpinning diagnostic angiography still apply to interventional studies.

Advancements in computed tomography, positron emission tomography, and magnetic resonance angiography have enabled noninvasive diagnosis of the heart and vascular system. Nonetheless, sophisticated invasive procedures continue to be utilized for diagnosis, serving as the foundation for the discipline of interventional radiology. New techniques for intervention are introduced every year. This presents a difficulty for the radiologists as well as the radiographers. To carry out these procedures safely and effectively, one needs to have a greater understanding of pharmacology as well as a constantly evolving set of technical skills and communication. Currently, diagnostic angiography has lost ground to interventional radiology as a distinct specialty.

The cardiovascular-interventional and cardiac-interventional technology examinations were the two postprimary advanced level exams that the American Registry of Radiologic Technologists (ARRT) introduced in January 2003 to replace its previous examination in this area. While the diagnostic aspect of the procedures is crucial to the overall care of the patient, the interventional (therapeutic) radiology field is quickly taking over as the main area of responsibility for radiographers working in the advanced procedure field. The comprehension and application of interventional procedures depend heavily on the skills acquired and honed in the diagnostic studies (Saine and Tyler, 2002; Youssef, 2008; Ikari et al, 2005; Campeau, L 1989; Ikari et al, 2010).

10.2. Types of Angiography

There are numerous angiography techniques that can be used to diagnose various medical issues.

- Computed tomography angiography (CTA) is a diagnostic technique that creates horizontal or axial images, or slices, of blood vessels using hardware, software, and X-rays.
- Through coronary angiography, the coronary arteries' interior can be seen. By using these images, stenoses in the arteries that may be the source of chest pain or even trigger a heart attack can be found.
- To measure blood flow, digital subtraction angiography (DSA) takes pictures of the brain's blood vessels.
- One procedure in nuclear medicine is radionuclide angiography. The examination of the target tissue is aided by a small quantity of radionuclide, such as a

radiopharmaceutical or radioactive tracer. Radionuclide angiography at rest evaluates the heart's pumping chambers.

- With pulmonary angiography, blood vessel abnormalities like stenosis, blockages, or aneurysms are imaged for assessment.
- Magnetic resonance imaging (MRI) and contrast dye are used in magnetic resonance angiography (MRA), which visualizes blood vessels. Medical professionals often use MRA to evaluate blood flow and examine soft tissues, such as the heart.
- Renal angiography also referred to as arteriography, uses imaging of the renal blood vessels to look for any abnormalities or blockages that may be affecting the kidneys' ability to receive blood (Table 10.1).

Table 10.1. A Few Studies Assessing High-Risk Plaque Features with Coronary Computed Tomography Angiography (CCTA)

First Author	Publication Year	Study Design	Patients (n)	Aim of the Study
Williams	2020	Multicenter randomized controlled trial	1769	To explore whether the quantification of low-attenuation plaque identified by CCTA enhances the ability to predict fatal or nonfatal MI when compared to traditional cardiovascular risk scores, Agatston scoring and the severity of obstructive CAD in stable patients presenting with chest pain.
Williams	2019	Multicenter randomized controlled trial	4146	To assess the prognostic implications of adverse coronary plaque characteristics with CCTA.
Puchner	2014	Multicenter randomized controlled trial	1000	To assess whether the identification of high-risk plaque features detected by CCTA in the emergency department can enhance the diagnostic accuracy of ACS beyond the presence of significant CAD and clinical risk assessment in patients experiencing acute chest pain but without objective evidence of myocardial ischemia or MI.

Otsuka	2013	Prospective study	960	To determine the predictive value of the napkin-ring sign detected by CCTA for future ACS events in patients with CAD.
Sun	2022	Prospective study	130	To examine the correlation between pericoronary inflammation and plaque morphology and components with CCTA in individuals with non-ST elevation ACS

MI: myocardial infarction; ACS: acute coronary syndrome; CAD: coronary artery disease.

Source: *Dell'Aversana S, Ascione R, Vitale RA, Cavaliere F, Porcaro P, Basile L, Napolitano G, Boccalatte M, Sibilio G, Esposito G, et al. CT Coronary Angiography: Technical Approach and Atherosclerotic Plaque Characterization. Journal of Clinical Medicine. 2023; 12(24):7615. https://doi.org/10.3390/jcm12247615.*

10.3. Techniques

Depending on the type of angiogram, the jugular or femoral vein is used to look at the right side of the heart and the venous system, and the femoral artery is most frequently used to look at the left side of the heart and the arterial system. A sort of contrast agent, which appears by absorbing the X-rays, is added to the blood to make it visible on the X-ray images using a system of guide wires and catheters (Figure 10.1).

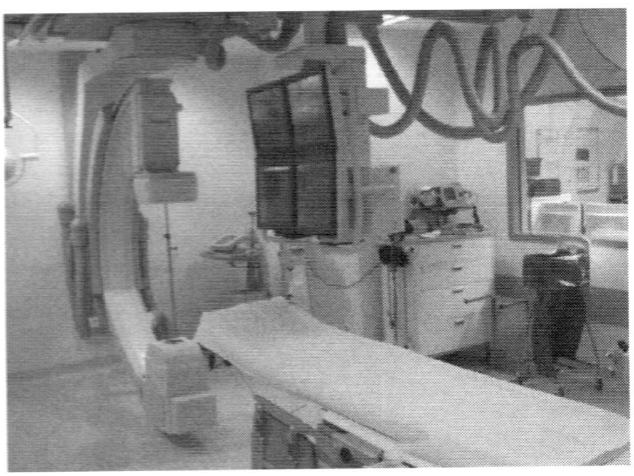

Figure 10.1. *Catheterization lab.*

Source: By Neoflash-Ownwork, CCBY-SA3.0, https://commons.wikimedia.org/w/index.php?curid=11370462.

The X-ray pictures that are captured can be still, in motion, or shown on film or an image intensifier. Digital subtraction angiography, or DSA, is the method typically used to obtain the images for all structures other than the heart. In this instance, pictures are typically captured at 2–3 frames per second, enabling the interventional radiologist to assess how well blood is flowing through a vessel or vessels. By using this method, the bones and other organs are "subtracted," leaving only the contrast agent-filled vessels visible. The heart images are captured without the use of a subtraction technique, at a rate of 15–30 frames per second. DSA cannot be used on the heart because it necessitates that the patient remain motionless. With the use of these two methods, the interventional radiologist or cardiologist can visually inspect the vessel for stenosis, or blockages or narrowings, which may be obstructing blood flow and producing pain (Figure 10.2).

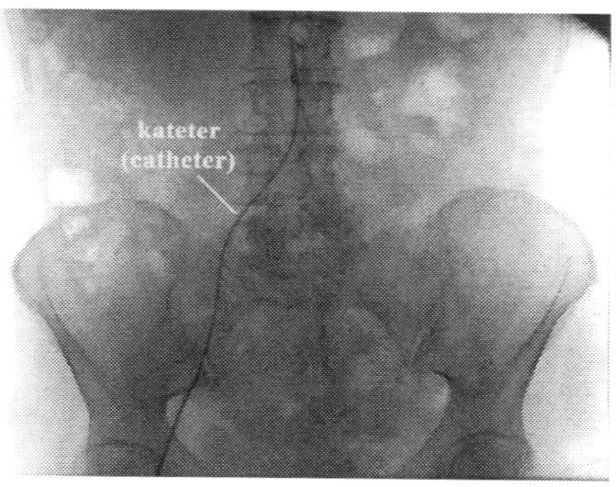

Figure 10.2. *Catheterization in selective angiography.*

Source: By Intermedichbo-Milorad Dimic MD, Nis, Serbia, CCBY-SA3.0, https://commons.wikimedia.org/w/index.php?curid=17771824.

To avoid access-site complications, the site of arterial entry is either manually compressed, stapled shut, or sutured after the procedure, if the femoral technique is used (Saine and Tyler, 2002; Youssef, 2008; Ikari et al, 2005; Campeau, L 1989; Ikari et al, 2010).

10.4. Angiographic Equipment

The versatility of angiographic equipment has increased significantly due to recent technological advancements in its design and construction, but these advancements have also raised costs and complexity. Numerous new factors need to be taken into account, regardless of whether one is thinking about installing a brand-new lab, renovating an existing lab, or just replacing a few parts. We go over these aspects in brief, focusing on the features that a contemporary angiographic facility must have, the power needs of the generators and tubes, generator switching and rectification, and the benefits and drawbacks of the recently released rotating C- and U-arm mounting units. It is assumed that visceral, peripheral, and interventional angiographic procedures will be the main uses of the laboratory.

10.4.1. Functional Requirements for Angiographic Laboratories

A wide range of diagnostic and interventional procedures must be possible in a 1980s angiographic laboratory. An angiographer's caseload primarily consists of peripheral artery "runoff" studies. A table shift device that enables sequential filming over the pelvis, thighs, knees, and calves with a stationary 14 x 14 inch (35.6 x 35.6 cm) film changer and a long-leg film changer combined with an X-ray tube mounted on the ceiling are required for this. Although it is only utilized in a very small percentage of situations, having the ability to film in biplane is highly desirable (e.g., studies of the aortic arch and inferior venacavagrams). The ability to magnify images with an angiography system is also regarded as very desirable.

One relatively new, very desirable feature is the ability to simultaneously orientate the X-ray tube and the imaging receptor (film changer or image intensifier) about a supine patient. It is now commonly acknowledged that cranial and/or caudal angulation of the X-ray beam is an essential component of coronary artery angiography; we have also discovered that these projections are highly valuable in abdominal imaging.

While not absolutely necessary, a 100 or 105 mm spot film camera is an expensive convenience. This eliminates the need to move the film changer and enables the angiographer to quickly acquire a series of films by manually injecting contrast material under fluoroscopic control. Finally, any new angiographic facility has to take digital imaging into consideration. According to preliminary reports, this new technique is a significant advancement in cardiovascular radiology and will have a big impact on radiologists' future approaches to vascular disease. There are still a lot of significant unanswered questions, though, like whether digital vascular imaging systems belong in dedicated fluoroscopic rooms or angiographic laboratories, what kind of systems are best, and if the very costly 14-inch (35.6 cm) image intensifiers are really required.

10.4.2. Power Requirements for X-ray Tubes and Generators

The fact that the power requirements for serial film angiography procedures have decreased significantly over the past ten years is one of the most significant factors in the current X-ray tube and generator technology. Serial film angiography was thought to require generators rated between 150 and 200 kW at the beginning of the 1970s. For a fast film sequence, larger focal spot (2.0 mm) X-ray tubes were usually utilized because small focal spot X-ray tubes could not withstand this level of loading.

For visceral and peripheral angiography, however, powerful generators and sizable focal spot X-ray tubes are no longer required or preferred. This is the outcome of two recent developments. The creation of rare earth screen-film systems is the first and most significant step. Before the development of rare earth systems, angiographic laboratories frequently employed screens like Kodak Xomatic Regular, which is made of barium strontium sulfate activated by europium. The speed of these screens was roughly twice that of par-speed screens. Presently on the market, rare earth screen-film systems can reach up to 12 times the par speed. No discernible loss of contrast or resolution has been made to achieve this remarkable increase in system speed.

The second innovation is the use of carbon fiber in serial film changer faceplates and angiographic tabletops. Compared to the materials previously used, carbon fiber transmits a significantly greater amount of the X-ray beam due to its low absorption. The combination of low-absorption tabletops, film changer plates, and rare earth screen-film systems has significantly decreased the power needs for angiographic facilities. Power outputs from generators greater than 85–100 kW are no longer required. Large focal spot X-ray tubes are also no longer necessary unless there are extremely rare circumstances. Even in large patients, focal spots with a nominal size of 0.6–0.7mm and a power rating of 40–60 kW are more than sufficient for the majority of abdominal angiography procedures. We advise that one X-ray tube in a lab set up for biplane angiography have a focal spot combination of 0.3–0.6 mm and the other a focal spot combination of 0.6–1.2 mm. Magnification angiography uses the 0.3 mm focal spot; these are typically rated at 10–15 kW. Large patients and digital vascular imaging of the abdomen would use the 1.2 mm focal spot, which is typically rated at 100–120 kW. The 0.6 mm focal spots are typically used in non-magnification angiograms that are standard.

The angiographer needs to consider other advantageous characteristics of angiographic X-ray tubes in addition to focal spot size. Adequate heat storage capacities and heat dissipation techniques are required for both the anode and tube housing. It is essential to have a relatively large focal track diameter (100 mm or more) and high-speed rotation (at least 9,000 rpm). A small focal spot size and enhanced heat distribution and dissipation within the target itself are made possible by a relatively small target angle. The target angle must, however, be sufficiently large to offer sufficient field coverage. A 10°–12° target angle is required to cover a 14 x 14 inch (35.6 x 35.6 cm) field at a 40 inch (101.6 cm) source-image distance; this would be regarded as the ideal target angle for angiographic X-ray tubes.

10.4.3. Generator Switching and Rectification Characteristics

Efficient and quick switching of the tube load is crucial in an angiographic generator, with the option of primary or secondary switching on either side of the high-voltage transformer. Secondary switching, though more complex and pricey, utilizes constant potential circuits with triode or tetrode switch tubes, or grid-controlled X-ray tubes. This method is best suited for cineangiographic labs requiring fast cine pulses and frequent exposures. Generators in non-cine angiographic labs can make do with a simpler three-phase, 12-pulse generator that incorporates silicon-controlled rectifiers for quick interrogation times. It is unnecessary to have secondary switching in these labs, as it could significantly increase the cost without adding much value.

10.4.4. Multiangulation Rotational Mounting Units: Advantages

The main manufacturers of X-ray equipment have created C- and U-arm units in recent years for mounting image intensifiers and X-ray tubes. As part of the process of outfitting new angiographic laboratories at the Brigham and Women's Hospital, researchers assessed four of these units (Philips Poly Diagnost UPI, CGR Arcomax, GE L/U System, and Siemens Angioskop). Comparable units have been designed by other businesses or are currently being designed. Every system has unique design elements, benefits, and disadvantages of its own. All of them have the same arrangement with the X-ray tube on one side of the C- or U-arm mount and the image intensifier and serial film changer on the other. The intensifier and changer are locked together so that one is positioned next to the X-ray beam and out of the way, and the other is centered towards the beam. When using serial filming for fluoroscopy, the two can be quickly switched out. If desired, a spot film camera can be installed on the image intensifier.

One of the main benefits of the new C- or U-arm mounting systems is that patients no longer need to be moved from the supine position to obtain oblique or sagittal projections. The patient can stay still on the angiographic table while the C or U arm is adjusted to provide various angles in different directions. This allows for a wide range of compound angles to be achieved, depending on the specific study and individual anatomy variations. Additionally, digital imaging quality is improved when the patient is relaxed and motionless in the supine position for the duration of the procedure.

The ability to quickly rotate the arm to obtain fluoroscopy anywhere between the direct frontal and direct lateral positions is another significant benefit of these units. When performing procedures like percutaneous cholangiography, common bile duct decompression, percutaneous nephrostomy, and abdominal biopsy that require inserting a needle through multiple tissue planes into deeply situated abdominal structures, fluoroscopy—whether at any angle or without requiring the patient to move—is especially helpful. During such procedures, accurate depth determination is useful, and it is obviously advantageous to be able to determine depth without moving the patient once the needle has been inserted. Similarly, the ability to fluoroscope and obtain films in multiple projections without moving the patient greatly facilitates the process of performing procedures such as tumor embolization and percutaneous transluminal angioplasty. This allows for the determination of the position of the catheter tip for both the lesion and the arterial bifurcations.

Quickly switching between the image intensifier and serial film changer is beneficial in angiography. This allows the angiographer to use fluoroscopy to accurately locate the center of the area of interest and adjust the angulation as needed. Once the centering and angling are determined, the image intensifier can be swiftly moved aside while the film changer automatically aligns itself with the X-ray beam for filming. This process ensures fast and accurate serial filming with minimal errors and time elapsed.

10.4.5. Multiangulation Rotational Mounting Units: Pitfalls

Despite the significant benefits that these C and U units offer, they have the following drawbacks.

10.4.5.1. Access to the Patient

There are various ways to mount these units on the ceiling or the floor. In certain systems, access to a patient's femoral or axillary regions may be impeded by the main beam of this mount or the crossbar portion of the C or U arm. The femoral approach is the main method used by most angiographers for visceral, peripheral, and interventional procedures. A lot of people also frequently employ the left axillary approach; others frequently use the translumbar approach instead of the axillary approach. In any case, the angiographer considering purchasing one of these devices needs to make sure that the main suspension beam's and the C or U arm's crossbar portion's configurations won't obstruct access to commonly used anatomic regions.

10.4.5.2. Rapidity and Convenience of Inversion of the Unit

Fluoroscoping, which involves filming with a second X-ray tube over the table and a film changer under it, is a technique most angiographers are familiar with. Fluoroscoping involves placing an X-ray tube under the table and an image intensifier over it. By doing this, the radiation exposure of the operator during fluoroscopy and the object-film distance during serial filming are reduced. To maintain this practice while utilizing a C- or U-arm mounting unit, it is evident that the process must begin with the fluoroscopy configuration of the "X-ray tube under," then be inverted to the filming configuration of the "X-ray tube over." This option is currently unavailable from one of the four units (GE); it can only be utilized with the image intensifier-film changer arm over the table and the X-ray tube under the table. The C or U arm can be inverted using the other three units, though the degree of difficulty and inconvenience will vary. Although the manufacturers emphasize the benefits of being able to invert these systems, in practice, inverting the unit can be difficult and time-consuming when patients are draped and have intravenous lines in place. When fluoroscopy or serial filming is required, it is more convenient—for us and other users of these units—to complete the process with the X-ray tube either over or under the table rather than attempting to invert the system each time.

This method avoids annoying delays during procedures, but it also has drawbacks of its own. Throughout the fluoroscopy procedure, the angiographer will be exposed to a slightly higher level of radiation because the X-ray tube will be above the table. In certain systems, the space needed to accommodate the combination of image intensifier and film changer beneath the angiographic table is so large that the table needs to be raised to the point where angiographers who are shorter than approximately 183 cm would find it difficult to perform procedures.

Furthermore, when the X-ray technologist tries to set the collimator for serial filming, the localizer light delineating the radiographic field won't be easily visible because the X-ray tube will be under the table the entire time. Also, because of the increased object-film distance when the changer is positioned over the patient, geometric unsharpness is introduced when filming posterior structures like the kidneys and aorta. If the angiographer plans to perform this maneuver in every situation, he must either accept these limitations or carefully assess the level of difficulty in inverting the unit.

10.4.5.3. Limitation in Choice of Serial Film Changers

The Elema Schonanden AOT is one of the most popular film changers. All C-on-U-arm systems are unable to accommodate this change due to its size and weight. Schonander Puck film changers are used by Siemens, GE, and Philips systems. A changer specifically made for this unit, the Maximax, is used by the CGR system. According to our observations, the Puck film changer is incredibly dependable, simple to load and unload, and conveniently card-programmed. In contrast to the AOT model, it does, however, have some shortcomings. It can only take three exposures per second (as opposed to six for the AOT), and the film magazines can only hold 20 films (as opposed to 30 for the AOT). Since the majority of angiographic studies don't call for more than 20 films or an exposure rate higher than three/sec, these aren't significant disadvantages. On the other hand, a greater filming rate might enhance an infrequent pulmonary arteriogram or aortic arch study. The primary disadvantage of using Puck film changers is that they are only useful for biplane filming, where the maximum exposure rate that can be achieved is only 1:5 films/sec. However, the Puck film changer is really good overall.

10.4.5.4. Fluoroscopic and Radiographic Coverage of the Lower Extremities for Peripheral Arteriography

In any angiographic laboratory, peripheral angiography is likely the most frequently used diagnostic procedure. All of the manufacturers claim that peripheral arteriography can be performed with a table shift device on their C- or U-arm systems. Nevertheless, in certain systems, the table's design, the location of the unit's main suspension beam, or the crossbar portion of the C or U arm all have an impact on how far the table can travel. The patient may need to be positioned on the table in one direction for fluoroscopy of the pelvis and abdomen during catheter insertion, then turned around to the opposite direction for serial filming during the peripheral runoff arteriogram in laboratories equipped only for single-plane filming, with the X-ray tube and changer mounted on the C or U arm. When the angiographer employs the left axillary approach, the issue is exacerbated, necessitating fluoroscopic and/or radiographic coverage from the shoulders to the ankles. A fully draped, catheterized patient is very difficult to turn around, and doing so almost certainly breaks sterile protocol. Laboratories that are set up for biplane filming and have a separate floor-mounted film changer and an extra X-ray tube mounted on the ceiling can significantly reduce this issue. These remove the requirement for the patient to change direction. The floor-mounted changer is usually placed between the C or U arm and the angiographic table base. The amount of available radiographic and fluoroscopic coverage for any C- or U-arm system should be carefully considered by the angiographer. Should this prove insufficient for peripheral arteriography, it will be imperative to incorporate an additional X-ray tube mounted on the ceiling and a floor-mounted film changer. This is one of the most compelling justifications for biplane capability in spite of the significantly higher cost.

10.4.5.5. Orientation of the Changer

With all four units, the film changer face moves in unison with the X-ray tube and stays perpendicular to the X-ray beam during standard angulation of the C or U arm in the transverse plane. In the Siemens, CGR, and GE systems, the film changer face stays perpendicular to the X-ray beam whether cranial or caudal angulation of the X-ray tube is used. With the Philips system, the film changer face stays parallel to the patient's long axis during cranial on caudal angulation rather than remaining perpendicular to the X-ray beam. This means that, depending on the degree of cranial or caudal angulation, the X-ray beam must inevitably strike the film changer face at an angle less than 90°. The image is somewhat distorted as a result. This distortion might not sit well with some angiographers. Our experience has shown that this is really a small drawback, offset by the fact that the film changer faceplate stays close to the patient's body the entire time, reducing object-film distance and increasing resolution.

10.4.5.6. Radiation Protection

Regarding the radiation exposure to the operator resulting from the use of these four units, relatively little is currently known. The fact that the X-ray tube was placed over the angiographic table for fluoroscopy instead of under it—due to convenience or necessity—may have a substantial impact on this. An unshielded X-ray tube and collimator are mounted together on one side of the C on U arm with the Siemens, GE, and CGR units. The lead housing of the Philips device encloses the collimator and X-ray tube. By decreasing leakage through the collimator and tube housing, this may improve protection. Mounting movable leaded glass shields—which can be swung to a desired position between the angiographer and the X-ray beam—on the ceiling or the unit itself varies depending on the manufacturer. Radiation safety is obviously very important when planning an angiographic laboratory, and more information is needed to assess how adequate the radiation safety is with each of these installations.

10.4.5.7. Generator Control Panel

The generator control panel's degree of flexibility varies greatly between manufacturers. While some units only permit step-by-step adjustments of 3–6 kV, others enable continuously variable kilovoltage selection.

The choice of milliampere-second (mAs) is likewise made in steps on certain units; neither the milliamperage nor the precise exposure time are indicated other than through the use of a chart. If an unintentionally high mAs is chosen, the device will automatically adjust by extending exposure time to an unacceptable degree.

Other units allow the user to select the desired duration of exposure; the resulting mAs is medicated after the milliamperage is automatically maximized in compliance with tube loading limits. With this kind of programming, one can make small changes to the radiography technique by changing the exposure time or the kilovoltage; the technologist determines the exposure time, which can never be unintentionally extended.

When choosing radiographic factors, technologists should try to minimize error and maximize flexibility in generator controls. Continuously variable voltage is preferable to step-only voltage selection because rare earth screens respond nonlinearly to changes in voltage. Additionally, rather than just allowing the selection of mAs, it is better for the control panel to allow the selection of a specific exposure time and to indicate the resulting mAs to be used for filming.

10.4.5.8. Collision Protection

During procedures, there is a significant risk of collision when manipulating these units. Angiogenous tables are often moved laterally, raised, or lowered. In the transverse plane, the C or U arms are rotated around the patient. It is possible to add caudal or cranial angulation. Parts of the C- or U-arm unit will almost certainly collide with the angiographic table, the table stand, the floor, other mounted accessories, or the unwary patient at some point during the procedure. Sensing equipment needs to be placed carefully and made with impact prevention or reduction in mind.

10.4.5.9. Location and Design of Unit Controls

To enable the angiographer or X-ray technologist to easily raise or lower the angiographic tabletop, shift it horizontally, raise or lower the C or U arm, rotate the arm in the transverse or sagittal plane, collimate the fluoroscopic beam, and choose different image intensifier modes, well-designed control devices are required at two separate locations in the angiographic laboratory. The ease of use and simplicity of operation of these controls varies significantly between the four units.

10.4.5.10. Room Size and Configuration

These units typically occupy a sizable amount of floor space and are rather large. A unit that is being considered for installation must be able to fit into the angiographic laboratory's designated size and shape. Planning for a second floor-mounted film changer and an additional ceiling-mounted X-ray tube is also necessary if biplane operation is being considered.

We think that overall, the benefits of the multiangulation rotational mounting units far exceed the disadvantages, despite the possibility of some unwanted features.

The increased adaptability offered by these units is especially crucial given the two significant developments in cardiovascular radiology over the last few years: the explosive growth of digital vascular imaging and interventional techniques. Their disadvantages can be significantly mitigated with careful preparation and consideration. The manufacturers are currently considering changes, enhancements, and even completely new designs that should further increase the efficacy of these systems (Saine and Tyler, 2002; Youssef, 2008; Ikari et al, 2005; Campeau, L 1989; Ikari et al, 2010).

10.5. Methods of Monitoring Patients

An angiography is a diagnostic procedure that checks for blood vessel blockages using X-ray images. Your doctor can see how blood flows through blood vessels in specific body parts thanks to this test. To determine the source of an artery or vein problem, they perform an angiography on your legs, kidneys, neck, heart, or other regions.

10.5.1. Indications

If you have symptoms that point to a blocked, damaged, or malformed artery, your doctor might advise angiography. An angiography test helps your doctor identify the extent of blood vessel damage and the cause of the issue. Your doctor can diagnose and/or treat the following conditions with the aid of an angiography test:

- Coronary artery disease
- Peripheral artery disease.
- Atherosclerosis
- Blood clots
- Aneurysm

During an angiography, your doctor will inject contrast dye into your body so that an X-ray machine can see it. Your blood vessel blockages and blood flow are depicted graphically on a screen.

10.5.2. Preparation

Your doctor might want to test your blood's clotting capacity before your angiography procedure. They also want to confirm that your kidneys are functioning normally. The night before your exam, after midnight, adhere to these instructions:

- Always get your doctor's approval before stopping any medication, especially anticoagulants and antiplatelet medications.
- If your healthcare professional approves:
- Avoid taking aspirin or any products containing aspirin.
- Do not take blood thinners for 72 hours before or 24 hours after the test.
- Do not take clopidogrel for five days before the scheduled date of the test.
- Take your other medicines as usual.
- If you have diabetes, find out when and how to take your medication, including insulin, by speaking with your doctor.

Observe all advice provided by your healthcare provider. On the day of your angiography, you'll need to:

- Keep your valuables at home, including jewelry.
- Make arrangements for someone you can trust to drive you home.
- Bring a list of the current medications and allergies.
- Inform your healthcare providers that you have diabetes.
- Change into a hospital gown and lie down on a specialized X-ray table.
- Consult with your healthcare provider to go over the guidelines, inquiries, and medical background.

10.5.3. During the Test

The location of the catheter will be made numb by the healthcare professional before the angiography procedure. Your blood vessels are accessed with a needle, and a wire is inserted through the needle. Carefully and slowly insert the catheter into your artery until the tip reaches the necessary examination area of the blood vessel. A tiny amount of dye or contrast material should be injected into the blood vessel and catheter. You might flush or feel the urge to urinate for the first few seconds after doing this. Get X-rays. See where the contrast agent travels on the X-ray screen to determine the direction and velocity of blood flow within your blood vessels.

If your physician finds a blockage, an angioplasty might be done right away. With this technique, the blockage is forced up against the arterial wall using a tiny balloon. If the angioplasty improves blood flow and leaves less than 30% of the blockage after the procedure, you might only need one.

You might need a stent if an angioplasty is unable to create an aperture big enough for blood to flow through. This tiny metal tube stays in your blood vessel to maintain its open state. This can be done right away by your provider after your angioplasty. If a stent is not the best option for a particular patient, bypass surgery is the suggested alternative.

10.5.4. After the Test

After removing the catheter, your medical professional will bandage the punctured area. To halt or prevent bleeding, they will apply pressure to the bandaged area for a minimum of fifteen minutes. You will need to stay in bed for four to six hours if the doctors insert the catheter through your leg. This lessens the possibility of bleeding from your incision. Your provider will evaluate you and go over at-home instructions with you before you head home.

10.5.5. Recovery

After your angiography, you ought to be able to check out of the hospital on the same day. For the next two days after you get back home, avoid bending over or stooping over anything heavier than 4 kg. This should stop any bleeding from the incision. After an angiography, some patients might have to stay the night in the hospital.

10.5.6. Complications

There are very few possible hazards connected to angiography. Nevertheless, issues may arise in the region where your healthcare provider made the skin incision to access your artery. Less than 1% of cases have angiography issues. These are the typical risks associated with an angiography procedure that pertain to the site of puncture:

- Bruises (common and go away in one to three weeks)
- Bleeding
- Infection
- Pain
- Kidney issues
- An allergic reaction to the contrast material (dye).
- Injury to blood vessels.
- A blood vessel blockage that could cause a heart attack or stroke (rarely).
- A blood vessel leak (rarely).

10.6. Basic Principles of Electrocardiography

An electrocardiogram, or ECG or EKG for short, is a medical test result that shows the electrical activity and rhythm of the heart during repeated cardiac cycles. The ECG strip, also known as ECG tracing, is grid paper on which it is printed. Electrocardiography is the process of creating an electrocardiogram. Using specialized electrodes over particular body parts, the cardiac impulses are recorded on the skin during this non-invasive medical procedure.

The primary goal of an ECG is to identify and treat any underlying heart structural abnormalities or cardiovascular problems. One of the most popular tests that cardiologists order to learn more about a patient's cardiac electrical functioning is electrocardiography.

10.6.1. Electrocardiogram Instrumentation

An ECG machine with a set of electrodes connected to a central signal processor via lead wires, a monitor, and a printer to display and print the ECG is used to perform an ECG test. A typical 12-lead ECG machine has 10 electrodes that are used to receive, gather, and transmit the electric potentials (biopotentials) from our bodies. Lead wires transport the biopotentials that the electrodes have collected to the central impulse processing device. The received biopotential is amplified, filtered, and processed by the central ECG machine to create ECG waves at predetermined intervals and segments. To create an ECG, the processed signals are printed on grid paper and shown on the monitor.

10.6.2. Principle of Electrocardiogram

The cardiac action potential and cardiac conduction are the foundation of the ECG. The cardiac action potential is produced by the SA node and is transmitted through the cardiac conduction pathway, changing the membrane voltage (potential) across the cardiomyocyte membrane. The cardiac cycle continues to run as a result of this alteration in the cardiac action potential. The cardiac impulse travels via the heart, permeates the surrounding tissue, and ultimately ends up on our skin. The electrodes of the ECG machine pick up this electric impulse in the skin and process it to create an ECG.

10.6.3. Procedure of Obtaining an Electrocardiogram

Assist the patient in falling asleep in a comfortable, relaxed position on a bed. Make sure there are no electrical or metallic items on the patient. Secure the electrodes in their designated spots. Ten electrodes are affixed to the patient's body at designated locations for a 12-lead ECG. The electrodes on each arm are called the RA, LA, RL, and LL electrodes. It is recommended to place the RA electrode on the right arm, the LA electrode on the left arm, the RL electrode on the right leg, and the LL electrode on the left leg (Figure 10.3).

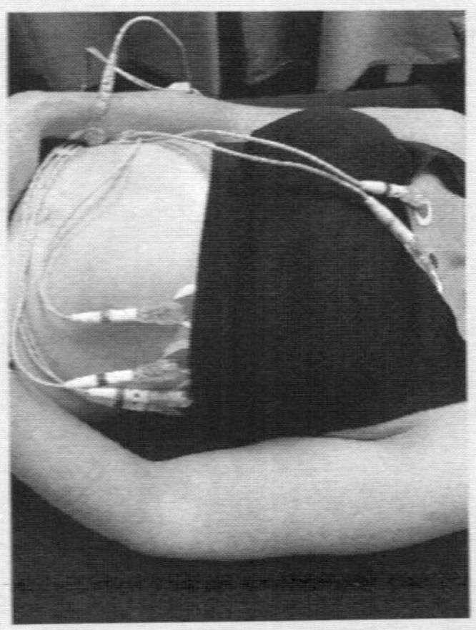

Figure 10.3. *A patient undergoing an ECG.*

Source: By Johnorchard-Ownwork, CCBY-SA4.0, https://commons.wikimedia.org/w/index.php?curid=91769052.

The six chest electrodes are numbered V1 through V6. Just to the right and left of the sternum, respectively, are the fourth intercostal spaces where the V1 and V2 are attached. The fifth intercostal space in the mid-clavicular line is where the V4 is attached. Attached between the V2 and V4 is the V3. In the left anterior axillary line, the V5 is attached horizontally to the left of the V4. In the mid-axillary line, the V6 is positioned horizontally to the left of the V5.

The ECG machine is turned on and the electrodes are connected to lead wires. The ECG machine is an automated device that creates an ECG by automatically recording cardiac electric impulse activity. The leads are cut off from the electrodes and the electrodes are detached after a sufficient ECG has been recorded.

10.6.4. Types of Electrocardiogram

These include:

- **Resting ECG:** This is the standard type of ECG commonly used for diagnostic purposes in hospitals. It is typically conducted with the patient lying still in a bed.
- **Exercise ECG:** It is the ECG recorded during physical activity, usually cycling a stationary bike or walking on a treadmill. This test, also known as a stress test, is used to track the heart's electrical activity when under physical stress.
- **Ambulatory ECG:** It is a kind of ECG that shows a heart's continuous electrical activity for at least 24 hours. In this kind, the patient wears a tiny, portable ECG device called a Holter monitor around their waist and is permitted to resume regular work for at least a day. The ECG is examined from the Holter

machine after the predetermined amount of time.

10.6.5. Waves in a Normal Electrocardiogram

The three normal waves are; the P-wave, the QRS-complex, and the T-wave.

- **P-wave:** Atrial depolarization can be seen in the ECG as the first minor upward wave. It is an illustration of the electrical activity that starts atrial systole, i.e., impulse that the SA node produces and sends right before the beginning of atrial systole.
- **QRS-Complex:** The second, larger, upright, triangular-shaped wave that is sharply steeper and represents rapid ventricular depolarization is called the QRS complex. The QRS complex is made up of three distinct waves: the S wave denotes the sharp descending deflection in the larger upright triangular wave of an ECG, the R wave the sharp ascending deflection, and the Q wave the initial downward deflection. The ventricular depolarization or ventricular systole phases of a cardiac cycle correspond with the QRS complex.
- **T-wave:** It is the last upward deflection in the shape of a dome that indicates ventricular repolarization. The U-wave, a low amplitude, hardly perceptible small upward deflection, appears in some ECGs immediately after the T-wave. This wave is thought to be caused by the repolarization of the interventricular septum.

10.6.6. Intervals in a Normal Electrocardiogram

The interval between the onsets of two waves in an ECG is measured and examined. These intervals of time correspond to the length of time impulses need to travel through the cardiac conduction pathway in order to initiate a synchronized cycle of the heart wall's depolarization and repolarization. These time periods are termed 'intervals' and there are two main intervals, viz. both the QT and PR intervals.

- **PR Interval:** The time interval between the start of the P-wave and the start of the QRS-complex on an ECG represents it. The PR interval is the amount of time the cardiac impulse needs to travel from the SA node to the ventricles via the AV bundle, atria, and ventricles. Usually, it takes between 120 and 200 milliseconds.
- **QT Interval:** In an ECG, it is shown as the interval between the beginning of the QRS complex and the conclusion of the T wave. It stands for the amount of time that passes between successive ventricular depolarization and repolarization. Typically, it lasts less than 440 milliseconds.

10.6.7. Segments in a Normal Electrocardiogram

Between two successive waves, there is a flat horizontal line, i.e., in an ECG, a "segment" is the transition between the end of one wave and the start of another. An ECG has two primary segments, namely both the ST and PR segments.

- **PR Segment:** The PR segment is the flat line that appears between the end of the P-wave and the start of the QRS complex. It is a representation of the interval of time between the ventricular and atrial systoles. It takes a little bit more time than 440 milliseconds.

- **ST Segment:** The electrically neutral region between the end of ventricular depolarization and the start of ventricular repolarization is represented by the flat line between the QRS complex and T wave. It typically lasts for 80 milliseconds.

10.6.8. Interpretation of ECG

Only trained medical personnel analyze and interpret an ECG. They focus mainly on the P wave, QRS complex, T wave, PR interval, QT interval, PR segment, and ST segment while reading an ECG. They study the elevation and depression of each wave, as well as the duration of the waves, segments, and intervals. Additionally, they analyze the heart rate, rhythm, and axis on an ECG. An ECG report is then interpreted based on the collective result of all these various components.

The following are the results of a normal ECG:

1. Heart Rate: Normal heart rate of 60 to 100 beats per minute
2. Heart Rhythm: Heart rhythm will be consistent and even
3. PR Interval: 0.12 to 0.20 seconds
4. QRS Duration: 0.06 to 0.10 seconds
5. QT Interval: 0.40 seconds
6. ST Segment: 0.08 seconds
7. P-wave
    i. Upright, uniform, and consistent before each QRS complex.
    ii. P duration < 0.12 seconds
    iii. P amplitude < 2.5 mm
8. T-wave: Upright in lead I, II, V3 to V6, and inverted in aVR.

10.6.9. Applications of ECG

- Identifying arrhythmias and associated heart conditions.
- Investigating the electrical activity of the heart and its cardiac cycle.
- Evaluating heart attacks and heart diseases.
- It is employed to assess recovery following cardiac surgery or medication.
- It is used in conjunction with ECHO to assess the heart's and the valves' overall structural and functional health. used to monitor the heart's response to stress.

10.6.10. Limitations of an ECG

- It only offers information regarding the electrical activity of the heart; it makes no mention of the anatomy of the heart.
- The body's electric potential, issues with the electrodes, and the presence of metallic or electrical objects nearby can all lead to false results in ECG reports.
- Because the interpretation of an ECG report is subjective, different healthcare professionals may report different results.
- The ECG only records electrical activity for a short while.
- Future cardiac events, the development of aberrant tissues and clots, and certain cardiac events unrelated to cardiac electric potential cannot be predicted by

it (Saine and Tyler, 2002; Youssef, 2008; Ikari et al, 2005; Campeau, L 1989; Ikari et al, 2010).

10.7. Establishing Vessel Access

In order to take blood or administer medication to a patient, a vascular access procedure involves inserting a flexible, sterile plastic tube called a catheter into a blood vessel. Chemotherapy, long-term IV feeding, intravenous (IV) antibiotic therapy, and blood transfusions are among the medical procedures that may require the use of a catheter. Vascular access offers a painless method of giving medicine or taking blood while sparing patients from the anxiety of frequent needle sticks.

Inform your physician of any potential pregnancy as well as any recent ailments, allergies, and prescription drugs you take, including aspirin and herbal supplements. It is possible that you will be instructed to cease taking blood thinners, aspirin, or nonsteroidal anti-inflammatory drugs (NSAIDs) a few days before your procedure. Additionally, you might be told to avoid eating or drinking anything for a few hours before. Wear loose, comfy clothes and leave your jewelry at home. You might be required to don a gown. Even though you will typically be discharged from the hospital after this procedure, you should still arrange for a ride home.

10.7.1. Vascular Access Procedures

A flexible, sterile thin plastic tube, known as a catheter, is inserted into a blood vessel during a vascular access procedure to enable efficient blood collection or delivery of drugs, blood products, or nourishment over a period of weeks, months, or even years.

Simple intravenous (IV) lines work well in short-term applications, but they are not appropriate for long-term use. A special, longer catheter known as a central venous catheter can be used when an IV line is required for an extended length of time and/or when a more secure venous access is required. The catheter can stay in place for a short while (days) or a long time (weeks to years), allowing for easy and frequent access over the required duration without requiring the patient to have additional skin punctures. To lower the risk of infection, the catheter is often implanted entirely or partially beneath the skin for longer-term access.

Vascular access procedures involve inserting a catheter under the skin into a vein, usually in the arms, legs, or neck, and then placing the catheter's tip into a large central vein that drains close to the heart.

10.7.2. Some Common Uses of the Procedure

Patients undergo vascular access procedures when they require:

- Intravenous antibiotic treatment.
- Medications.
- Chemotherapy, or anti-cancer drugs.
- Long-term intravenous (IV) feeding for nutritional support.
- Repeated drawing of blood samples.
- Hemodialysis is a procedure used to treat individuals with malfunctioning kidneys. It involves taking blood out of the body, cleaning it of waste and excess fluid, and then putting it back into the body using a specialized machine and tubing.

Access catheters may also be used for:

- Blood transfusions.
- Patients who are difficult to keep or administer a basic, functional IV line.

For similar reasons, vascular access procedures are also frequently carried out in children using similar techniques and child-sized devices. Children may need vascular access procedures for the following reasons, for example:

- Intravenous antibiotic treatment.
- Chemotherapy.
- Medications:
  - when the child is not able to safely swallow medication.
  - that are more effective when given by IV such as heart (cardiac) medications.
- Long term intravenous (IV) feeding for nutritional support.
- Hemodialysis.
- Blood transfusions.
- Children who have difficulty receiving or maintaining a simple functional IV line.
- The need for frequent and repeated drawing of blood samples (Harold and Dauerman, 2007; Hon et al, 2010).

10.7.3. Preparation

Your doctor may perform blood tests before your procedure to assess kidney function and determine whether or not your blood clots normally. All of the medications you take, including herbal supplements, should be disclosed to your doctor. Enumerate all allergies, with a focus on those to contrast agents, general anesthesia, and local anesthetic. Before your procedure, your doctor might advise you to stop taking blood thinners, aspirin, or nonsteroidal anti-inflammatory drugs (NSAIDs). If a woman is pregnant, she should always disclose this to her doctor and the technician. To prevent radioactively exposing the fetus during pregnancy, doctors won't do many tests. If an X-ray is required, the physician will take measures to reduce the infant's exposure to radiation.

You'll get detailed instructions on how to get ready, along with any adjustments you need to make to your regular medication regimen. In addition to prescription drugs, your doctor might advise you to fast for a few hours before the procedure. Make arrangements for a ride home following your procedure. For the exam, you might have to take off some clothes and/ or change into a gown. Take off any jewelry, eyeglasses, removable dental appliances, and any metal objects or clothing that could obstruct the X-ray images.

10.7.4. Equipment Used

Vascular access catheters, guide wires, X-ray and ultrasound machines, and needles are used in this procedure. A radiographic table, one or more X-ray tubes, and a video monitor are usually used for this examination. X-rays are transformed into video images via fluoroscopy. It is used by doctors to monitor and direct procedures. The video is generated by the X-ray machine and a detector that is hung over the examination table.

With the aid of the X-ray equipment, the catheter and wire can be safely advanced and the catheter tip can be precisely positioned to maximize the catheter's functionality. Ultrasound scanners are comprised of a transducer that scans the body, a video display screen, and a console with a computer and electronics. The patient is not exposed to radiation during an ultrasound.

A vein that is suitable for the implantation of a catheter is evaluated and identified using ultrasound. Additionally, it gives the interventional radiologist the capacity to locate suitable veins, some of which may be deeper and larger than veins that are visible or feelable on the skin's surface. To enhance image quality, transducer-skin contact is improved with the use of ultrasound gel. When performing a venous puncture (or access), an interventional radiologist can advance the needle straight into the vein with the aid of ultrasound guidance, which offers real-time or live visualization. By doing so, the interventional radiologist can reduce the risk of potential complications like bleeding and increase the likelihood that the venous puncture will be successful.

A vascular access catheter is more resilient and resistant to infection than the catheter used in a typical intravenous (IV) line. The way these catheters are made allows them to reach into the main central vein that is closest to the heart. Depending on their intended purpose, catheters differ in size, length, and lumen count.

The major types are as follows:

- A peripherally inserted central catheter, or PICC, is a lengthy catheter that inserts into the major vein (i.e., inferior or superior vena cava) close to the heart from an arm or leg vein. It usually offers central IV access for a few weeks, but it can stay in place for several months. When a catheter is positioned so that its tip stays in a sizable vein but does not extend into the largest central vein, it is referred to as a "midline catheter." Some may be suitable for use with CT contrast injections (manufactured for forceful contrast injections), and they may have one or two lumens.
- A non-tunneled central catheter is intended to be inserted via a comparatively large, more central vein, such as the femoral vein in the groin or the jugular vein in the neck. It may have a larger caliber than a PICC. The entry point of the vein used is not far from the skin exit point of a non-tunneled central catheter.
- A cuff that promotes tissue growth around a tunneled catheter may help keep it in place inside the body. Catheters that are tunneled come in various sizes and varieties. A catheter that is tunneled is safe and simple to use. The catheter can stay more securely in place for longer periods of time because the tunnel and cuff reduce the chance of catheter infection.
- Similar to tunneled catheters, a port catheter, also known as a subcutaneous implantable port, is a device that consists of a catheter attached to a small reservoir that is inserted beneath the skin. The catheter and reservoir are positioned entirely beneath the skin. Every time the catheter is used, the patient's skin is punctured; however, once the placement incision heals, there are no limitations on bathing or showering.

Additional equipment, such as an intravenous line (IV), an ultrasound machine, and blood pressure and heart rate monitors, may be used during this procedure (Harold and Dauerman, 2007; Hon et al, 2010).

10.7.5. Performing the Procedure

The overlying skin where the vascular catheter is to be inserted is cleaned and covered with a sterile surgical drape after the best location for the procedure has been determined. Before the procedure begins, the operator and assistant will put on sterile gowns and gloves. Vascular access procedures are typically carried out in an operating room or an interventional radiology suite by a specially trained interventional radiologist. At your bedside, a midline catheter and certain PICC lines might be inserted without the use of imaging guidance. These are threaded through a sizable vein in the upper arm and inserted through a vein close to the elbow.

These operations can be carried out either as an inpatient or an outpatient. The medical professional or nurse will place you on your back. In order to administer sedative medication intravenously before, during, or after the procedure, a nurse or technologist may place an intravenous (IV) line into a vein in your hand or arm. Usually, sedative drugs are not needed for PICC implantation. Your physician will apply a local anesthetic to numb the area. Before the area gets numb, it might burn or sting for a short while.

The doctor will make a very small skin incision at the site.

- **PICC:** A small needle is inserted into the arm vein and a small guide wire is advanced into the large central vein, known as the superior vena cava, under X-ray (fluoroscopy) guidance by the doctor, physician assistant, or nurse in order to place a PICC line. After that, the catheter is positioned by passing it over the guide wire. Next, the guide wire is taken out. In the event that X-ray guidance is not used, a chest X-ray is taken after insertion to verify the location of the catheter tip.
- **Non-tunneled Central Catheter:** A comparatively larger vein, such as the femoral vein in the groin or the jugular vein in the neck, is used to insert these catheters.
- **Tunneled Catheter:** The doctor will make one small skin incision, usually in the lower neck, to place a tunneled catheter. The jugular vein at the base of the neck is typically punctured with a needle under ultrasound guidance, and under X-ray guidance (fluoroscopy), a small guide wire is advanced into the large central vein known as the superior vena cava. A tunnel beneath the skin is then created by making a second, smaller incision beneath the first. The catheter is inserted through the tunnel and into the vein using X-ray guidance. The tip of the catheter is inserted into the superior vena cava, which is the largest vein. The cuff is positioned beneath the skin in the catheter's tunneled path. It is usually composed of Dacron®. To help keep the catheter firmly in place, the doctor will finally sew up the end of the tunnel. Usually, the stitches don't need to be taken out until the catheter is removed.
- **Port Catheter:** Generally, two incisions are needed to implant a subcutaneous port (unless it's in the arm, in which case one incision may be enough). Underneath the skin is the port reservoir. A tiny skin incision is made, a little pocket is made beneath the skin for the port, and the incision is slightly longer than the device's diameter. The remainder of the process is comparable to inserting a central catheter through a tunnel. Upon completion of the procedure, a small, elevated area remains on your body at the reservoir site. The port ends in a sizable central

vein in the chest after passing through an access site in a vein of your arm, shoulder, or neck. Using a specialized needle, it is possible to repeatedly puncture the silicone covering the reservoir to gain access. Most implanted port types have a reservoir septum with a useful lifetime of roughly 1,000 punctures.

Incisions are secured with surgical glue, stitches, or specialized tape. If X-ray (fluoroscopy) was used during the placement procedure, an X-ray may be taken afterwards to make sure the catheter is positioned correctly, but it is usually not required. After that, the vascular access catheter that was implanted is operational. Before you leave for home, the nurse or doctor will take out your IV line. A smaller catheter and equipment suitable for the patient's size may be used for pediatric patients. The X-ray equipment settings will be changed to suitably lower the radiation dose needed to guide the catheter placement because children are smaller than adults.

Deeper sedation is commonly used for pediatric procedures, sometimes with the help of an anesthesiologist. It might be necessary for your child to fast for up to six hours prior to the procedure. Detailed instructions will be provided to you based on your child's age. Inform your doctor about any medications, latex allergies, X-ray dye allergies, and your child's past experiences with sedation. Tell your doctor about any past vascular access device placements, similar surgical procedures, or unique anatomical features for your child so they can determine the ideal spot for the device. Your child might have a preference for which arm to use if a PICC line needs to be inserted. You can talk to the doctor about this beforehand.

10.7.6. During the Procedure

Your body will have devices attached by the doctor or nurse to track your blood pressure and heart rate. When the nurse injects the local anesthetic and puts the IV line needle into your vein, you may experience a slight pinch. The site of the skin incision feels the most sensation. The physician will apply a local anesthetic to numb this area. When the doctor places the catheter in an artery or vein, you might feel pressure. You won't experience severe discomfort, though.

You will experience comfort, sedation, and relaxation if sedation is used during the procedure. The extent of your sedation will determine whether or not you stay awake. When the needle is inserted into the vein and the tunnel is formed, you might experience some pressure. Talk to the doctor or nurse if this starts to hurt so they can administer more local anesthetic. In the event that the arm is utilized to implant a PICC line, an upper arm tourniquet will be applied. To assist with the initial venous puncture and to help dilate the vein, a tourniquet may be used.

To place the catheter, you will need to lie flat for thirty to forty-five minutes. After the procedure, you should recover at home for the rest of the day if you are not spending the night at the hospital. The following day, you can carry on with your regular activities, but you shouldn't lift anything heavy. You might have soreness, bruising, and swelling in your shoulder, neck, or chest after a subcutaneous port or tunneled catheter is inserted, but these side effects go away in a few days. Painkillers might be useful at this point.

You will be given instructions on how to take care of the vascular access device that is specific to you and your incision(s). It's crucial to keep the catheter site dry and clean during the first week. Some doctors, but not all of them, will advise sponge bathing the area surrounding the catheter site, followed by cleaning it with peroxide, applying an antibiotic ointment, and bandaging it. After a week, you might be able to take a shower while covering the catheter site with a piece of plastic wrap. Swimming or taking a bath should not be done while the incision is submerged in water. Heparin solution flushing may be recommended for your catheter to help prevent blood clots from forming and obstructing it.

You should call the physician or nurse if you have any questions about your vascular access device or if:

- the device malfunctions.
- there is bleeding at the insertion site.
- you develop a fever.
- you notice redness, increased swelling, tenderness, warmth or fluid drainage at the catheter insertion site.

Usually, a medical professional removes vascular access catheters. Similar to how an IV is removed, nurses or technologists can remove PICC and non-tunneled central catheters and cover the site with a Band-Aid. A doctor will remove port catheters and tunneled catheters. Local anesthetic is used to numb the skin in order to remove these catheters. The port catheter must be removed through an incision. Removal is an out-patient procedure that takes less than an hour to complete. Until the incision heals completely after removal, the skin must be kept dry.

To ensure that your catheter is positioned correctly, your interventional radiologist will use X-ray imaging during the placement procedure or a chest X-ray taken right after the procedure. Your doctor will also use a needle, syringe, or catheter to inject fluid to test the functionality of your vascular access device (Harold and Dauerman, 2007; Hon et al, 2010).

10.7.7. Benefits

- With a central catheter, infusions of medication or nutritional substances are possible without the risks associated with intravenous (IV) therapy, such as local tissue damage from toxic drug leaks.
- Under many circumstances, inserting this kind of tube offers a straightforward and painless way to take blood or administer medication, nutrients, or both.
- The patient is spared the stress and discomfort of multiple needle sticks thanks to vascular access devices.
- When a patient needs to repeatedly enter the venous circulation over an extended period of time for any reason, the vascular access device is a very helpful solution. There are numerous designs available that are appropriate for various situations.
- Vascular access device placement is an excellent option for patients needing chemotherapy or other long-term care. Their arm veins won't get severely scarred, and they won't require an IV line to be inserted for every treatment.
- When medications or fluids that irritate the vein wall are required, a PICC is a great help. This method can be used to administer a variety of products, such as blood products and antibiotics. Frequent blood draws and IV feedings are two more uses for the catheter.
- Following implantation, a vascular access device may be used right away. Certain varieties can keep up their good performance for a year or more.

- When not in use, the devices are simply removed. For patients with severe kidney disease, a catheter may be the only means of gaining access to the circulatory system for hemodialysis.

10.7.8. Risks

Vascular access devices come with two types of risks: those that happen during or soon after placement and delayed risks that happen just because the device is inside your body. Some of the risks connected to implanting a vascular access device are as follows:

- There are risks associated with any procedure that involves inserting a catheter into a blood vessel. These dangers include bleeding or bruises at the puncture site, infection, and harm to the blood vessel. To reduce these risks, the physician will take appropriate measures.
- Soon after the catheter is inserted, an infection may appear at the site of the incision. If you closely adhere to the instructions regarding the incisions' healing care, the risk is reduced.
- There could be bleeding or hemorrhaging. By having a blood test beforehand to ensure that your blood clots normally, this risk can be reduced. The procedure might be delayed or you might get medicine or blood products to help with blood clotting if your blood is too thin.
- An extremely rare ailment known as a pneumothorax—a buildup of air in the chest that could result in the collapse of one lung—can strike a patient. This can happen if a vein in the neck or chest is used to insert a catheter or port, but not if an arm vein is used. When ultrasound or fluoroscopy is used to guide catheter placement, the risk is reduced. Significant reductions in the risk of pneumothorax occur when these catheters are placed by interventional radiologists under the guidance of appropriate imaging.
- While the catheter is being inserted, there may be a brief disruption to the heart's regular rhythm. During the procedure, the issue is readily identified and resolved by modifying the position of the catheter.
- Seldom will the catheter enter an artery as opposed to a vein. This will require the removal of the catheter. The artery then usually heals on its own, but on rare occasions, surgery is required to repair it.

10.7.8.1. Delayed Risks

- There are two possible delayed infection types: a bloodstream infection or a skin infection at the catheter or port insertion site. Following port placement, infections are less frequent. Washing your hands and the hands of anyone else who will be handling the device before flushing it or cleaning the insertion site can reduce the chance of a delayed infection. Every time the dressing is changed, the area needs to be thoroughly examined. Those with low white blood cell counts are more susceptible to infection.
- A break or hole in the catheter

could cause fluid to leak. By not always clamping the catheter in the same location and by never flushing it with excessive force, breaks can be prevented. Two crucial first aid steps are as follows: 1) place a sterile gauze pad on the skin to cover the break; and 2) clamp the catheter between the damaged portion and the skin insertion site. Although internal catheter fractures are uncommon, when they do occur, an X-ray of the chest will reveal the issue. Most of the time, open surgery is not necessary to remove the broken fragment.

- It's possible for the catheter to come loose by accident. The catheter could come out if it is not properly fastened to the skin. In the event that this occurs, call your doctor right away and apply pressure to the incision site with a sterile dressing.
- Breathlessness or chest pain could result from an emergency caused by a lot of air in the catheter. Should you experience dyspnea or chest pain as a result of air being forced into your vein via the catheter, you should immediately clamp the catheter, turn over onto your left side, and dial your local emergency telephone number. By making sure the catheter cap is tightened and by clamping the catheter both before and after syringe insertion, this issue can be avoided.
- A fibrin sheath or clot of blood can obstruct any kind of vascular access catheter. By carefully following directions for flushing the catheter, you can reduce the risk. Sometimes a medication injection can clear an occluded or closed catheter; other times, the catheter needs to be removed or replaced with a new one. On rare occasions, an additional interventional radiology procedure can "strip" the catheter and restore it to normal function.
- There could be swelling in the arm, shoulder, neck, or head if the vein where the catheter is positioned gets occluded, or closed off. If this happens, give your doctor a call right away. Sometimes removing the catheter is necessary to treat the clot, but it can also be treated with a blood thinner.
- Patients may occasionally feel as though their heartbeat is skipped or irregular, which could be connected to the catheter. Make a call to your doctor if this happens. To alleviate this, the catheter tip might need to be slightly readjusted.

10.7.9. Limitations of Vascular Access Procedures

While some varieties of central venous catheters can last for months or even years, most catheters need to be replaced due to poor functioning after a predetermined amount of time. Most implanted port types have a reservoir septum that lasts only roughly 1,000 punctures, making them unsuitable for patients who need IV access on a regular basis. Certain patients have extremely weak veins that make them unsuitable for the implantation of catheters. This usually happens when these access veins have been used for a long period of time (years of intravenous feeding, etc.). In these patients, finding a vein suitable for catheter implantation may be extremely challenging, necessitating the use of unusual venous entry sites (e.g., either via the liver or the back) (Harold and Dauerman, 2007; Hon et al, 2010).

10.8. Vessel Puncture Closure Devices

A vascular closure device is often a segment of collagen, a fibrous protein present in skin, bone, and connective tissue, a metallic clip, or a suture, which is a stitch used to quickly seal a tiny puncture in an artery following an angiography. The imaging of blood vessels that can be seen on real-time X-ray images or pictures is known as angiography. This aids in highlighting anomalies or providing direction for medical care. The femoral artery, a sizable artery that passes through the area of the groin, is frequently used for arterial access. A specialized physician must use a tiny needle to puncture the artery through the skin in order to gain access through this artery. Then, the puncture site is used to insert a plastic sheath or tube into the artery.

It will be necessary to remove the plastic sheath that allows access to the femoral artery after the angiographic procedure is finished. The artery will then have a tiny hole in it that is equal to the size of the plastic sheath. If treatment is not given, the hole will keep bleeding. Usually, the doctor or nurse will apply manual compression, placing their fingers directly over the location of the artery's hole, to stop the blood flow from it.

Depending on the size of the plastic sheath inserted into the artery, manual compression is typically very effective but may take ten to fifteen minutes or more. After the plastic sheath is removed, patients undergoing manual compression must lie flat in bed with their hips straight for at least four hours. Devices for vascular closure offer a substitute for manual compression. There is no need for continuous compression because these devices immediately seal the femoral artery access site.

10.8.1. Personnel

Proceduralists (such as vascular surgeons), first assistants (residents, fellows, Cath lab technicians, physician assistants), radiology technicians, and nursing staff are needed for the procedure. Depending on the precise nature of the procedure, the anesthesiologist may or may not be present.

10.8.2. Preparation

For the procedure, both groins should be prepared and draped. In order to have a baseline examination for comparison and to make sure the lower extremity's pulse does not change after the vascular access closure device is applied, we typically advise performing a thorough pulse exam prior to beginning the procedure. The pedal signals are marked with a pen and a Doppler device.

10.8.3. Technique or Treatment

It is important to remember a few general guidelines for all vascular access closure devices. Together with the assessment of anatomic landmarks and fluoroscopic guidance, the common femoral artery should be accessed under ultrasonographic guidance. For first access, a micropuncture kit should be utilized. The puncture site should be below the inguinal ligament and the most superior aspect of the femoral head. It should also avoid puncturing the superficial and deep femoral arteries, as well as any area of the artery that is heavily calcified. After inserting the micropuncture needle and wire, we typically nick the skin at the access site with a scalpel. Tissues are dispersed down to the artery's level using a hemostat. By removing extra tissue between the skin and the artery, this step aids in the later placement of the closure mechanism. The micropuncture wire is taken out after the 4F micropuncture catheter is positioned. To ensure that the access is placed appropriately, that the vessel is suitable for the closure device (particularly in terms of size and arterial plaque), and to rule out any complications from the access, such as dissection or perforation, a femoral angiogram is obtained with the image intensifier set to the appropriate obliquity (Figure 10.4).

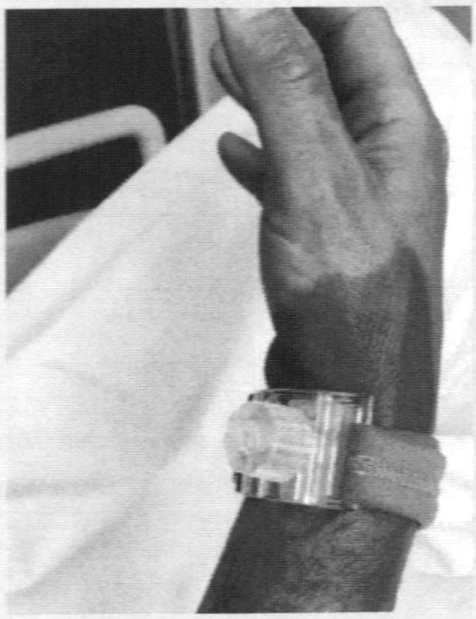

Figure 10.4. *A vascular closure device.*

Source: By Oyoyoy-Ownwork, CCBY-SA4.0, https://commons.wikimedia.org/w/index.php?curid=131586248.

10.8.4. Complications

There are three categories of complications related to vascular access closure devices.

- **Ischemic:** Vascular access closure devices can cause lower extremity ischemia, which may be associated with distal embolization or access artery stenosis or occlusion. It is crucial to choose a device based on the features of the access artery in order to reduce this kind of problem. Open surgical exploration is typically used to treat these complications. In certain instances, endovascular techniques have also been utilized.
- **Hemorrhagic:** If the device is inserted into a vessel that has undesirable features, like dense calcifications, or if it is positioned anatomically incorrectly (above the inguinal ligament), there is a greater chance of hemorrhagic complications. Increased age, an interventional procedure, and end-stage renal disease are additional factors that can raise the risk of bleeding. Continuous bleeding resulting from malfunctioning devices can cause anemia and hemodynamic instability, necessitating the conversion to open surgical femoral exploration, especially if wire access is lost. Alternatively, manual compression may be used while allowing the heparin to wear off or giving protamine to reverse the heparin that was given during the procedure if the sheath size used was small and the patient is hemodynamically stable. Pseudoaneurysm development from the access site can also result from incomplete closure. Open surgical exploration or ultrasound-guided thrombin injection are the two possible management options for this pseudoaneurysm, depending on the imaging characteristics and clinical circumstances.
- **Infectious:** Vascular access closure devices introduce foreign materials (like polyethylene glycol, nitinol, and braided sutures) into the body, which seldom acts as a vector for

infection. Sterilization techniques should be followed closely throughout the process to reduce the risk of infectious complications from closure devices.

10.8.5. Clinical Significance

Today's proceduralist has access to a vast array of vascular access closure devices to help maintain hemostasis at the vascular access site. It is advisable for the proceduralist to become acquainted with the appropriate uses and avoidance of certain devices. Comparing these devices to the conventional manual compression method, it is evident that the former can facilitate patient discharge and ambulation sooner. Normally, we keep patients on bed rest for four to six hours following manual compression; however, if a vascular closure device has been used, this period of time is shortened to one to two hours. It should be highlighted, though, that no single gadget has shown to be unquestionably better. Furthermore, compared to manual compression, the use of closure devices has not led to a decrease in vascular complications. These devices have been used at other locations, including the brachial/subclavian arteries, even though they were intended and approved for use in the common femoral artery.

Vascular closure devices are now available after a variety of percutaneous procedures. In order to stop bleeding, these devices offer an alternative to manual compression. Due to their frequent use, healthcare professionals—including invasive cardiologists—need to be conversant with these devices. The majority of these devices operate in a similar way, but to make sure there is no bleeding, the patient must still be monitored for 30 to 120 minutes. There is little to no difference between these devices, according to small case series, and between 80 and 100% of vessel closures are successful (Harold and Dauerman, 2007; Hon et al, 2010)

A Closer Look

Coronary Angiography

An X-ray is used during a coronary angiogram test to examine the coronary arteries, which are the blood vessels that supply the heart. Usually, the goal is to determine whether a blood vessel is blocked or narrowed. The most common method for diagnosing coronary artery disease is a coronary angiogram. A coronary angiography is a component of the cardiac catheterization group, which is a broad category of cardiac exams and procedures. One or more catheters—thin, flexible tubes—are used during cardiac catheterization. The tubes are inserted into the body's main blood vessels, including the heart. A tiny skin incision is necessary for the test. To clear any clogged arteries, angioplasty and stenting can be performed during a coronary angiography.

A computed tomography (CT) scanner may be utilized to examine the heart's blood vessels. It is not necessary to insert tubes inside the body for this kind of angiogram. A coronary CT angiogram is what it's known as (CCTA). It could be carried out to assess a patient's need for cardiac catheterization. During a CT angiogram, a vessel narrowing or blockage cannot be treated. The catheter-based kind of coronary angiography has to be performed if the test reveals a blocked or constricted artery. A coronary angiography is performed to check for heart blood vessel constriction or blockage.

If you have angina, or chest pain, your medical team may recommend a coronary angiography. Issues with blood vessels. Congenital heart defect is the term for a heart condition you were born with a disease of the heart valves requiring surgery.

Usually, other noninvasive cardiac tests are performed before an angiography. These tests could consist of a stress test, an echocardiogram, or an electrocardiogram.

- **Risks:** Risks are associated with coronary angiography because it involves the heart and blood vessels. However, significant issues are uncommon. Risks and issues that could arise include:
  - Blood vessel injury.
  - Excessive bleeding.
  - Heart attack.
  - Infection.
  - Irregular heart rhythms, called arrhythmias.
  - Kidney damage due to the dye used during the test.
  - Reactions to the dye or medicines used during the test.
  - Stroke.

- **How you Prepare:** A coronary angiography may occasionally be performed in an emergency. Maybe not enough time to get ready. Your healthcare team will provide you with preparation instructions when the test is scheduled in advance. These instructions are usually included in general guidelines:
    - For a few hours prior to the test, refrain from eating or drinking anything. The time that you should cease eating and drinking is determined by your care team.
    - Make sure you can take your prescription medications. When you visit the hospital, bring a list of your medications.
    - Don't forget to include their dosages. If you have diabetes, let your care team know. Before having a coronary angiography, you might require insulin or another medication.
- **What You Can Expect:**
    - **Before the Procedure:** A catheterization laboratory is a room in a hospital or medical center where a coronary angiography is performed. Many refer to it as a Cath lab. Your medical team discusses your medications and allergies with you prior to the test. After changing into a hospital gown, you go pee if necessary. Don't wear jewelry, hairpins, contacts, or eyeglasses.

      The medical staff takes your pulse and blood pressure. Electrodes are sticky patches that are applied to your arms, legs, and sometimes your chest. Your heartbeat is captured by the patches. They remain in place during the whole test and for some time after. A medical practitioner might trim a small patch of hair from the region where a catheter—a flexible tube—is going to be inserted. After cleaning, the area is made numb.
    - **During the Procedure:** A coronary angiography is performed while you are lying on a table. To keep you securely on the table, straps cross your legs and chest. An IV is inserted by a medical professional into a vein in your hand or forearm. Sedative medication is injected through the IV. The medication promotes calmness and relaxation during the examination or procedure. It might put you to sleep. Your overall health and the reason for the coronary angiography will determine how much sedation you require. You might be semi-conscious or completely conscious. Alternatively, a mix of medications may be administered to induce a sedative-like state in you. We refer to this as general anesthesia.

      To access an artery, the physician performs an incision, a tiny cut. This wound could occur in the wrist or leg. A catheter, which is a thin, flexible tube, is inserted into the artery and guided to the heart. It shouldn't be sensed by your body in any way. Once the catheter is positioned correctly, dye enters the heart's blood vessels through the tube. The movement of the dye is observed through X-ray images. We refer to these pictures as angiograms. A blood vessel may be blocked or constricted if the dye is unable to pass through it.

      It could take an hour or more to finish an easy coronary angiography. It depends on whether concurrent cardiac testing and treatments are performed. Should a blockage be discovered, the artery may be widened by expanding a balloon that is inserted through the catheter. To maintain the artery open, a stent—a mesh tube—may be inserted.

The catheter is taken out of the body after the examination or procedure is finished. The small incision can be sealed with a clamp or tiny plug.

- **After the Procedure:** You are brought to a recovery area following a coronary angiography. A medical team monitors your vital signs, including blood pressure, oxygen saturation, and heart rate. If the catheter was inserted in your leg, you will need to lie flat for a few hours. This lessens the chance of bleeding. There's a chance that the catheter site will hurt for a while. There might be a small bump and a bruise. A coronary angiography can result in some patients returning home the same day. Others, based on the test results, may spend a day or longer in the hospital.

Here are some general guidelines to help you recover:

- Drink lots of water to help your body eliminate the dye.
- For a few days, refrain from heavy lifting and intense exercise.
- Find out when you can take a shower or bath from your medical team.
- As instructed by your healthcare team, take your medications.

Your care team tells you when you can return to work and daily activities.

Call your health care professional's office if you have:

- Breathlessness or pain in the chest. bleeding, freshly developed bruises, swelling, or worsening pain at the catheter site.
- Signs and symptoms of an infection, like fever.
- Seepage or a color shift in the vicinity of the cut.
- Depending on the color of your skin, this could be a shade of red, purple, or brown.
- A shift in the arm or leg used for the test's temperature or color.
- One arm or leg feels weak or numb.

If the area where the catheter was inserted continues to bleed and does not stop under pressure, contact your local emergency number.

- Results: The coronary artery flow is depicted on a coronary angiogram. The test results can be used by a medical practitioner to determine whether an artery is blocked or narrowed. Find out how much of the heart's blood flow is restricted. Check for atherosclerosis, a condition where fats, cholesterol, and other substances accumulate in and on the walls of the arteries. Examine the outcomes of earlier cardiac surgeries.

Your care team can better plan the best course of action for treating your condition with this knowledge.

Summary

- Angiography is a general term for the radiographic examination of the blood vessels. These studies are used to image pathologic and physiologic changes in visceral, cerebral, peripheral, and cardiac anatomy by injecting a contrast agent into specific portions of the vascular system.
- A variety of angiography procedures are available that can be harnessed to diagnose different medical conditions such as computed tomography angiography, coronary angiography, digital subtraction angiography, radionuclide angiography, etc.
- Depending on the type of angiogram, access to the blood vessels is gained most commonly through the femoral artery, to look at the left side of the heart and at the arterial system; or the jugular or femoral vein, to look at the right side of the heart and at the venous system. Using a system of guide wires and catheters, a type of contrast agent (which shows up by absorbing the X-rays), is added to the blood to make it visible on the X-ray images.
- Recent technologic developments in the design and construction of angiographic equipment have added substantially to its versatility but have also increased the cost and complexity.
- One of the most important considerations in current X-ray tube and generator technology is the fact that power requirements for serial film angiographic procedures have diminished considerably during the past decade. In the early 1970s, it was believed that 150–200 kW generators were required for serial film angiography. Because small focal spot X-ray tubes could not tolerate this degree of loading for a rapid film sequence, larger focal spot (2.0 mm) X-ray tubes were routinely used.
- An angiography is a diagnostic procedure that uses X-ray images to check blockages in your blood vessels. This test allows your healthcare provider to see how blood circulates in blood vessels in particular areas of your body. They use an angiography of your heart, neck, kidneys, legs, or other areas to locate the source of an artery or vein issue.
- Electrocardiogram, commonly known as ECG or EKG is a medical test report indicating the heart's electrical activity and rhythm during repeated cardiac cycles. It is printed on grid paper called the ECG strip or ECG tracing.
- In an ECG, the time period between the beginnings of two waves is measured and analyzed. These time periods represent the time required by impulses to transmit in the cardiac conduction pathway causing a coordinated cycle of depolarization and repolarization of the heart's wall.
- A vascular access procedure inserts a flexible, sterile plastic tube called a catheter into a blood vessel to allow blood to be drawn from or medication to be delivered into a patient's bloodstream. A catheter may be used for intravenous (IV) antibiotic treatment and/or other medications, chemotherapy, long-term IV feeding and blood transfusions. Vascular access spares patients the stress of repeated needle sticks and provides a painless way to draw blood or deliver medication.

References

1. Chow, J., Tan, C. H., Tin, A. S., Ong, S. H., Tan, V. H., Goh, Y. S., Gan, H. W., Tan, K. S., Lingamanaicker, J. (2012). Feasibility of transradial coronary angiography and intervention using a single Ikari left guiding catheter for ST elevation myocardial infarction. *Journal of Interventional Cardiology, 25*, 235–244.
2. Clark, T. M. (2002). Scanning laser ophthalmoscopes. In P. J. Saine & M. E. Tyler (Eds.), *Ophthalmic Photography: Retinal Photography, Angiography and Electronic Imaging* (2nd ed., pp. 306–321). Boston: Butterworth-Heinemann.
3. Dauerman, H. L., et al. (2007). Vascular closure devices: The second decade. Journal of the American College of Cardiology, Vol. 50, No. 17, 2007, © 2007 by the American College of Cardiology Foundation ISSN 0735-1097/07/$32.00, Published by Elsevier Inc. doi:10.1016/j.jacc.2007.07.028.
4. Hon, L. Q., Ganeshan, A., Thomas, S. M., Warakaulle, D., Jagdish, J., & Uberoi, R. (2010). An overview of vascular closure devices: What every radiologist should know. *European Journal of Radiology, 73*(1), 181–190. https://doi.org/10.1016/j.ejrad.2008.09.023.
5. Ijichi, T., & Ikari, Y. (2013). Transradial coronary angiography with virtual 1 French, sheathless 3 French catheter. *Catheterization and Cardiovascular Interventions, 82*, E676–E677.
6. Ikari, Y., Masuda, N., Matsukage, T., Ogata, N., Nakazawa, G., Tanabe, T., & Morino, Y. (2009). Backup force of guiding catheters for the right coronary artery in transfemoral and transradial interventions. *Journal of Invasive Cardiology, 21*, 570–574.
7. Ikari, Y., Matsukage, T., Yoshimachi, F., Masutani, M., & Saito, S. (2010). Transradial and slender percutaneous coronary intervention: Less invasive strategy in PCI. *Cardiovascular Intervention and Therapeutics, 25*, 60–64.
8. Ikari, Y., Nagaoka, M., Kim, J. Y., Morino, Y., & Tanabe, T. (2005). The physics of guiding catheters for the left coronary artery in transfemoral and transradial interventions. *Journal of Invasive Cardiology, 17*, 636–641.
9. Ikari, Y., Nakajima, H., Iijima, R., Aoki, J., Tanabe, K., Nakayama, T., Miyazawa, A., Hatori, M., Kyouno, H., Tanimoto, S., Amiya, E., Nakazawa, G., Onuma, Y., & Hara, K. (2004). Initial characterization of Ikari Guide catheter for transradial coronary intervention. *Journal of Invasive Cardiology, 16*, 65–68.
10. Ishiguro, H., Murohara, T., & Ikari, Y. (2011). The feasibility of using Ikari left catheter via the right radial approach in a patient with dextrocardia for better guiding support. *Journal of Invasive Cardiology, 23*, E288–E290.
11. Kabachinski, J. (2005). DICOM: Key concepts—Part I. *Biomedical Instrumentation & Technology, 39*, 214–216.
12. Campeau, L (1989). "Percutaneous radial artery approach for coronary angiography". Catheterization and Cardiovascular Diagnosis. 16 (1): 3–7. doi:10.1002/ccd.1810160103. PMID 2912567.
13. Lin, C. J., Fang, H. Y., Chen, T. H., & Wu, C. J. (2013). Transradial percutaneous coronary intervention for chronic total occlusion using sheathless technique and retrograde approach. *Catheterization and Cardiovascular Interventions, 82*, E206–`E210.

14. Nakashima, M., Ikari, Y., Aoki, J., Tanabe, K., Tanimoto, S., & Hara, K. (2015). Intravascular ultrasound-guided chronic total occlusion wiring technique using 6 Fr catheters via bilateral transradial approach. *Cardiovascular Intervention and Therapeutics, 30*, 68–71.
15. Repanas, T., Christopoulos, G., & Brilakis, E. S. (2015). Administration of viper slide for treating severe radial artery spasm: Case report and systematic review of the literature. *Cardiovascular Revascularization Medicine, 16*, 243–245.
16. Robertson, L., Andras, A., Colgan, F., & Jackson, R. (2016). Vascular closure devices for femoral arterial puncture site haemostasis. *Cochrane Database of Systematic Reviews, 3*, CD009541. https://doi.org/10.1002/14651858.CD009541.pub2.
17. Saine, P. J., & Tyler, M. E. (Eds.). (2002). *Ophthalmic Photography: Retinal Photography, Angiography and Electronic Imaging* (2nd ed., pp. 247–248). Boston: Butterworth-Heinemann.
18. Scheinert, D., et al. (2007). The safety and efficacy of an extravascular, water-soluble sealant for vascular closure: Initial clinical results for Mynx. *Catheterization and Cardiovascular Interventions, 70*, 627–633.
19. Torii, S., Fujii, T., Murakami, T., Nakazawa, G., Ijichi, T., Nakano, M., Ohno, Y., Shinozaki, N., Yoshimachi, F., & Ikari, Y. (2017). Impact of a single universal guiding catheter on door-to-balloon time in primary transradial coronary intervention for ST segment elevation myocardial infarction. *Cardiovascular Intervention and Therapeutics, 32*, 114–119.
20. Torii, S., Masuda, N., & Ikari, Y. (2016). Retrograde approach via left internal mammary artery using a 5 Fr guiding catheter. *Cardiovascular Intervention and Therapeutics, 31*, 156–160.
21. Wu, E. B., & Ikari, Y. (2013). Stingray balloon used in slender percutaneous coronary intervention for chronic total occlusion. *Journal of Invasive Cardiology, 25*, E155–E158.
22. Yamada, T., Mizuguchi, Y., Taniguchi, N., Hata, T., Nakajima, S., & Takahashi, A. (2014). Mother-child aspiration technique. *International Heart Journal, 55*, 455–458.
23. Youssef, A. A., Hsieh, Y. K., Cheng, C. I., & Wu, C. J. (2008). A single transradial guiding catheter for right and left coronary angiography and intervention. *Euro Intervention, 3*, 475–481.

INDEX

E

F

G

H

I

K

L

M

N

FSC
www.fsc.org
MIX
Papier | Fördert
gute Waldnutzung
FSC® C083411

Kolibri 360 GmbH
Ferdinand-Jühlke-Straße 7
99095 Erfurt, Deutschland
produktsicherheit@kolibri360.de